Advances in Medical Discourse Analysis: Oral and Written Contexts

Linguistic Insights

Studies in Language and Communication

Edited by Maurizio Gotti,
University of Bergamo

Volume 45

PETER LANG
Bern · Berlin · Bruxelles · Frankfurt am Main · New York · Oxford · Wien

Maurizio Gotti & Françoise Salager-Meyer (eds)

Advances in Medical Discourse Analysis: Oral and Written Contexts

PETER LANG
Bern · Berlin · Bruxelles · Frankfurt am Main · New York · Oxford · Wien

Bibliographic information published by Die Deutsche Bibliothek
Die Deutsche Bibliothek lists this publication in the Deutsche Nationalbibliografie; detailed bibliographic data is available on the Internet at ‹http://dnb.ddb.de›.

British Library and Library of Congress Cataloguing-in-Publication Data:
A catalogue record for this book is available from *The British Library,* Great Britain, and from *The Library of Congress,* USA

Published with a grant from Università degli Studi di Bergamo (Italy), Dipartimento di Lingue, Letterature e Culture Comparate.

ISSN 1424-8689
ISBN 3-03911-185-X
US-ISBN 0-8204-8382-6

Hochfeldstrasse 32, Postfach 746, CH-3000 Bern 9, Switzerland
info@peterlang.com, www.peterlang.com, www.peterlang.net

Contents

Medical Discourse in Written Contexts

MAURIZIO GOTTI / FRANÇOISE SALAGER-MEYER

Introduction

1. Medical discourse analysis

Medicine is both an *area of knowledge* (of body systems, their diseases and treatments) and the applied practice of that knowledge to medical *praxis*. This is why medicine is said to be both a science and an art, the science (and technology) being the evidential basis for solving clinical problems, and the art being the application of this medical knowledge combined with intuition and clinical judgment to determine the best diagnosis and treatment plan for each patient.

Human societies have developed different systems of healthcare practice since at least the beginning of recorded history. The earliest type of medicine in most cultures was the use of plants (herbalism) and animal parts. This was usually employed along with 'magic' of various kinds in which animism (the notion of inanimate objects having spirits), shamanism (the vesting of an individual with mystic powers), and divination (the attainment of truth through magic) played a major role.

The practice of medicine developed gradually, and separately, in ancient Egypt, China, India, Greece, Persia and elsewhere. The main shift in medical thinking was the gradual rejection in the early 15th century of what could be called 'the traditional authority approach' to science and medicine according to which the claims of prominent personalities were not to be discussed; they were, on the contrary, adopted as absolute truth (cf. Taatvitsainen / Pahta 2004). Before the 17th century the doctrines of the ancient world dominated the theory and practice of Western medicine. Galenism, for example, taught that diseases resulted from an imbalance in the 'four humours', and that treatment with bloodletting and purging would re-establish equilibrium.

Thinkers like Vesalius led the way in improving or even rejecting the theories of great authorities from the past such as Galen, Hippocrates and Avicenna. Of course, the weakening of the Church's power over society made such new attitudes towards knowledge possible. During the 17th century, for example, a new approach to medicine, based on observation and experimentation, increasingly gained acceptance and challenged the *status quo* (Porter1997). From this 'modern' ideology, came Thomas Willis' detailed account of the central nervous system (Garrison 1929), Francis Glisson and colleagues' pioneering work on rickets (Nagy 1988), the first attempt to transfuse blood (Nagy 1988), and an increasing acceptance of Harvey's work on the circulatory system (Webster 1974).

Medicine, as it is practised nowadays, developed largely in the late 18th and early 19th centuries in England, Germany and France, through the work of such figures as Rudolph Virchow, Jean Martin Charcot and Claude Bernard. Scientific medicine (also called, *inter alia*, allopathic, conventional, evidence-based, orthodox medicine or biomedicine in opposition to complementary/alternative medicine referred to as 'unscientific' or unorthodox) yields testable and replicable results for publication in research papers (see Piqué / Posteguillo, Flottum, and Divasson / Pérez, this volume), review articles and meta-analyses (see Mungra, this volume), editorials (see Carnet / Magnet, this volume). Evidence-based medicine replaced the early western medical traditions which were based, *inter alia*, on herbalism, the 'four humours' and other pre-modern theories.

Since the existence of human society, medicine has thus occupied a prominent place in all cultures and times, because it represents a common concern of all human beings: their health and lives. This is why the delivery of high quality, affordable access to healthcare is at the top of the political agenda in most parts of the world. Never before has medicine played such an important, absorbing and fundamental function as that observed today.

Central to medical practice is one of the key factors for successful treatment, especially of chronic diseases, that is, the doctor-patient relationship and interactions (Hughes 1994). Other health professionals (e.g., nurses) also establish relationships with patients and perform interventions from their particular perspectives (see Candlin, this volume). Doctors and patients interact in an intimate and very complex way, as all the papers in the first part of this volume clearly show. Following the great technological advances in medicine over the last 40 years, many aspects of the relationship between doctor and patient have changed considerably, as the general practitioner has been replaced by a wider range of specialists and sub-specialists.

This doctor-patient relationship can be analyzed from many perspectives: from an ethical angle (see Barton, this volume), in terms of how it serves the goals of non-maleficence, beneficence, autonomy and justice, from a cross-cultural/cross linguistic standpoint (see Guido and Roberts, this Volume), from a gender perspective (see Menz / Lalouschek, this volume) and obviously from a cross-speciality viewpoint (see Ribeiro / Souza Pinto and Sarangi / Howell, this volume). Many other issues could be added to this list. Different societies, periods and cultures assign different values to different priorities; in the past 30 years, for example, medical care in the Western world has increasingly emphasized patient autonomy in decision making.

The doctor-patient relationship and process can also be analyzed as a social power relationship (e.g. Foucault 1963), or economic transactions. Physicians have gradually been accorded higher status and respect over the last century, and have been entrusted with the control of access to prescription medicines as a public health measure. This has produced a concentration of power which entails both advantages and disadvantages for specific categories of patients in particular settings. A further twist has occurred in the last 25 years as the cost of medical care has risen, and third parties (insurance companies or government agencies) often demand a share of decision-making power, thus reducing the freedom of choice of both doctors and patients in many ways.

We claimed above that never before has medicine played such an important, absorbing and fundamental function. Proof of this development is abundant but we will only cite two aspects here. The first is the growing number of medical journals published annually worldwide, and the second the recent appearance of non-medical journals devoted to the (linguistic, socio-linguistic, socio-historical, etc.) study of medical discourse.

By the end of the 1980s, some 2 million medical papers in seven different languages were published by about 25,000 (conventional) medical journals, 15,000 of which were considered 'serious' journals. By the year 2000, over 5 million medical papers were published annually (Cooter 2000). This hyperinflation of information is mostly due to the fact that each discipline is subject to a sub-division every 10 years, which in turn leads to the creation of new specialized journals (Régent 2000). If we add to this figure the 500 or so journals in nursing and dentistry, the final figure is 10 million health-related papers published each year.

Not only 'conventional' but also unconventional medical journals (Brodin / Danell 2005) are steadily on the increase. Indeed, complementary and alternative medical therapies (CAM) have attracted increased national attention from the media, the medical community, government agencies and the public (see Salager-Meyer *et al.*, this volume). Surveys performed in the USA and elsewhere suggest that CAM is popular throughout the industrialized world (Goldbeck-Wood *et al.* 1996, Eisenberg *et al.* 1998), and the number of CAM papers published both in CAM journals and in conventional medical journals such as *JAMA, BMJ* and the *Annals of Internal Medicine*, is growing at a very fast rate (Brodin / Danell 2005).

As for the publication of non-medical journals devoted to the study of written (and, to a much lesser extent, oral) medical discourse, the first title is the *EMP* [English for Medical Purposes] *Newsletter* published by the University of Kuwait back in the 1980s. We must also mention the e-journal *Panace@* (written in Spanish, but accepting papers written in four other languages), which was launched in September 2000 and is entirely devoted to the discussion of issues related to the translation, history and development of medical language. *Social Science and Medicine* and the interdisciplinary journal of healthcare, ethics and society *Communication and Medicine* are two additional examples of the growing importance of the study of medical discourse. *Communication and Medicine* aims to consolidate different traditions of discourse and communication research, for an improved understanding of the psychosocial, cultural and ethical aspects of healthcare in contemporary societies; it is targeted at an interdisciplinary audience of healthcare professionals and researchers as well as students in the medical, social and human sciences.

The journals *The Annual Review of Applied Linguistics, English for Specific Purposes, Historical Pragmatics, LSP and Professional Communication,* and *Journal of English for Academic Purposes* – all devoted to the analysis of scientific discourse – publish an increasing number of linguistic, diachronic, socio-historical and cross-linguistic analyses of oral and/or written medical discourse. A sample of such studies, written by international scholars working in the field, is offered in the second part of this book.

Lastly, the fact that the second edition of the *Encyclopedia for Language and Linguistics* (Brown 2006) features a special section entitled *Medicine and Language* which, for the first time, brings together several perspectives on this relatively new research area, is proof to the applied linguistic community's growing awareness of the importance of the analysis of medical discourse.

2. The contents of the book

The volume is divided into two parts, devoted respectively to the analysis of oral and written medical discourse. The first part opens with ELLEN BARTON's examination of discussions between physicians and the families of terminally ill patients in intensive care units in American hospitals. She argues that an ethics of consensus in these discussions is actively co-constructed (or not) as a trajectory of alignment by both physicians and families, partly by raising and negotiating ethical concerns about end-of-life decisions. She concludes that applied linguistics and discourse analysis provide a valuable approach and methodology for the interpretation of discussions of ethical issues and concerns.

HUGO BOWLES reviews the contribution of Conversation Analysis (CA) to the study of medical discourse. In particular, his chapter takes into account the latest literature in order to assess the place of CA in current health communication research, and suggests future areas of interest for researchers working on medical discourse from a CA perspective. He argues that it is in applied and interdisciplinary areas that CA research will most usefully be able to inform health communication studies.

SALLY CANDLIN's chapter questions the conventional wisdom of western medicine, the utility of the bio-medical model and the dominance of health professionals in healthcare delivery to adult patients. Underpinning the discussion is an acknowledgment of the ethical issues guiding professional practice at local and policy-making levels. Evidence in support of this argument is taken from situated discourse in the nursing assessment, analysed according to the principles of CA. Her analysis of audio-recorded interactions demonstrates that observation, examination and data analysis are only meaningful if explanatory value is assigned to the text.

MARIA GRAZIA GUIDO explores the ways in which past traumatic experiences of war and torture are first represented in the narratives of West African refugees and later reported and investigated in the specialized discourse of Psychiatry. More specifically, she analyses the cognitive and discursive incongruities identified in the ways native trauma narratives are conventionally textualised into medical registers. Guido's analysis leads her to conclude that the ætiology associated with trauma-diagnostic constructs in African contexts can in fact encompass a multiplicity of factors including natural/physical as well as supernatural/spiritual and even socio-political causes.

RICK IEDEMA's contribution analyses two recent studies from New South Wales (Australia): the first was an analysis of written reports on clinical errors or 'critical incidents' (CIRs); the second focused on clinicians responding to these incident reports with so-called 'root cause analysis' (RCA) in order to discover the rationale of practice that leads clinicians to make such errors. The chapter outlines the main discursive features of CIRs and RCAs and explains the increasing significance of these text types in contemporary healthcare organizations, explaining how the intensification of knowledge practices and relationships affects modern medicine through such self-reflexive techniques as CIR and RCA.

FLORIAN MENZ and JOHANNA LALOUSCHEK investigate how physicians reconstruct the clinical history of patients admitted to a cardiology ward, discussing whether the description of 'chest pain' differs according to its causes and patient gender. Their analysis shows that support from physicians can enhance patients' ability to describe the kind and course of symptoms, making them aware of the fact that, in such a setting, patients rather than physicians are the experts when it comes to describe a pain.

BRANCA TELLES RIBEIRO and DIANA SOUZA PINTO's chapter investigates how and why the medical model still prevails in psychiatric and teaching settings. Its general plan for the construction of the interview can be gleaned by looking at institutional framings when a doctor asks for information or clarifications, introduces and closes topics. These queries frequently interrupt the patient's narratives and interfere with the doctor's assessment. In a discussion of interviews conducted by a neuro-psychiatrist and subsequent research interviews involving the psychiatrist and a researcher, critical viewpoints and narratives attest to complex professional alignments vis-à-vis institutional discourse on the one hand, and personal stances on the other, thus revealing a three-way tension between professional, institutional and personal discourses.

CELIA ROBERTS' chapter focuses on the impact of globalisation on the increasing diversity of doctor-patient consultations in British cities. In particular, it examines continuities and discontinuities in the detail of day-to-day talk between family doctors and patients from a range of ethnic and linguistic backgrounds. On one side, the analysis shows that, despite the discursive and professional changes of late modernity, much of what happens in the consultation is continuous with the past. On the other side, discontinuities arising in today's global cities in the organisational processes of a 'new work order' are reflected in new discoursal features that can be traced in medical talk. The analysis of a few videorecordings of family doctor consultations shows that the changing landscape and emerging discontinuities in healthcare produce new discourses which require health professionals to be and act in new ways.

SRIKANT SARANGI and LUCY BROOKES-HOWELL offer an account of how genetic counselling case notes are a result of situated interaction. Their analytic focus is on the counsellors' choice of trajectory which lies at the basis of case notes entries. In particular, they examine links between the talk component in counselling and its textual realisations in case records, highlighting the insights that may be gleaned into the professional practice and overall aims of genetic counselling.

The second part of the volume is devoted to medical discourse in written texts. DIDIER CARNET and ANNE MAGNET's investigation of medical journal editorials enables them to identify two types of editorial: those published in journals that address general practitioners and the scientific community in general, and those in journals addressing specialists, where editors comment on or highlight research articles published in the same issue. This chapter analyses the first type, which appears to be a fully original genre, at the crossroads between scientific and general journalistic discourse. The evidence collected points to potential similarities of this genre with editorials in quality newspapers and magazines, from a linguistic as well as a discursive point of view.

The focus of KJERSTI FLØTTUM's chapter is on personal and polyphonic expressions in academic research articles, which show how and to what extent such texts differ linguistically and rhetorically from research articles in economics and linguistics. Due consideration is also given to the similarities and differences between articles written in different languages (English, French and Norwegian). The results of the analysis suggest that disciplinary factors are more important than language, though variables such as age, position, subdisciplines, subject and journal guidelines may constitute additional explanatory factors.

DAVID R. HALL's contribution takes into account the language of medical leaflets written for people other than the traditional learned intermediaries (doctors, pharmacists and other healthcare workers) to assess their degree of readability and impact on the potential 'empowerment' of readers. This issue is explored bearing in mind the problems involved in the drafting of documents that attempt to link professional and lay discourse, leading to the conclusion that empowerment is not always a consequence of greater availability of information: in fact, the original intention of those who lobby for greater transparency is often used for other purposes, so that under the cloak of empowerment control remains in the hands of the powerful.

The objective of ISABEL K. LEÓN and LOURDES DIVASSON's study is to analyse noun-phrase postmodification structures, both qualitatively and quantitatively, in a corpus of biomedical research papers. Their approach is both syntactic and rhetorical, with a grammatical analysis of lexical and morphosyntactic noun-phrase features followed by the identification of plausible connections between these features, the communicative function of research papers and their rhetorical sections. The results point to the conclusion that there is indeed a close connection between some of the structural features identified in postmodification and the communicative function of the research paper's rhetorical sections.

SUSAN MCKAY concentrates on health magazines articles written for two target groups commonly considered 'at risk' (teenage girls and men) and looks at how such texts construct risk messages associated with the main causes of morbidity and mortality in these groups. McKay's analysis points out that both types of magazine are attuned with their respective audiences, their identity and assumed sensibility to health issues. The language of teenage girl magazines employs imitative speech, mimicking their code and incorporating it into the discursive structures of the texts to reflect the conversation-like quality of advice from peers. Men's magazines also use an imitative register designed to reflect the vernacular of its readers. Its use of humour and irony works in anticipation of reader resistance to health advice while its pragmatism and appeal to rationality evoke business-like risk discourse.

PHILIPPA MUNGRA investigates the macrostructure and the rhetorical moves of research articles in medical journals. In particular, she analyses the standard moves and steps most found in review papers from two types of synoptic publications, namely systematic reviews and meta-analyses. The structure of these introductory texts is shown to follow closely Swales' (1990) CARS model for primary research articles. Similar conclusions are reached for the Methods and Results sections. The study also shows that the main orientation of secondary research articles is to furnish robust data in order to justify therapeutic decisions in treatment or risk reduction, as commonly observed in preventive medicine.

PÄIVI PAHTA looks at the use of amplifiers in various types of written medical texts, from scientific discourse among professionals to popularized accounts for a general readership. She first provides a quantitative overview of macrolevel tendencies and then identifies individual features for a more discrete microlevel investigation. Her analysis reveals an intricate, multifaceted pattern of variation, with the use of amplifiers influenced by a complex web of overlapping social, situational and linguistic factors, including target audiences, discipline-approved practices and generic conventions, domain-specific communicative roles, written and spoken modes of communication, and co-occurrence of lexical clusters.

Peer-assessment is the object of JORDI PIQUÉ-ANGORDANS and SANTIAGO POSTEGUILLO's chapter. They examine whether positive/ negative assessment remains stable across medical English written genres or undergoes significant variations. In written academic research, positive/ negative reporting items appear to be a common linguistic resource, although they are not employed consistently across different medical texts in English. Furthermore, the study of reporting expressions across such texts suggests that the use of these linguistic items also varies according to which article section is considered.

FRANÇOISE SALAGER-MEYER, MARIA ANGELES ALCARAZ ARIZA, MARYELIS PABÓN and NAHIRANA ZAMBRANO discuss the genre of acknowledgements in two medical corpora: one taken from scientific/conventional medicine research articles and the other from complementary/alternative medicine research articles. Their findings corroborate the view that the acknowledgement space is the only site in a research paper where science can be portrayed as a dialogic process, thus revealing the complex web of interpersonal debts which the construction of knowledge implies. There are important differences between the modalities of acknowledgments in the two corpora and these greatly depend on the recency of complementary/ alternative medicine, which requires less space and far fewer contributors, acknowledgees and sources of funding, when compared to scientific/conventional medical research papers.

The aim of IRMA TAAVITSAINEN's study is to probe the earliest phase of metadiscursive practices in English medical writing. By combining corpus linguistic methodology with discourse analysis she identifies overt expressions of textual guidance and comments on the evolving text, in order to uncover social-discoursal practices in scientific writing from the Late Medieval period. She also discusses how and to what extent features that may operate at the metatextual level are used, and whether any patterns reflecting the Scholastic thought-style are discernable. This bottom-up empirical study shows that Middle English practices deviate from modern conventions and that the taxonomies applied to modern metadiscourse need to be adapted for earlier texts.

LAURA WRIGHT analyses a request for medical supplies from London to the Island of St Helena written by a doctor in 1715. The list is extremely interesting not only because it shows what drugs, herbs and equipment were deemed essential or desirable for treating the island's population, but also because it gives the medical nomenclature, symbols and abbreviations of the period. In order to discover what sources this doctor might have consulted, either from his own library in St. Helena, or during his apprenticeship in London, three kinds of medical works are surveyed: the authoritative, professional lists of drugs published by accredited apothecaries and doctors; popular household books used by the populace; and the publications of William Salmon, a prolific author whose work would have been read and used by doctors at that time. Although it seems that all three kinds were in use, the medical language of this sea-faring doctor seems to have been mainly influenced by Salmon's works. This shows that, whilst Salmon's actual contribution to medical knowledge may have been minimal, he played a major role in the global dissemination of medical literature.

As shown by this overview, the volume offers a considerable variety of themes, data and research methods which are clearly representative of the eclectic interest in medical discourse and of the wide range of approaches developed for its analysis. Our hope is that this wide range of theoretical frameworks, methodologies and orientations will allow readers to gain a clear and detailed picture of current trends in medical discourse analysis.

References

Brodin, Jenny-Ann / Danell, Richard 2005. Sprititualised Medicine? A Bibliometric Study of Complementary and Alternative

Medicine (CAM). Paper delivered at the 4th EASST Conference. Paris. August.

Brown, Keith (ed.) [2]2006. *Encyclopedia of Language and Linguistics*. London: Elsevier.

Cooter, Michael 2000. News Notes. *European Science Editions* 26/2, 67.

Eisenberg, David / Davis, R. / Ettner, S. / Appel, S. / Wilkey, S. / Rompay, M.V. / Kessler, R. 1998. Trends in Alternative Medicine Use in the United States (1990-1997). *Journal of the American Medical Association* 28/18, 1569-76.

Foucault, Michel 1963. *Naissance de la Clinique: Une Archéologie du Regard Médical*. Paris. Presses Universitaires de France.

Garrison, Fielding H. 1929. *An Introduction to the History of Medicine*. Philadelphia: W.B. Saunders.

Goldbeck-Wood, Sandra / Dorozinski, Alexandre / Lie, Leiv G. 1996. Complementary Medicine is Booming Worldwide. *British Medical Journal* 13, 131-3.

Hughes, John 1994. *Organization and Information at the Bed-Side: The Experience of the Medical Division of Labor by University Hospitals' Inpatients*. Ph.D Dissertation. University of Chicago. Department of Sociology.

Nagy, Doreen 1988. *Popular Medicine in 17th Century England*. Bowling Green, Ohio: Bowling Green State University Popular Press.

Porter, Roy 1997. *The Greatest Benefit to Mankind*. London: Harper Collins.

Régent, Odile 2000. Pratiques de communication en médecine. *Langages* 105, 66-75.

Swales, John 1990. *Genre Analysis: English in Academic and Research Settings*. Cambridge: Cambridge University Press.

Taavitsainen, Irma / Pahta, Päivi 2004. *Medical and Scientific Writing in Late Medieval English*. Cambridge: Cambridge University Press.

Webster, Charles 1974. *The Intellectiual Revolution of the Seventeenth Century*. London: Routledge.

Medical Discourse in Oral Contexts

ELLEN BARTON

Trajectories of Alignment and the Situated Ethics of End-of-Life Discussions in American Medicine

1. Introduction

Sarangi and Roberts set an interdisciplinary goal of developing "an ethics of practical relevance" (1999: 2) for joint work in applied linguistics and medical communication. Such an ethics would focus on communicative situations and events that involve medical decision-making with ethical dimensions through the discourse analysis of naturally-occurring instances of these interactions. In contrast to research on ethics that sets out a normative (that is, prescriptive) decision-making procedure that physicians and patients or surrogates ought to follow (Beauchamp / Childress 2001), a discourse analysis describes the interplay of ethical issues and concerns in decision-making as it actually happens in and across encounters between physicians, patients, and families (Solomon 2005). This kind of discourse analysis offers a descriptive approach to ethics by showing how ethical issues emerge in decision-making as situated in the discourse of particular communicative events (Barton / Sarangi 2005).

Following this approach, the research reported here looks at one particular communicative event in end-of-life care in American medicine – the end-of-life (EOL) discussion between physicians and families of terminally ill patients in intensive care.[1] In American hospitals, one of every five patients dies in an ICU (intensive care

1 Although a study of EOL care and communication across languages and cultures would be fascinating and important, that would be far beyond the scope of a single chapter. I limit myself to American medicine in this chapter because my data come from an intensive care unit in an American hospital. For one cross-cultural comparison (the United States and New Zealand), see Cassell (2005).

unit) (Angus / Bonato / Linde-Zwirble *et al.* 2004), and this number is expected to increase as the population ages and the technology of medicine continues to advance in its ability to support life in critically ill patients (Prendergast / Luce 1997). In ICUs, the majority of deaths involve the decision to withhold or withdraw life support and other aggressive measures aimed at cure in order to provide palliative care aimed at comfort for the end of life (Curtis / Rubenfeld 2001). This decision is the focus of a recognized communicative event – the EOL discussion where physicians typically consult with families in order to proceed within a negotiated consensus to change the goals of treatment from therapeutic to palliative care (Shannon 2001; Levy 2001; Curtis / Patrick 2001; Curtis / Patrick / Shannon *et al.* 2001; Curtis / Engelberg / Wenrich *et al.* 2002; Cassell 2005; Kaufman 2005). In this chapter, after presenting some background information about this research (section 2), I present a discourse analysis of a corpus of EOL discussions and argue that an ethics of consensus in these discussions is actively co-constructed (or not co-constructed) as a trajectory of alignment by both physicians and families, in part by raising and negotiating ethical concerns about EOL decision-making: specifically, I show how the concept of medical futility, defined as treatment that will not benefit the patient (Schneiderman / Jecker / Johnson 1996: 669), emerges as an ethical principle in decision-making for both physicians and families and how a trajectory of consensual alignment with respect to medical futility can be assumed, negotiated, or blocked (section 3). I then consider this empirical description of ethical decision-making with respect to current models of bioethics, and conclude by suggesting that applied linguistics and discourse analysis provide a valuable approach and method for the development of a descriptive ethics of practical relevance that is grounded in the way that participants in medical decision-making actually attend to their ethical issues and concerns (section 4).

2. Background

The research reported here is part of a larger team project.[2] It draws upon an ethnographic study of life and death in intensive care at a large, urban teaching hospital, here called Midwestern Hospital (Cassell 2005), and develops a discourse analysis of a corpus of 20 recorded and transcribed EOL discussions that took place in the Surgical Intensive Care Unit (SICU) at Midwestern Hospital. In this corpus, 14 discussions reached a decision to withdraw life support, and 6 discussions did not. The discourse analysis of the data was inductive, looking to describe the recurring structural organization of EOL discussions as well as the variations in discussions across the corpus (Schiffrin / Tannen / Hamilton 2001; Johnstone 2000; Sarangi / Roberts 1999).[3]

In previous work on this corpus (Barton / Aldridge / Trimble / Vidovic 2005), we described the four structural phases within the EOL discussion, each with a particular set of functions in the progression of the discussion toward a decision to withdraw life support: the Opening (Phase 1), where physicians as well as families co-construct the traditional authority of a medical encounter with the physician in the interactional and decision-making lead; the

---

2 This research was supported in part by a grant from the National Institutes of Health for the project entitled SICU Care at the End of Life, Timothy Buchman, MD PhD, Principal Investigator (NR05124), at Washington University, St. Louis, MO. The project was reviewed and approved by the site IRB (Washington University Medical Center HSC #99-0310). My use of the corpus of EOL discussions was also reviewed and approved by Wayne State University (HIC #125802B3E). Participants' confidentiality was protected through the use of pseudonyms: initials for physicians, and category labels for family members (Son, Dtr/daughter, Fam/family member, relationship to patient unknown). I would like to thank Tim Buchman and Joan Cassell for making this corpus available to me and for commenting in detail on many drafts of my work.

3 For ease of exposition, excerpts from the transcripts are regularized in spelling and punctuation for intonation (. for falling; , for continuing; ? for rising). Incomplete words are noted with -, and utterances with --. Latching is signified by ==. Deleted material is indicated by [...]. Unless relevant to the analysis, overlap, back channels and other features were not included in the excerpts.

Description of Current Status (Phase 2), which functions to establish the terminal status of the patient and imply the futility of continued treatment; the Decision-Making (Phase 3), which functions to effect a holistic decision to withdraw life support; and the Logistics of Dying (Phase 4), which functions to describe the specifics of dying in the SICU and to revisit issues arising in the previous phases. In this work, we argue that it is Phase 2 that is crucial in the functional progression of the EOL discussion because it is here that physicians and families interactionally establish a consensus that the patient is dying, which makes it reasonable that continuing further treatment, including life support, would be futile and only prolong the patient's suffering. In other words, if Phase 2 of the discussion does not interactionally establish a consensus concerning terminal status and medical futility among the physician(s) and family members, the decision to withdraw life support does not take place. In interaction, as will be shown in the analysis below, families have and use multiple means for verifying the determination of medical futility and for participating in the decision to withdraw life support. Further, it is in interaction that the ethical basis for this decision emerges, for both physicians and families.

3. Trajectories of alignment and emerging ethics in interaction

Before beginning this analysis, it is important to note that the EOL discussion is not the only communicative event in EOL care. Like most medical communication in American hospitals, EOL communication is both multiply sourced and systematically discontinuous. Some EOL communication is what is called bedside communication, where any number of different professionals and individuals (physicians, nurses, technicians, social workers, chaplains, and other staff members) talk informally to families in short exchanges or lengthier updates on the patient's condition throughout an ICU course. The EOL discussion, however, is recognized as a more formal communicative event: it is scheduled, held in a conference room, and conducted, at Midwestern Hospital, by the attending physician in charge of the unit for the week. The actual decision-making, however, may be more serial than simultaneous, and more medical than familial: in her ethnography of this unit, Cassell (2005) notes that EOL discussions were not convened unless the physician had determined that it was medically appropriate to discuss the withdrawal of futile treatment, a practice also noted by Kaufman (2005) and Anspach (2003) in their ethnographies of ICUs. This medical decision-making prevailed more often than not – 14 out of 20 discussions in this corpus – but not without considerable interaction to build (or block) consensus.

In the following subsections, I describe several different trajectories of the EOL discussion where the participants in the discourse do or do not co-construct the decision to end life support based on medical futility, and I argue that these trajectories illustrate the co-construction of the ethical principles that govern this decision, not only on the part of physicians but also on the part of families. I present a description of three different trajectories of interaction in Phase 2 and Phase 3 of the discussion: overt or assumed alignment (3.1), negotiated alignment (3.2), and blocked alignment (3.3). I also describe the ethical principles that re-emerge in Phase 4 of the discussion (3.4).

3.1. Overt and assumed alignment

Sometimes the EOL discussion proceeds within a trajectory of interactional alignment throughout. Phase 2 of the discussion typically ends with a summary section that more or less directly establishes the terminal status of the patient and thereby implies the futility of continued medical treatment. When there is overt agreement to the summary statements ending Phase 2, physicians then move to Phase 3 of the discussion, which first establishes the patient's wishes as the framework for decision-making and then effects a holistic decision to withdraw life support. The following example illustrates such an aligned movement from Phase 2 to Phase 3:

(1) Dr. E: [*Phase 2 summary*] [W]e don't think she's ever going to get better. We can keep her body alive on the machine for a very long period of time, but==
Dtr: ==but she is going now.
Dr. E: [*Phase 3 decision-making*] And it sounds like that's not what she would want.
Dtr: No.
Dr. E: Everybody is in agreement with that and that's what Dr. [X] has said as well. [...] [B]ased upon what everybody said, her to her doctors and all of you to me, it sounds like it's not what she would want.
Dtr: No. (Jordan)

Using the contrastive term *but* as a latched pivot, which, perhaps, symbolizes the contrast between life and death, the physician and daughter jointly construct a summary statement that is a fairly direct statement of medical futility and terminal status in the lay language of dying, with the daughter using the cliché that *she's going now*. With this consensus interactionally established, the physician moves the discussion into Phase 3 by expressing the patient's wishes as a holistic decision-making statement, again in lay language (*that's not what she would want*). Here, too, the daughter provides overt agreement with the confirming negative *no*, thereby aligning herself with the inferential reference of the pronoun *that* as the decision to withdraw life support in order to let the patient die. The physician then overtly establishes this decision as a consensus three times by noting that *everybody is in agreement*, that another physician involved in the care is in agreement, and even specifying that *what everybody said* included the patient (*her to her doctors*) as well as the family (*all of you to me*). The decision statement is repeated here, too, along with a second instance of the daughter's aligned response.

In the corpus of the 14 EOL discussions that made a decision to withdraw life support, four were in overt alignment, with families using positive back channels and statements of agreement. Two other discussions were arguably in assumed alignment, in that the discussion progressed to a decision, although the family did not express alignment overtly, instead remaining silent (there is no video data to see whether there was non-verbal alignment). I place these two discussions in this category because the two discussions, although monologic, showed no signs of interactional trouble, moving smoothly through all four phases.

In sum, what the physicians choose to emphasize in an aligned progression to decision-making, primarily through the discourse strategies of repetition and accounts of agreement and understanding, is the consensus of all parties that the patient's status is terminal and the decision is to end treatments that are futile, including life support. The ethical principle that emerges in these interactions thus is consensus.

3.2. Negotiated alignment

A greater number of EOL discussions that progressed to a decision to withdraw life support, however, did so by negotiating medical futility as the basis for decision-making. In the six discussions that were in overt or assumed alignment, medical futility seemed to be accepted as established through a physician's monologue, and the central ethical concern was the consensus of all parties, also as constructed primarily by the physician. In discussions with negotiated alignment, however, the central ethical concern that emerges is medical futility; in other words, futility must be established as a necessary condition for consensus. The primary discourse strategy for this negotiation of medical futility was a recursive recycling of Phase 2 after Phase 3 had begun, and both families and physicians utilized this strategy. In the corpus, eight discussions that made an EOL decision recycled Phase 2; in six discussions the family initiated a recycled Phase 2, and in two discussions the physicians did.

In discussions that negotiated alignment, Phase 2 was recycled within Phase 3, sometimes at great length and often more than one time, before decision-making. The following example illustrates the two most frequent recurring concerns raised by families in a recycled Phase 2, a verification of terminal status and a review of the course of treatment:

(2) Dr. E: [*Phase 3 beginning*] Based upon our conversations of a few weeks ago [...] it seems clear to me that what you were telling us was that Mrs. [Norris] would not want to live in the hospital if she were going to be prolonged on machines with no real chance of recovery. [...]

Fam: She does not want to be brain dead. That's what you're talking about, isn't it? She's had two strokes in her brain like thing [*CAT scan*]. And you're talking about her more likely being brain dead. [...]
Fam: Is this the first CAT scan we've had done on her? [...]
Fam: So that's not something you would do in the beginning. [...]
Fam: Is that a normal thing?
Dr. E: Yes. [...] But back to where we are right now, we have two things which sound like this is not as she would want to live. [...] Either one of them [*the strokes or the infection*] would lead me to think that the appropriate thing to do would be for us to turn the ventilator down to the same air as you and I are breathing and stop giving her support with machines and let nature take its course.
Fam: [*Beginning of Phase 4 logistics*] When you do that, are you going to be able to keep her from having any pain? (Norris)

After the physician initiates Phase 3 within the framework of the patient's wishes as the bid for decision-making, the initial response of the family seems to indicate alignment (*She does not want to be brain dead*). Even though consensus concerning terminal status appears to be established, this family recycles Phase 2 by asking questions about treatments that have not worked, treatments that have become futile. After this recycled Phase 2, when the physician again makes a Phase 3 bid for holistic decision-making (*the appropriate thing to do would be ... [to] let nature take its course*), this time the family exhibits alignment by moving to Phase 4 and asking a question about the logistics of dying that presume the decision is to withdraw life support is in effect (the reference of *that* in *when you do that*).

Interestingly, it is not only families who recycle Phase 2 when they apparently want to negotiate decision-making through a repetition of the establishment of terminal status and medical futility. In two discussions, physicians recycled Phase 2 after Phase 3 had begun (in one discussion the physician seems to recycle Phase 2 after what appeared to be precipitous decision-making on the part of the family; see Barton *et al.* 2005). In the other discussion, the physician seems to use recycling Phase 2 as a discourse strategy in response to a lack of uptake on the part of the family to the bid for Phase 3 decision-making:

(3a) Dr. I: [*Phase 3 beginning*] I think that we have to look from the perspective of what Mrs. [Quorn] herself and what she would want to have done were she to know what she was faced with--

> [...] It is likely that-- um-- if we continue to provide aggressive support as we are not that um-- things are going to-- um-- ah-- languish to the extent that-- that may have improvements one day and-- and-- and-- and decreases the next day-- um-- over a fairly long time?
> And-- I think that-- that I-- I guess what-- what we need to sit and really look at carefully is whether or not that is something that she would want for what we perceive to be a very, very unlikely positive outcome. [...] I mean, there are aggressive approaches that we could continue to pursue. It would involve, you know, at a minimum a big operation in the next couple days-- ah-- that she may not survive the operation, but assuming that she survived-- even survived the operation, neither one of us in our experience believe[s] that she will ever make it out of the hospital-- um-- back to the state that she was in before she got here. [...] Um-- I would like to take a good look at the wound this afternoon. (Quorn)

This lengthy monologue begins with two bids for decision-making, but they contrast notably in fluency. The first is a fluent deployment of the frame of the patient's wishes and a bid for decision-making (*what she would want to have done*). After this first bid receives no uptake, though, the second bid is markedly dysfluent, with many hesitation markers and a question about *languish[ing]* in the ICU that also receives no response. Without uptake to either bid, the physician again bids for decision-making, this time assessing the outcome even more directly (*a very, very unlikely positive outcome*). At this point, however, perhaps in response to the interactional trouble, he recycles a Phase 2 description of medical problems and their possible treatment. These treatment options include *a big operation*, one that *she may not [even] survive* in order to *return to the state she was in*. Nevertheless, the physician offers to re-evaluate the patient for treatment (*take a good look at the wound*). After more discussion of the problematic consequences of continued aggressive treatment in yet another bid for decision-making, the family does express alignment:

(3b) Dtr: Um-- she does not want that. She does not want to be on the vent, she does not want to be prolonged. (Quorn)

Only after a full recycling of the Phase 2 description of the patient's medical problems and a full discussion of what would likely be futile treatments does this daughter express her mother's wishes not *to be prolonged.* In this discussion, then, decision-making does not take place until the daughter seems satisfied that a full consideration of medical treatment has taken place. This decision is thus based on the specific treatments that will be withheld as well as the life support that will be withdrawn.

In sum, when physicians and families negotiate alignment to decision-making, they often do so by recycling and repeating the Phase 2 description of medical problems, repetitively establishing that the status of the patient is terminal and that further treatments would be futile. In most discussions medical futility is established primarily with respect to the withdrawal of life support, as in (2), but some discussions, such as (3), establish medical futility by talking in detail about specific treatments. The negotiation of decision-making thus takes place as families and physicians raise their concerns until they seem satisfied that the decision to withdraw life support is ethical based in large part on the verification of medical futility. In the trajectory of negotiated decision-making, neither families nor physicians indicate alignment is in place for decision-making until medical futility is established to their satisfaction, suggesting that it is a primary ethical concern.

3.3. Blocked alignment

As noted above, six EOL discussions did not progress to a decision to withdraw life support. All of these discussions included multiple recyclings of Phase 2 as described above, along with multiple bids for Phase 3 decision-making on the part of physicians, but negotiation did not arrive at a consensus. Families use a variety of discourse strategies to block the inferences of terminal status and medical futility as well as the alignment to decision-making, including silence, as shown above in (3a), as well as neutral continuers and topic acknowledgments without topic development in terms of the inferences suggested by the physician, as in the following example:

(4) Dr I: [*Phase 2*] She is requiring a lot of medications to support her blood pressure.
Dtr: Mm-hmm.

Dr. I: And the picture seems to be one of very severe sepsis, that is a severe infection in the blood and ah, it seems like that sepsis is affecting multiple organ systems. [...] Um, her kidneys--
Dtr: Yes.
Dr. I: And ah, her hepatic-- her liver system and the ability of her blood to clot and behave normally. So when someone in the-- experiences all of these, um, complications of the sepsis in the face of the strong medications that we are using, um, [*Phase 3*] we feel like it is important to try to touch base with the family and clarify the goals of treatment and what you imagined the goals of treating her to be.
Dtr: OK.
Dr. I: Does that make sense? What questions can I answer to help that make sense?
Dtr: ((silence)) (Flushing)

In this Phase 2-Phase 3 sequence, the physician mentions a series of medical problems, including blood pressure, sepsis, and multiple organ failure, but the daughter uses neutral continuers (*mm-hmm* and *yes* with falling intonation) and the topic acknowledgment *OK* with no uptake of the Phase 2 inferences that the problems add up to terminal status and that a Phase 3 decision to withdraw life support under palliative care might become *the goals of treat[ment]*. The physician here then resorts to a rather desperate bid for the acknowledgment of the inferences that would *make sense* in this situation, but the family member again blocks both the inference to terminal status and the bid for decision-making with her silence.

In terms of the ethical principles that emerge in EOL discussions, the most intriguing discourse strategy that families use to block alignment is the expression of hope. In effect, expressions of hope orient the discussion away from ending treatment and toward the possibilities of continuing medical treatment, which thereby makes EOL decision-making ethically impossible.

In all six of the non-decision-making encounters, there are expressions of hope in a Phase 2 that effectively block the inferences that the patient's status is terminal and that further treatment would be futile. Hope seems to be related to two situations: the possible return of consciousness, and/or the possible positive outcomes of treatment. In the following examples, the Swanson family in (5) uses an expression of hope for consciousness to block the inference of terminal status in Phase 2, and the Flushing family in (6) similarly uses an expression of hope for response to treatment in a recycled Phase 2:

(5) Dr. U: How do you think he's doing at the moment?
Wife: Well, one thing, when I call his name, he responds. [...] Yesterday he kind of opened his eyes when [his son] was here. And so actually I think he must realize that it's us. (Swanson)

(6) Dr. I: What is your understanding about what brought her in to see Dr. S. (in the) first place?
Dtr: Um well I took her to emergency about one month ago.
[*Lengthy description of course of care*]
So we get that out-- if we can get the infection take care of, get on top of it-- which will help the rest of her grow stronger. (Flushing)

By blocking the inferences of terminal status and futile treatment, these expressions of hope make it impossible to make an ethical decision to end life support: where there is hope of the return of personhood or improvement toward survival, the situation is not one of medical futility, and medical futility is necessary to an ethical decision to withdraw life support.

But it is not only family members who offer expressions of hope that block the progression of the discussion toward decision-making. Physicians, too, indirectly express hope by offering treatment options such as continued ICU care, as in (7):

(7) Dr. E: Again, this is not something-- if he is to get better, he is not going to get better rapidly. So if I say to you in the next couple of days-- if there's hope, that doesn't mean that A, he's going to live, or B, or mean that he's going to magically wake up and get off the ventilator like people do on TV. It would just mean that we take it on day to day if it is reasonable to fight another day. (Farmer)

But offering continued ICU care *if there's hope*, even with the expectation that the patient will not ultimately survive or improve, leaves the course of care open-ended. As Cassell (2005) notes, however, taking things day by day and continuing ICU care, especially ventilator life support, often leads to prolonged courses of futile care.

Sometimes physicians offer or even order additional treatment, as in (8), which also blocks the inferences necessary to ethical EOL decision-making:

(8) Dr. U: Um-- one of the options that we would like to talk about potentially is whether or not we should do a tracheostomy which would-- um-- allow us basically-- ah-- leave him on the breathing machine but have him in a-- in a position where he could be more comfortable and-- and awake. (Farmer)

While the patient is still being treated actively, especially if it would allow a return to consciousness (*comfortable and awake*), EOL decision-making cannot ethically take place.

In sum, expressions of hope change the ethical perspective on the situation of a patient by blocking the inference that the patient's status is terminal. More specifically, offering treatment options or even discussing treatment options blocks the inference that further treatment would be futile. Sometimes it is families that refuse to align themselves with the interactional trajectory toward decision-making, as in (7), and other times it is physicians that depart from the trajectory toward decision-making by offering treatment, as in (8). By re-orienting the EOL discussion away from medical futility and toward treatment and possible improvement or survival, however, families and physicians cannot ethically proceed to EOL decision-making. In all six non-decision-making discussions in the corpus, the discussion included either expressions of hope, discussions of treatment options, or both.

3.4. Co-constructing the ethics of palliative care

Once the parties in decision-making discussions are in interactional alignment with respect to the terminal status of the patient and the futility of continued treatment (Phase 2) and the decision to withdraw life support has been made holistically in lay language (Phase 3), Phase 4 of the discussion turns to the logistics of dying in the ICU. Phase 4 is the longest and most interactive phase of the EOL discussion, and one of the functional accomplishments of this phase is that physicians and families co-construct a combined medical-lay discourse of palliative care. In other words, physicians use terminology from medicine to make explicit the consequences of the decision to withdraw life support by telling families exactly how death will take place, noting specifically that the time frame of dying is always uncertain:

(9) Dr. E: And so what we will do, we'll stop everything except for pain medication and sedation medicine. I told you yesterday, I can tell all of you, so I'm going to tell all of you that we can make her comfortable and we can make her pain free. You have my guarantee on that. We'll turn her to the same oxygen that you and I are breathing off the ventilator, we won't restart dialysis so that it will be natural [...] with dignity. [...] I honestly don't know right now whether this is going to take an hour or two days. [...] (Schilling)

Through repetition throughout Phase 4, physicians construct the key concepts of death within palliative care: comfort, defined as being pain free; natural, defined as the absence of excessive technology; in sum, death with dignity. The specification of an uncertain time frame is the most frequent topic of Phase 4.

Even after the logistics of death are described by physicians in terms of palliative care, families routinely check the claim that patients will not suffer any pain:

(10) Dr. U: I will make sure that he never feels short of breath. I will make sure that he is never uncomfortable.
Wife: All that I am scared about, I just do not want him to [*wake up*]--
Dr. U: I promise you-- this much I can promise 100% that he will have no anxiety and no shortness of breath and no discomfort. (Kuster)

In Phase 4, families are repeatedly assured that palliative care is truly comfort care, in terms of physical pain as well as psychic consciousness.

Both physicians and families bring up additional ethical concerns related to palliative care in Phase 4. For instance, attention to consciousness is the second most frequent topic in Phase 4. Even in overtly aligned discussions in Phase 2 and Phase 3, physicians explain the level of consciousness that ethically licenses the use of palliative care in Phase 4:

(11) Dr. E: I can guarantee you [...] that he will be pain free, that he will be comfortable. He will not know what's going on. He already doesn't know what's going on. If he was able to understand what was going on, if there was any chance that he could understand what was going on, I wouldn't be having this conversation with you right now. (Gordon)

Families, too, ask questions about their concerns regarding consciousness in Phase 4:

(12) Fam: But she moving. She moving her legs, she kind of opened her eyes.
Dr. E: She has. I'm not telling you that she's brain dead, she has some brain function. She can move, but she is in a very, very deep sleep. (Jordan)

(13) Dtr: And when they suctioned him though and--When they suctioned him in his mouth, he shut his mouth and moved away.
Dr. U: OK as any of us would do that-- that is a reflex and you can see that from a dog or a fish or a frog. (Hunt)

Although the final comparison is not a flattering one, it describes the remaining brain activity as reflex rather than thought. The absence of conscious personhood, then, is an important ethical principle underlying the move to palliative care.

Physicians also do deliberate interactional work to draw an ethical distinction between the withdrawal of life support and the practice of euthanasia:

(14) Dr. I: So the plan would be to have her pass away as peacefully and naturally and comfortably as possible while she's in the hospital. [...] So that we're not hastening her death. [...] That's a real important point.
Fam: I understand it; that's what I want.
Dr. I: This is a very different process than euthanasia or anything like that, where you actively contribute to somebody dying, somebody who would otherwise not die. This is a very different-- (Paulson)

Related to the topic of time lines, physicians emphasize that palliative care does not hasten the process of death, which would be euthanasia.

In sum, there is a close connection between the ethical concerns raised in Phase 2 and Phase 4, although the mode of interaction shifts. In Phase 2, physicians are the dominant interlocutor, and their determination of medical futility is expressed monologically. In Phase

4, families are the dominant interlocutor, and their concerns about medical futility are raised through questions and satisfied through dialogue. It is possible to view this as an emerging ethics that is distributed across the entire EOL discussion. Physicians present medical futility as an implication of the terminal status of the patient in Phase 2, presumably to their own clinical and ethical satisfaction. Sometimes the physician's articulation seems sufficient for families as expressed in overt or assumed alignment. When it is not, families negotiate the physician's determination of medical futility before decision-making by recycling Phase 2 recursively within Phase 3. Even after the decision is made (or not), however, both physicians and families revisit key ethical principles in Phase 4, including medical futility and personhood. An ethics of consensus is thus co-constructed across multiple dimensions and in different phases of the EOL discussion to withdraw life support and allow the patient to die.

4. Ethics emerging in interaction

By and large, the ethical principles that emerge in the interaction of EOL discussions are centrally concerned with the consensus of all parties that the patient's status is terminal based on a determination of medical futility. This consensus emerges in a trajectory of alignment, sometimes after considerable negotiation, that allows the decision to move to palliative care. However, even sustained negotiation aimed at establishing consensus does not always lead to decision-making; families have a number of discourse strategies to block a trajectory of alignment and thus the progression to decision-making. In particular, one of these strategies is to counter bids for decision-making with expressions of hope, which effectively blocks EOL decision-making by making this decision ethically impossible.

In the literature of bioethics, this description of EOL decision-making is in considerable conflict with the dominant model of principalism, where the balance among principles of autonomy, beneficence, non-malfeasance, and justice are prescribed as the only way to arrive at an ethical decision (Beauchamp / Childress 2001). It is not that these principles do not emerge at all in actual EOL discussions: there is considerable attention to beneficence, particularly in the review of the patient's course of aggressive treatment that took place in the ICU, and the principle of non-malfeasance (do no harm) is central in the discussion and its decision since futile care can be seen to be harmful to the patient in that it prolongs suffering. And although this sample of EOL discussions is too small to make any claims about justice, the discussions, in this corpus at least, did not vary notably according to gender, ethnicity, or socioeconomic class. In terms of principles, it is interesting to note that the beneficence and non-malfeasance, and, to a more culturally relative extent, justice, are longstanding principles of medical ethics back to Hippocrates (Lloyd 1950). This research, however, contributes to an ongoing critique of autonomy as the contemporary operationalization of ethical decision-making.

Autonomy is defined as the right of patients to self-determination in medical care, in particular by making their own medical decisions and treatment choices based upon their personal values and beliefs or the understanding of these values by a surrogate decision-maker (Beauchamp / Childress 2001; Kapp 2001). Perhaps because it is the principle that they added to contemporary medical ethics, many bioethicists see autonomy in absolute terms: "Respect for autonomy is not a mere *ideal* in health care, it is a professional *obligation*" (Beauchamp / Childress 2001: 63 [authors' emphasis]). But Schneider (1998: 1) argues that "this triumph of autonomy in bioethics" is a questionable victory, since his research on medical decision-making shows that patients and families are not necessarily eager to exercise their right to autonomy, seemingly preferring a professional model of advice and recommendation. In the EOL discussions described above, autonomy was not overtly practiced. In fact, as can be seen in the description of Phase 3, decision-making does not even take place in explicit form; rather, it takes place in terms of a trajectory of alignment across the entire discussion. Further, the trajectory of non-alignment in discussions that did not end in a decision to withdraw life support was not blocked because the principle of autonomy was not in effect; in fact, what was not in effect was consensus. What this discourse analysis of EOL discussion shows is that both physicians and families seem deeply concerned with ethical issues, but they attended more specifically to the ethical dimensions of the particular decision at hand, and more generally to an ethics of consensus rather than autonomy.

This research, then, suggests a set of contributions that discourse analysis and applied linguistics can make to the literature of bioethics and to the development of ethical practices of decision-making in interaction. First, and perhaps most importantly, it suggests that bioethics can be broadened and, perhaps, deepened by looking for the actual ethical concerns that both physicians and families bring to decision-making. Second, it is able to identify and describe these concerns as they emerge in interaction: in EOL decision-making, for instance, medical futility is seen as crucial, with its related concerns about suffering, consciousness, personhood, and dignity. Third, it points to consensus and the importance of interaction in negotiating that consensus as a key dimension of ethical decision-making, an inter-relatedness among medical professionals and families that is ignored in a primary focus on the autonomy of the individual. Finally, it allows a legitimate preference of both physicians and families for the maintenance of a professional model of medicine, one that allows parties, if they choose, to assume the trust of a fiduciary relationship between physician and patient that incorporates an ethics of consensus underlying medical decision-making.

References

Angus, Derek / Bonato, Amber / Linde-Zwible, Walter *et al.* 2004. Use of Intensive Care at the End of Life in the United States: An Epidemiologic Study. *Critical Care Medicine* 32, 638-643.

Anspach, Renee 2003. *Deciding Who Lives: Fateful Choices in the Intensive-Care Nursery*. Berkeley: University of California Press.

Barton, Ellen / Aldridge, M. / Trimble, Thomas / Vidovic, Justin 2005. Structure and Variation in End-of-Life Discussions in the

Surgical Intensive Care Unit. *Communication & Medicine* 2, 1-21.

Barton, Ellen / Sarangi, Srikant 2005. Autonomy-in-Interaction: Decision-Making in Palliative Care. Paper presented at COMET-VELIM 2005, University of Sydney, Australia.

Beauchamp, Tom / Childress, James ^{5}2001. *Principles of Bioethics*. Oxford: Oxford University Press.

Cassell, Joan 2005. *Life and Death in Intensive Care*. Philadelphia: Temple University Press.

Curtis, J. Randall / Engelberg, Ruth / Wenrich, Marjorie *et al.* 2002. Studying Communication about EOL Care during the ICU Family Conference: Development of a Framework. *Journal of Critical Care Medicine* 17, 47-160.

Curtis, J. Randall / Patrick, Donald 2001. How to Discuss Dying and Death in the ICU. In Curtis / Rubenfeld (eds), 85-102.

Curtis, J. Randall / Patrick, Donald / Shannon, Sarah *et al.* 2001. The Family Conference as a Focus to Improve Communication about EOL Care in the Intensive Care Unit: Opportunities for Improvement. *Critical Care Medicine* 29, N26-N33.

Curtis, J. Randall / Rubenfeld, Gordon (eds) 2001. *Managing Death in the ICU*. New York: Oxford University Press.

Johnstone, Barbara 2000. *Qualitative Methods in Sociolinguistics*. New York: Oxford University Press.

Kapp, Mitchell 2001. Legal Liability Anxiety in the ICU. In Curtis / Rubenfeld (eds), 231-244.

Kaufman, Sharon 2005. *...And a Time to Die: How American Hospitals Shape the End of Life*. New York: Scribner.

Levy, Mitchell 2001. Making a Personal Relationship with Death. In Curtis / Rubenfeld (eds), 31-36.

Lloyd, G.E.R. (ed.) 1950. *Hippocratic Writings*. London: Penguin.

Prendergast, T. J / Luce, J. M. 1997. Increasing Incidence of Withholding and Withdrawal of Life Support from the Critically Ill. *American Journal of Respiration* 155, 15-20.

Sarangi, Srikant / Roberts, Celia 1999. The Dynamics of Interactional and Institutional Orders in Work-Related Settings. In Sarangi, Srikant / Roberts, Celia (eds) *Talk, Work and Institutional Order: Discourse in Medical, Mediation and Management Settings*. Berlin: Mouton de Gruyter, 1-60.

Schiffrin, Deborah / Tannen, Deborah / Hamilton, Heidi (eds) 2001. *The Handbook of Discourse Analysis*. Malden, MA: Blackwell.

Schneider, Carl 1998. *The Practice of Autonomy: Patients, Doctors, and Medical Decisions*. New York: Oxford University Press.

Schneidermann, Lawrence / Jecker, Nancy / Jonsen, Albert 1996. Medical Futility: Response to Critiques. *Annals of Internal Medicine* 125, 669-674.

Shannon, Sarah 2001. Helping Families Prepare for and Cope with a Death in the ICU. In Curtis / Rubenfeld (eds), 165-182.

Solomon, Marilyn 2005. Realizing Bioethics' Goals in Practice: Ten Ways 'Is' can Help 'Ought'. *Hastings Center Report* 35, 40-47.

HUGO BOWLES

Conversation Analysis and Health Communication: Updating a Developing Relationship

1. Introduction

Although, as Dudley Evans (2004: 206) has noted, studies of talk in professional domains have received much less attention than research on written genres, medicine is the one professional domain in which oral talk has continued to be researched in some depth. This is partly due to the fact that the importance of communication in the health services is increasingly recognised, and this has given rise to interest in communication studies at the level of medical school teaching and curriculum development with educational journals such as *Medical Education* now devoting considerable space to issues of health communication. However, perhaps the main reason for the pre-eminence of oral research in medical domains compared to other areas of professional talk is the attention which has traditionally been devoted to medical communication from the conversation analysis (CA) perspective, which has been the dominant paradigm for the analysis of talk over the last 40 years. Much of the early CA research in the 1960s was carried out in the area of medical talk – a tradition which has continued until the present day through the work of CA scholars such as Heritage and Maynard.

However, although the status of CA research within medical discourse is a consolidated one, there is no doubt that the direction of this research is changing (Heritage 1999: 73). The aim of this chapter is to analyse this shift by tracing the development of CA research in medical discourse. The literature, particularly that of the last 10 years, will be examined in order to establish the place of CA in current health communication research and to use this overview to suggest future areas of interest and development for researchers working on medical discourse from the CA perspective and, vice-versa, those interested in using CA to inform their own medical oral discourse research. It will be argued that it is in applied and interdisciplinary areas that CA research will most usefully be able to inform studies of health communication.

In developing these ideas, this chapter will be structured in two parts. The first part (§ 2) will discuss the methodology of CA and how it relates to the study of medical oral discourse, and the second part (§3) will focus on applied and cross-disciplinary CA research in health communication.

2. CA methodology

Conversation analysis has its historical roots in ethnomethodology and shares with it a desire to show how the organisation of social interaction makes manifest the structures of social institutions. A detailed history of the early development of CA can be found in Heritage (1984) and CA methodology has been described in detail in a number of recent accounts such as those by Ten Have (1999, 2001a). The account of CA methodology outlined in § 2.1 and 2.2 is based on more detailed summaries in Hutchby / Wooffitt (1998) and Seedhouse (2004).

2.1. CA and institutional talk

The object of research of CA is generally described as 'talk-in-interaction' and its main focus is "to discover how participants understand and respond to one another in their turns at talk, with a central focus on how sequences of action are generated". (Hutchby / Wooffitt 1998: 14). By analysing language in terms of social action, CA practitioners are looking at the way in which interaction is organised through talk, rather than looking at it in terms of linguistic categories such as speech events or speech acts. Given CA's emphasis on the organisational structure of talk, *a priori* issues of power, gender, race do not form part of the analysis. Seedhouse describes the analytical process as follows:

> CA is concerned with uncovering the underlying *machinery* which enables interactants to achieve this organisation and order [...]. This does *not* mean that CA provides access to participants' cognitive or psychological states. Rather, it means that analysts trace how participants analyse and interpret each others' actions and develop a shared understanding of the progress of the interaction. (Seedhouse forthcoming)

Within this overall framework, which seeks to analyse the machinery of interaction, CA has also produced its own methodology for the analysis of institutional talk. In this methodology it takes a view of the institutional context. Seedhouse defines it as follows:

> CA has a dynamic, complex, highly empirical perspective on context. Contributions are *context-shaped* in that they cannot be adequately understood except by reference to the sequential environment in which they occur and in which the participants design them to occur. Contributions are *context-renewing* in that they inevitably form part of the sequential environment in which a next contribution will occur. As Heritage (1984: 242) puts it, "The context of a next action is repeatedly renewed with every current action", and is transformable at any moment. (Seedhouse 2004: 43)

This CA view of context as dynamic and continually renewed contrasts with the traditional static idea of institutional context. In CA terms, the fact that a conversation takes place in a doctor's surgery does not make it a 'medical' conversation. One can have an ordinary chat in a doctor's surgery just as one can have a medical conversation in a supermarket. In the same way, the medical status of the participants in the talk does not necessarily characterise the talk as medical. Talk between a doctor and a patient may have the characteristics of ordinary conversation rather than the typical patterns of doctor–patient interaction. Hutchby and Wooffitt have pointed out a distinction between formal and non-formal types of institutional talk describing formal types as "more traditional and ceremonial" and non-formal types as "more loosely structured, but still task-oriented, lay/professional encounters" (1998: 148). Clearly, however, it is not the relative formality of a functional context which characterises it as medical. A medical lecture to students or a demonstration in a teaching hospital ward by a consultant, for example, may be formal whereas a standard consultation with a family doctor would be described as informal. Nor is it possible in CA to characterise talk as institutional by virtue of the fact that it extends over time between the same participants in the same place. Different phases of an interaction tend to have different characteristics depending on its sequential development and it is for this reason that CA studies concentrate on defining the interaction within phases of talk, such as opening or closing sequences.

The idea, then, of a 'medical' context is not an *a priori* category in CA research. Instead CA regards different institutions as having different institutional aims and organisations of the interaction appropriate to those aims. So the characterisation of talk as institutional thus depends on the extent to which interaction is organised in accordance with institutional aims. In Schegloff's (1992) words, institutional talk is a 'speech-exchange system' in which participants orient towards particular aspects of context. The nature of this system can only be revealed in the extent to which orientation to institutional aims is revealed as being *procedurally relevant* by the participants themselves. The aim of the CA researcher is thus to determine which elements of contexts are relevant to the interactants at any point in the interaction. This is a problematic task, as Schegloff explains:

> Even if we can show by analysis of the details of the interaction that some characterisation of the context of the setting in which the talk is going on (e.g. 'in the hospital') is relevant to the parties, that they are oriented to the setting so characterised, there remains another problem, and that is to show how the context or the setting (the local social structure) in that aspect, is procedurally consequential to the talk. How does the fact that the talk is being conducted in some setting (e.g. 'the hospital') issue in any consequence for the shape, form, trajectory, content or character of the interaction that the parties conduct? And what is the mechanism by which the context-so-understood has determinate consequences of the talk? (Schegloff 1992: 111)

In order to answer these questions, CA analysts need to "provide evidence of the work setting's relevance to the participants in the interaction being examined, and a description of the practices in which its procedural consequentiality is displayed" (Schegloff 1992: 117). It is for this reason that CA-based articles on medical discourse may invoke both a particular 'activity type' (Levinson 1992), for example a 'doctor–patient interview', and the particular social action taking place within it, for example, 'breaking bad news', 'managing optimism' or 'delivering and receiving diagnoses' (see § 2.2, 3.1, 3.2 for further discussion and examples).

2.2. The CA method – How is the analysis carried out?

CA uses naturally occurring data of verbal and, increasingly, of non-verbal communication. This data is closely transcribed using a highly detailed system and subjected to close turn-by-turn analysis, in which no detail of the interaction is *a priori* regarded as insignificant. The main focus of this turn-by-turn analysis is for the analyst to answer the question, for each turn, 'why that, in that way, at that moment?'. Sacks *et al.* (1974) described the turn-taking system as a system based on turn constructional units and transitional relevant points. Speakers may opt to carry out specific social actions at these points or may choose not to. As shown in §2.1, the organisation of turn-taking in institutional settings will be constrained and related to the institutional goal; in an interview between doctor and patient, for example, there are certain identifiable turn-taking patterns of this kind (see § 3.1 for further examples and discussion).

There are a number of tools which CA analysts use to help them examine turn-taking. The first is the concept of the *adjacency pair*. These are paired utterances (e.g. question-answer) in which the production of the second part is required by (or made *conditionally relevant* by) the first part. Consider the following example, of an opening sequence of an encounter between a health visitor (HV) and a first time mother (M), taken from Heritage / Sefi (1992: 379):

HV: 1 and you feel- (0.3) you're alright ba:thing
(.) her?
M: 1 I haven't bathed her ye:t
HV: 2 haven't you really
M: 2 no:. she had a bath when she came home from hospital

In this case, Heritage and Sefi analyse the adjacency pair within the overall framework of the entire opening sequence, describing the HV's initial inquiry as being projected towards an affirmative 'no problem' response and that the mother's negative reply indicates 'a potentially problematic state of affairs', which becomes the focus of subsequent analysis. This example illustrates how a CA study might aim to show how patients' answers to doctors' questions are organised within an overall design.

Another important tool is the idea of *preference*. In general, acceptance is a preferred or affiliative action, which is conducive to social solidarity, and rejection such as the negative reply of the mother in the above example is a dispreferred or disaffiliative one, which requires greater explanation or mitigation. As will be illustrated in §3.1, medical oral discourse reveals particular preference patterns in particular interactive situations.

Another important conversational practice is *repair*, which has been described as "the major, though not the sole, resource for parties to talk-in-interaction for displaying that they are dealing with trouble or problems in speaking, hearing or understanding the talk" (Schegloff *et al.* 2002: 25). Since repair is particularly prominent in contexts in which there is trouble in understanding a speaker's talk, issues of fluency / disfluency occurring in same-turn repair are becoming increasingly researched and their relevance for intercultural medical discourse and medical training are illustrated in § 3.1.

An aspect of CA methodology which is particularly relevant for medical discourse is the question of *quantitative* and *qualitative* methods. Traditionally, CA has been a qualitative research method which relies heavily on close case-by-case analysis of individual conversations. For this reason quantitative methods in CA are frowned upon – "the focus on quantification tends to lead the analyst away from considering closely, on a case-by-case basis, how participants themselves are orienting to one another's actions" (Hutchby / Wooffitt 1998: 116). Schegloff (1992) has also warned against the dangers of generalising from data that are only valid in one particular case in one particular circumstance.

However, given the emphasis on sequencing and pattern-seeking in much CA work, this essentially qualitative approach does not mean that quantity can be ignored or that generalisations cannot be made. Indeed, although qualitative research is still very much to the forefront, the use of statistics in the analysis of medical talk is on the increase. Stivers (2003), for example, identifies particular treatment recommendation formats and then uses a statistical approach to test whether parents are more or less likely to have reported receiving a treatment depending upon the treatment recommendation format used. Perkins (1995: 373) includes quantitative analysis in her research on aphasic patients because "it has the major advantage of facilitating comparison which is important in the evaluation in the effectiveness of therapy".

Finally, CA methodology is making increasing use of videorecorded evidence. This has produced an increase in the amount of attention now being paid to the role of non-verbal cues in the organisation of medical talk. Research into non-verbal interaction in medical settings has focused on the role of laughter (Haakana 2002), silence (Ten Have 1991a), body movement (Modaff 2003), gaze (Robinson 1998), gestures in the expression of pain (Heath 2002), amongst others. A significant example of this type of research is the recent work by Beach, Pigeron and Good (2003) on the way in which cancer patients respond to doctors' depiction of their symptoms. Beach *et al.* analyse the role of both verbal (hesitations, repairs and restarts) and non verbal aspects (gaze, grimacing, smiling) within an overall three-part structure (doctor description of symptoms – patient response – doctor response).

It should be noted that the increased use of statistics and the analysis of non-verbal aspects of interaction is one of the main reasons for the increase in CA-based studies in the applied sphere. This will be further discussed in § 3.2.

3. Medical discourse and applied conversation analysis

As §2 has suggested, the CA approach requires medical interaction to be studied as an activity type with a strong focus on the analysis of its characteristic phases and sequential moves and the social action that they generate. We will now look in more detail at what these activity types might be.

3.1. Medical activity types

The *doctor–patient interview* is the activity type which has been most studied within CA. It has a number of sequential phases, which traditionally run from history-taking through to physical examination (Stivers / Heritage 2001; Robinson / Stivers 2001), and CA researchers have examined different aspects of each of these phases. For example, close attention has been paid to different aspects of the way in which doctors and patients interact during the interview to 'do diagnosis' (Heath 1992; Maynard 1992; Gill / Maynard 1995), to deliver and receive good and bad news (Maynard 1991a, 1991c, 1997a, 1997b, 2003; Peräkylä 1998; Maynard / Frankel 2003), to negotiate prescription requests (Robinson 2001), to deal with test results (Pomerantz / Rintel 2004) or to discuss taboo subjects such as death (Lutfey / Maynard 1998), disability (Parry 2004) or sexuality (Weijts *et al.* 1993).

Particular doctor–patient *formats* have also been examined in some detail. For example, question-answer sequences have been studied in the doctor–patient interview by Frankel (1990; 1995) and Gill (1998) and in the history-taking phase by Stivers and Heritage (2001) and Boyd and Heritage (2005), who have identified ways in which doctors structure their questions to favour certain kinds of response. Other settings such as the psychotherapy interview (Czyewski 1995) or the psychiatric interview (Bergmann 1992; Mellinger 1995; see also Telles Ribeiro and Souza Pinto this volume) have been shown to involve specific interactional devices in the organisation of the interview format.

The most recent CA research on doctor–patient studies is in a collection by Heritage and Maynard (2005), the contents of which are summarised in Maynard and Heritage (2005). The main thread running through the collection is that doctor–patient interaction is analysable as a set of problem-solving exercises by both parties in which both are faced with what Maynard and Heritage (2005: 431) call 'sociomedical dilemmas' which include the framing and presentation of the encounter.

As well as looking at the interactional patterns of particular formats such as history-taking or the delivery of diagnosis, which are general formats that are likely to occur across a number of medical settings, researchers have looked at the way in which particular formats are generated in particular settings, particularly those areas of medicine which oblige interactants to take on particular *institutional roles* or to which interactants orient in a particular way. In particular the relation between format and *identity* has also been discussed by Ten Have (1995). This work is related to his earlier work (1991b) on *role differences* and the consequence of *asymetrical power relations* for medical discourse (see also Maynard 1991b).

The object of this kind of role study includes different kinds of interaction: first it includes interaction in settings such as the intensive care unit (Robillard 1994) or anaesthetic room (Pilnick / Hindmarsh 1999) in which doctors and patients may take on particular roles. Alternatively it might include settings in which a doctor may not even be involved such as the pharmacy, in which the pharmacist takes on a dual role of informant and adviser (Pilnick 1998, 1999).

A third possibility is the particular roles that are implied when the patient is essentially a third party to the talk; these include settings such as the pediatric clinic in which the role of the parent in the presentation of the child's problem (Stivers 2001) or deciding treatment (Stivers 2002) is a significant factor in orienting the talk about the patient, or even the veterinary clinic, in which a commentary prior to diagnosis (Stivers 1998) and talk 'with and about' animals (Roberts 2004) impose a different interactional structure from that of the standard doctor–patient interview.

Finally, there are studies of an institutional role (e.g. 'the doctor') stemming from a different disciplinary and cultural background. This is the case of Ruusuvuori's (forthcoming) CA-based comparison between doctor–patient interaction taking place in general practice and homeopathic consultations.

As well as doctor-carer-patient talk, there has been considerable recent CA interest in the talk of the patients themselves. Interaction *between patients* has been analysed by Arminen (1998) in a study of therapeutic interaction in Alcoholic Anonymous meetings. Alongside doctor–patient and patient-patient talk, there are also CA studies of *medical expert/non-expert* talk. The most notable of these are the studies of 'lay diagnosis' by Jones (2001), Beach (2001a, 2001b) and Ten Have (2001b). This area of talk, occurring between non-specialists and 'about medicine' is a growing area of CA research – a growth which is perhaps part of the widening of the research area which Candlin and Candlin (2003) have invoked for health care research in general.

Apart from two studies of meetings between health visitors and new mothers at home (Heritage / Sefi 1992; Heritage / Lindstrom 1998), there has been little CA work on what might be termed *paramedical* talk. i.e. talk involving paramedical personnel, which is a type of interaction, as Candlin and Candlin (2003) point out, that is particularly important for health service delivery. Nursing interaction, for example, is described by Candlin and Candlin (2003: 144) as "a key site of engagement" and they regard the lack of research on nursing interaction as an area which needs to be urgently developed, particularly in the intercultural sphere.

3.2. Applied conversation analysis and medical discourse

Applied conversation analysis is a significant area of growth in the analysis of talk and we trace here its development in the area of medical discourse. The notion of applied CA has been addressed by Ten Have (2001a) and in a recent collection by Richards and Seedhouse (2005), and the areas in which the relationship between CA and applied linguistics can be developed have been set out in a review article by Schegloff *et al.* (2002). Seedhouse (forthcoming), following Schegloff, argues that CA and applied linguistics are moving closer together, summarising this growing link as follows:

> Applied linguistics, which has its roots in language, finds its realisation through action, so a method of inquiry that brings together these two aspects as part of a coherent programme of investigation and description offers a perspective to which applied linguists should be particularly receptive. (Seedhouse forthcoming)

Seedhouse cites support from a number of CA researchers, notably comments by Heritage (1999: 73) – "part of the claim of any framework worth its salt is that it can sustain 'applied' research of various kinds" – and Drew (2005: xv) – "A few years ago, I would have said that AL and CA were wide apart; but now I think [...] that there is an increasing convergence between the two."

The area of applied medical CA research has been identified by Heritage (1999) as a likely area of development. If there is to be a convergence of CA with medical discourse, what direction and what form the application should take? According to Richards (2005), the model of application which is most consistent with the nature of CA is that of description leading to informed action. If this is the case, then we need to ask what areas of medical communication might this model of 'CA description leading to informed action' be applied to. The recent research suggests that the areas most ripe for development are medical training, speech pathology and intercultural discourse in medical domains.

3.2.1. Medical training

The relationship between CA and medical training can be classified in terms of CA studies *of* medical training, and the use of CA *within* a medical training programme. As regards the former, the talk of the medical training process has been revealed by Pomerantz (2003), in a study of modelling techniques, and by Zemel (2003) in a case study of surgical instruction in the operating theatre. Zemel's work in particular has revealed the complexity of the talk, showing how medical training is often simultaneous and multi-layered, with a surgeon teaching anatomy to medical students while at the same time demonstrating surgical techniques to trainee surgeons, all within the context of attending to the patient being operated on and the staff present in the operating theatre. The utility of this kind of study is to show at what point during the training process, interaction between trainer and trainee becomes problematic and perhaps ineffective.

As regards the use of CA *within* a medical training programme, Barnes (2005) has pointed out that training in medical communication, which has historically tended to concentrate on communication by participants in talk on an individual basis, is greatly enriched by CA's insistence that medical discourse is a collaborative construct between interactants. In her view, CA description can inform medical training firstly by identifying the problematic areas in medical talk and then by recommending solutions to the problem. This problem-solution type of description can then be used as material for trainers and trainees during medical training. Some early examples of CA-informed types of medical training are described in Booth and Perkins (1999) and Tapsell (2000). Maynard and Heritage (2005: 433) also stress the importance of how, in the pedagogical sphere, trainees need to be sensitised to the cooperative and co-constructed nature of doctor–patient talk by carrying out their own recordings and analysis of talk. They describe a method developed by Halkowski (2005) for helping medical students to analyse problematic areas of recorded doctor–patient interaction from a CA perspective.

The relationship between CA and the medical education curriculum is also discussed in Maynard and Heritage (2005) who argue that conversation analysis fits best with certain types of approach to medical education, namely patient-centred, biopsycho-social and relationship-centred approaches.

3.2.2. Speech pathology

Like medical communication trainers, speech pathology researchers are making increasing use of CA data and the relationship between CA and speech pathology has been recently discussed in Schegloff (2003). According to Hesketh and Sage (1999), this upsurge of interest in CA data stems from the way in which CA-informed descriptions shed light on the effects of communication impairment in a meaningful and realistic manner. This has been particularly true in the areas of *aphasia* and in the area of *stammering research*.

With regard to aphasia, there have been some highly succcessful applications of CA research, with a special issue of *Aphasiology* (1999, vol.13) being devoted to the subject. Of particular importance is the use of CA as an assessment tool for aphasia, discussed in Booth and Perkins (1999). The role of CA in stammering research has been discussed in Acton (2004), who argues that it is important, not just to examine the articulation of the individual stammerer but to examine how stammering unfolds during interaction and how participants deal with it. She argues that CA, with its strong interactional focus, is an appropriate framework for this kind of research because it is able "to draw attention to the relationship of stammerers' conversations to the organisational constraints of ordinary conversation" (2004: 35).

3.2.3. Intercultural medical discourse

As Candlin and Candlin (2003) have noted, communication in contexts of linguistic and cultural diversity is highly complex and this kind of intercultural communication is becoming an increasingly common phenomenon in societies with high rates of immigration. Since CA is applicable to any kind of talk, it is suggested that it is as helpful for diagnosing when and how problematic talk occurs interculturally as it does for talk between native speakers of a particular language.

In this respect CA research has the same utility for intercultural discourse as it does for speech pathology. Seedhouse describes this similarity as follows:

> CA research reinforces a shift away from a linguistic deficit model focussed on individual performance towards a model in which communicative competence is seen to be co-constructed. In this model, many of the interactional competencies of L2 students, non-native speakers and speech-disordered patients can only be revealed through painstaking CA analysis. (Seedhouse forthcoming)

Recent CA studies of medical intercultural talk in Gardner and Wagner (2004) and Mondada (2004) reveal how the issue of identity is particularly important. For example, Mondada's study of the interaction of surgeons at an international conference indicates that the identity of speakers as NNS was of less significance than their identity as 'experts', 'seniors' or 'juniors'.

CA studies of intercultural talk are also likely to have an effect on the teaching of special purpose language teaching in medicine, both in terms of what they reveal about the nature of NS-NNS talk and by comparison with talk between native speakers (Schegloff *et al.* 2002). The specific relationship between CA and LSP is addressed in a collection by Bowles and Seedhouse (forthcoming).

4. Conclusion – The future of CA and medical discourse

In conclusion, the present analysis of the development of the relationship between CA and medical discourse has shown a number of reasons why CA is likely to continue to expand in medical fields. The first is because CA is by its very nature interdisciplinary. As Schegloff (1992: 104) has remarked, "if it is not a distinctive discipline of its own (which it may well turn out to be), CA is at a point where linguistics and sociology (and several other disciplines, anthropology and psychology, among them) meet". CA thus lends itself to interdisciplinary research by providing raw data and a methodology – what Barnes (2005: 115) calls "a systematic approach for empirical investigations" – for other disciplines to use.

A second reason why the medical areas to which CA can be applied will continue to widen is methodological. As has already been shown, this is partly because CA is making increasing use of visual evidence, and partly because it is making greater use of both quantitative and qualitative methods. In areas such as medical communication skills training and speech pathology, where more qualitative CA research methods have been in use for some time, there is a move towards a more quantitative, data-driven approach in an effort to achieve greater validity of results. On the other hand, in more linguistic fields, such as intercultural medical discourse and the teaching of language for medical purposes, there is a move towards using qualitative CA research as a basis for the description of medical talk by identifying patterns in individual interactions and looking for them across a wider corpus. Use of this twin-track approach, involving quantitative and qualitative analysis working in harness, is on the increase in applied linguistics generally and is regarded by Acton (2004) as being likely to increase in applied medical CA.

A third reason is the applicability of CA to a wide variety of medical situations. As has been shown, CA is applicable to multiparty encounters involving multiple interactions and practices, and different kinds of participants, including different health care professionals, trainees and patients.

In what areas of medical discourse is applied CA likely to expand? Barnes argues that the future direction of the relationship between CA and medical discourse will depend on the way in which healthcare practices themselves change and expand within societies. She has identified a number of areas in which this might occur:

> In the future as health care continues to be decentralised and dispersed among a range of 'experts', the remit of health communication research may widen. We may then see the inclusion of studies in even more non-traditional sites, such as the UK's nurse-led service NHS direct, radio or television 'phone-ins' with health care 'experts', peer-run social support self-help groups or telephone lines, troubles-tellings about illness to friends and families, calls to workplaces to explain absenteeism, interaction and work practices in alternative medicine. (Barnes 2005: 115)

Given its interdisciplinary nature, methodologically adaptable characteristics and applicability to all forms of talk, it would seem that CA is well placed to keep up with this predicted diversification of health care settings and practices and the kind of discourse which they are likely to produce.

References

Acton, Ciaran 2004. A Conversation Analytic Perspective on Stammering: Some Reflections and Observations. *Stammering Research* 1/3, 249-270.

Arminen, Ilkka 1998. *Therapeutic Interaction: A Study of Mutual Help in the Meetings of Alcoholics Anonymous*. Helsinki: The Finnish Foundation for Alcohol Studies.

Barnes, Rebecca 2005. Conversation Analysis: A Practical Resource in the Health Care Setting. *Medical Education* 39, 113-115.

Beach, Wayne 2001a. *Lay Diagnosis*. Special issue in honour of the late Robert Hopper. *Text* 21/1-2.

Beach, Wayne 2001b. Introduction: Diagnosing Lay Diagnosis. *Text* 21/1-2, 13-18.

Beach, Wayne / Pigeron, Elisa / Good, Jeffrey 2003. Describing and Responding to Cancer Symptoms: The Interactional Embodiment of 'Fear'. Paper given at the 2003 convention of the International Communication Association.

Bergmann, Jorg 1992. Veiled Morality: Notes on Discretion in Psychiatry. In Drew / Heritage (eds), 137-162.

Booth, Susan / Perkins, Lisa 1999. The Use of Conversation Analysis to Guide Individualized Advice to Carers and Evaluate Change in Aphasia: A Case Study. *Aphasiology* 13, 283-303.

Bowles, Hugo / Seedhouse, Paul forthcoming. *Conversation Analysis and LSP*. Bern: Peter Lang.

Boyd, Elizabeth / Heritage, John 2005. Taking the Patient's Medical History: Questioning during Comprehensive History Taking. In Heritage / Maynard (eds).

Candlin, Christopher / Candlin, Sally 2003. Health Care Communication: A Problematic Site for Applied Linguistics Research. *Annual Review of Applied Linguistics* 23, 134-154.

Czyzewski, Marek 1995. Mm hm Tokens as Interactional Sevices in the Psychotherapeutic In-take Interview. In Ten Have, Paul / G. Psathas (eds) *Situated Order: Studies in the Social Organization of Talk and Embodied Activities*. Washington DC: University Press of America, 73-90.

Drew, Paul 2005. Foreword: Applied Linguistics and Conversation Analysis. In Richards / Seedhouse (eds), xiv-xx.

Drew, Paul / Heritage, John (eds) 1992. *Talk at Work: Interaction in Institutional Settings*. Cambridge: Cambridge University Press.

Dudley-Evans, Tony 2004. Genre Analysis. In K. Malmkjaer (ed.) *The Linguistics Encyclopedia*. London: Routledge, 205-208.

Frankel, Richard 1990. Talking in Interviews: A Dispreference for Patient-initiated Questions in Physician–Patient Encounters. In G. Psathas (ed.) *Interactional Competence*. Washington: University Press of America, 231-62.

Frankel, Richard 1995. Some Answers about Questions in Clinical Interviews. In G. Morris / R. Chenail (eds) *The Talk of the Clinic: Explorations in the Analysis of Medical and Therapeutic Discourse*. Hillsdale NJ: Lawrence Erlbaum, 49-70.

Gardner, Rod / Wagner, Johannes (eds) 2004. *Second Language Conversations*. London: Continuum.

Gill, Virginia Teas / Douglas Maynard 1995. On 'Labelling' in Actual Interaction: Delivering and Receiving Diagnoses of Developmental Disabilities. *Social Problems* 42, 11-33.

Gill, Virginia Teas 1998. Doing Attributions in Medical Interaction: Patients' Explanations for Illness and Doctors' Responses. *Social Psychology Quarterly* 61, 322-360.

Glenn, P. / LeBaron, C. / Mandelbaum, J. (eds) 2003. *Studies in Language and Social Interaction: Essays in Honor of Robert Hopper*. Mahwah NJ: Lawrence Erlbaum.

Haakana, Markku 2002. Laughter in Medical Interaction: From Quantification to Analysis, and Back. *Journal of Sociolinguistics* 6, 207-35.

Halkowski, Tim 2005. Realising the Illness: Patients' Narratives of Symptom Discovery. In Heritage / Maynard (eds).

Heath, Christian 1992. The Delivery and Reception of Diagnosis in the General Practice Consultation. In Drew / Heritage (eds), 235-67.

Heath, Christian 2002. Demonstrative Suffering: The Gestural (Re)embodiment of Symptoms. *Journal of Communication* 52, 597-617.

Heritage, John 1984. *Garfinkel and Ethnomethodology*. Cambridge: Polity Press.

Heritage, John 1999. Conversation Analysis at Century's End: Practices of Talk-in-interaction, their Distributions and their Outcomes. *Research on Language and Social Interaction* 31, 69-76.

Heritage, John / Lindstrom, Anna 1998. Motherhood, Medicine and Morality: Scenes from a Medical Encounter. *Research on Language and Social Interaction* 31, 397-438.

Heritage, John / Maynard, Douglas 2005 *Communication in Medical Care: Interaction between Primary Care Physicians and Patients*. Cambridge: Cambridge University Press.

Heritage, John / Sefi, Sue 1992. Dilemmas of Advice: Aspects of the Delivery and Reception of Advice in Interactions between Health Visitors and First-time Mothers. In Drew / Heritage (eds), 359-417.

Hesketh, Anne / Sage, Karen 1999. Conversation Analysis – Overview. *Aphasiology* 13, 4-5.

Hutchby, Ian / Wooffitt, Robin 1998. *Conversation Analysis*. Cambridge: Polity Press.

Jones, Charlotte 2001. Missing Assessments: Lay and Professional Orientations in Medical Interviews. *Text* 21, 113-150.

Levinson, Stephen 1992. Activity Types and Language. In Drew / Heritage (eds), 66-100.

Lutfey, Karen / Maynard, Douglas 1998. Bad News in Oncology: How Physician and Patient Talk about Death and Dying without Using those Words. *Social Psychology Quarterly* 61, 321-341.

Maynard, Douglas 1991a. Bearing Bad News in Clinical Settings. In B. Dervin (ed.) *Progress in Communication Sciences*. Norwood NJ: Ablex, 143-72.

Maynard, Douglas 1991b. On the Interactional and Institutional Bases of Asymmetry in Clinical Discourse. *American Journal of Sociology* 97, 448-95.

Maynard, Douglas 1991c. The Perspective-display Series and the Delivery and Receipt of Diagnostic News. In D. Boden / D. Zimmerman (eds) *Talk and Social Structure: Studies in Ethnomethodology and Conversation Analysis*. Cambridge: Polity Press, 162-92.

Maynard, Douglas 1992. On Clinicians Co-implicating Recipients' Perspective in the Delivery of Diagnostic News. In Drew / Heritage (eds), 331-58.

Maynard, Douglas 1997a. The News Delivery Sequence: Bad News and Good News in Conversational Interaction. *Research on Language and Social Interaction* 30, 93-130.

Maynard, Douglas 1997b. Structural Aspects of Bad News and Good News in Conversational Interaction. In A. Marcarino (ed.) *Analisi della conversazione e prospettive di ricerca in etnometodologia*. Urbino: Edizioni QuattroVenti, 59-76.

Maynard, Douglas 2003. *Bad News, Good News: Conversational Order in Everyday Talk and Clinical Settings*. Chicago: University of Chicago Press.

Maynard, Douglas / Frankel, Richard 2003. Indeterminacy and Uncertainty in the Delivery of Diagnostic News in Internal Medicine: A Single Case Analysis. In Glenn / LeBaron / Mandelbaum (eds), 393-410.

Maynard, Douglas / Heritage, John 2005. Conversation Analysis, Doctor–Patient Interaction and Medical Communication. *Medical Education* 39, 428-435.

Mellinger, Wayne 1995. Talk, Power and Professionals: Partial Repeats as Challenges in the Psychiatric Interview. In J. Siegried (ed) *Therapeutic and Everyday Discourse as Behavior Change: Toward a Microanalysis in Psychotherapy Process Research*. Norwood NJ: Ablex, 391-418.

Modaff, Daniel 2003. Body Movement in the Transition from Opening to Task in Doctor–Patient Interviews. In Glenn / LeBaron / Mandelbaum (eds), 411-22.

Mondada, Lorenza 2004. Ways of 'Doing Being Plurilingual' in International Work Meetings. In Gardner / Wagner (eds), 27-60.

Parry, Ruth 2004. The Interactional Management of Patients' Physical Incompetence: A Conversation Analytic Study of Physiotherapy Interactions. *Sociology of Health and Illness* 26, 976-1007.

Peräkylä, Anssi 1998. Authority and Intersubjectivity: The Delivery of Diagnosis in Primary Health Care. *Social Psychology Quarterly* 61, 301-20.

Perkins, Lisa 1995. Applying Conversation Analysis to Aphasia: Clinical Implications and Analytic Issues. *European Journal of Disorders of Communication* 30, 372-383.

Pilnick, Alison 1998. 'Why didn't you just say that?': Dealing with Issues of Asymmetry, Knowledge and Competence in the Pharmacist/Client Encounter. *Sociology of Health and Illness* 20/1, 29-51.

Pilnick, Alison 1999. Patient Counselling by Pharmacists: Advice, Information or Instruction?. *The Sociological Quarterly* 40/4, 613-622.

Pilnick, Alison / Hindmarsh, Jon 1999. 'When you wake up, it'll all be over': Communication in the Anaesthetic Room. *Symbolic Interaction* 22, 345-60.

Pomerantz, Anita 2003. Modeling as a Teaching Strategy in Clinical Training: When does it Work?. In Glenn / LeBaron / Mandelbaum (eds), 381-91.

Pomerantz, Anita / Rintel, Sean 2004. Practices for Reporting and Responding to Test Results During Medical Consultations:

Enacting the Roles of Paternalism and Independent Expertise. *Discourse Studies* 6, 9-26.

Richards, Keith 2005. Introduction. In Richards / Seedhouse (eds), 1-18.

Richards, Keith / Seedhouse, Paul (eds) 2005. *Applying Conversation Analysis*. Basingstoke: Palgrave Macmillan.

Roberts, Felicia 2004. Speaking to and for Animals in a Veterinary Clinic: A Practice for Managing Interpersonal Interaction. *Research on Language & Social Interaction* 37, 421-47.

Robillard, Albert 1994. Communication Problems in the Intensive Care Unit. *Qualitative Sociology* 17, 383-95.

Robinson, Jeffrey 1998. Getting down to Business: Talk, Gaze and Bodily Orientation during Openings of Doctor–Patient Consultations. *Human Communication Research* 25, 97-123.

Robinson, Jeffrey 2001. Asymmetry in Action: Sequential Resources in the Negotiation of a Prescription Request. *Text* 21, 19-54.

Robinson, Jeffrey / Stivers, Tanya 2001. Achieving Activity Transitions in Primary-care Encounters: From History Taking to Physical Examination. *Human Communication Research 27*, 253-298.

Ruusuvuori, Johanna forthcoming. 'Empathy' and 'Sympathy' in Action: Attending to Patients' Troubles in Finnish Homeopathic and General Practice Consultations. *Social Psychology Quarterly*.

Sacks, Harvey / Schegloff, Emanuel / Jefferson, Gail 1974. A Simplest Systematics for the Organization of Turn Taking for Conversation. *Language* 50/4, 696-735.

Schegloff, Emanuel 1992. On Talk and its Institutional Occasions. In Drew / Heritage (eds), 101-134.

Schegloff, Emanuel 2003. Conservation Analysis and Communication Disorders. In C. Goodwin (ed.) *Conversation and Brain Damage*. New York: Oxford University Press, 21-55.

Schegloff, Emanuel / Koshik, Irene / Jacoby, Sally / Olsher, David 2002. Conversation Analysis and Applied Linguistics. *Annual Review of Applied Linguistics* 22, 3-31.

Seedhouse, Paul 2004. *The Interactional Architecture of the Language Classroom*. Oxford: Blackwell.

Seedhouse, Paul forthcoming. Conversation Analysis and Language Learning. *Language Teaching.*

Stivers, Tanya 1998. Pre-diagnostic Commentary in Veterinarian-Client Interaction. *Research on Language and Social Interaction* 31, 241-77.

Stivers, Tanya 2001. Negotiating who Presents the Problem: Next Speaker Selection in Pediatric Encounters. *Journal of Communication* 51/2, 1-31.

Stivers, Tanya 2002. Participating in Decisions about Treatment: Overt Parent Pressure for Antibiotic Medication in Pediatric Encounters. *Social Science & Medicine* 54, 111-30.

Stivers, Tanya 2003. Treatment Recommendation: An Exploration of Design Variation. Paper given at the 2003 convention of the International Communication Association.

Stivers, Tanya / Heritage, John 2001. Breaking the Sequential Mold: Answering 'More than the Question' During Comprehensive History Taking. *Text* 21, 151-185.

Tapsell, Linda 2000. Using Applied Conversation Analysis to Teach Novice Dietitians History Taking Skills. *Human Studies* 23, 281-307.

Ten Have, Paul 1991a. The Doctor is Silent: Observations on Episodes without Vocal Receipt during Medical Consultations. In B. Conein / M. de Fornel / L. Quéré (eds) *Les formes de la conversation*, vol 2. Issy-les-Moulineaux: CNET, 55-76.

Ten Have, Paul 1991b. Talk and Institution: A Reconsideration of the 'Asymmetry' of Doctor–Patient Interaction. In D. Boden / D.H. Zimmerman (eds) *Talk and Social Structure: Studies in Ethnomethodology and Conversation Analysis.* Cambridge: Polity Press, 138-63.

Ten Have, Paul 1995. Formatting the Consultation: Communication Formats and Constituted Identities. In E. Huls / J. Klatter-Folmer (eds) *Artikelen van de Tweede Sociolingustische Conferentie*. Eburon Delft, 245-68.

Ten Have, Paul 1999. *Doing Conversation Analysis: A Practical Guide*. London: Sage.

Ten Have, Paul 2001a. Applied Conversation Analysis. In A. McHoul / M. Rapley (eds) *How to Analyse Talk in Institutional Settings: A Casebook of Methods*. London: Continuum, 3-11.

Ten Have, Paul 2001b. Lay Diagnosis in Interaction. *Text* 21, 251-260.

Weijts, Wies / Houtkoop, Hanneke / Mullen, Patricia 1993. Talking Delicacy: Speaking about Sexuality during Gynaecological Consultations. *Sociology of Health and Illness* 15, 259-78.

Zemel, Alan 2003. Teaching Surgery: The Achievement of Multiple Instructional Outcomes in the Operating Room. Paper given at the 2003 convention of the International Communication Association.

SALLY CANDLIN

Constructing Knowledge, Understanding and Meaning Between Patients and Nurses

1. Introduction

The traditional western bio-medical model of health care, resulting in the dominance of health professionals in the professional patient relationship, is one which is challenged by many professionals as well as by the general public. This dominance refers not necessarily to an interpersonal relationship invested with powerful asymmetries, but to an acknowledgment that health professionals are representatives of an institution which the patient has approached with health needs. These representatives include members of the nursing profession who are then placed immediately *a fortiori* in a more dominant position. Such dominance relates both to the *habitus* and the *capital* of the nurse (Bourdieu 1991) and the *members' resources* upon which both participants in any interaction draw (Fairclough 1989: 24), i.e. what "people have in their heads and draw upon when they produce and interpret texts – including their knowledge of language, representations of the natural and social worlds they inhabit, values, beliefs, assumptions and so on". For the nurse, members' resources (MR) include professional education, experience and expertise, and also access to health care services/personnel facilitated by membership of the professional and bureaucratic institutions.

In this chapter I propose that the caring process is more meaningful and acceptable to the patient, and the consequent health outcomes enhanced, when the situation is one not of dominance of the nurse over the patient, but one which is egalitarian in nature. This demands that the relationship which develops is one where the patient's contribution to the discourse is considered by both participants to be vital: where the patient is seen to understand and share in goal identification, participates appropriately in the care processes and treatment, and is an active partner in care rather than a passive recipient.

2. Cultural considerations

It is a truism to state that patients and health care professionals do not always share the same values and belief systems. Neither do they necessarily identify the same health-related goals. In contemporary society it is likely they not only do not share a common history, economic, educational and social backgrounds but frequently belong to different ethnic groups. This presents a complex situation demanding that interlocutors appreciate individual differences, particularly as they relate to beliefs about health and illness; beliefs which are often culturally determined. I argue that if the nurse, as the partner who is a representative of an institution, and therefore with the greater potential to be dominant, aims to develop a therapeutic relationship where mutually defined and agreed goals are met, she must first develop an in-depth knowledge of the patient's health beliefs, past health experiences and current expectations.

Accordingly, nurses need to acknowledge that nursing is a culture as clearly defined as a culture based on ethnicity (cf. Roberts / Sarangi 1995). Similarly, she must recognise that the patient is a member of a culture – one which is derived not necessarily from membership of an ethnic group, but from a social historical world with its own values, beliefs, customs, conventions, habits and practices: what Thompson (1990) would call the 'descriptive conception of culture'. S. Candlin (1993: 31) cites Thompson's definition of the culture or group or society as "the array of beliefs, customs, ideas and values, as well as material artefacts, objects and instruments which are acquired by individuals as members of the group or society" (Thompson 1990: 123). Because health beliefs are deeply embedded in the individual's culture and history (cf. Helman 1990) a successful nurse-patient relationship first requires that participants explore and understand each other's cultural health beliefs and understanding. The nurse must be aware that culture is represented by meaningful symbols that include behaviours and language use. She must also recognise that a patient is not able to enter and share in another's world/culture unless the symbolic representations can be interpreted and made meaningful. However, the meaning and value given to any symbolic form by one person is not of necessity the same as that given to it by another. This then impacts on the interpretation of any utterance. Interpretation involves not only understanding the overt message and rules of the culture (whether the culture is that of the health care system, the particular hospital, or the institution of nursing), but also of its hidden symbols and their symbolic value. These symbols within nursing are grounded in a long history of the institution and, along with the profession itself, are continually evolving. They are symbols based on a unique body of knowledge, and are represented linguistically partly by the specialised lexicon which has the potential to effectively subordinate a patient in any nurse-patient interaction. The language is the language of the institution of which the patient is not a member. An understanding by participants, and certainly by the nurse, of the differences is a pre-requisite if she is to discover ways to enter into the other's world and deliver culturally sensitive nursing care (Leininger 1985).

2.1. Application to the identification of nursing goals

Because the beliefs and values of both individuals and institutions are as disparate as those of ethnic groups, the goals identified by institutional members are neither necessarily shared nor agreed by participants. Nursing goals are multiple and the means whereby they are negotiated and accomplished within the institutional context may be complex and multi-faceted. To highlight one factor, such as cultural considerations, and ignore factors such as age, gender, education and other individual variables, is to ignore the holistic nature of the individual and of nursing care. However, not to acknowledge the disparity in cultural beliefs leaves the way clear for the dominant group's voice to be heard over the less dominant group or individual, thus having the potential to re-enforce ideologically-based practices (cf. Sarangi 1996). It follows from this that the autonomy of the patient might be threatened. The nurse is then faced with the task of not only facilitating mutual nursing goal identification, but also of ensuring that the patient's social goals are met so that care is sensitive, appropriate and acceptable. This care, in turn, is based in part and importantly, upon the successful achievement of communication goals so that appropriate information is elicited, and the nature and meaning of the nursing care for the individual is understood. The activities whereby these goals are identified include the health assessment of individual patients. This is a nursing activity which is based partly on interactions between the nurse and patient. The process within the health care system in which interactions takes place (represented in Figure 1) demonstrates the dominance of the concept of culture and communication in the health care system. This model provides the background and framework for the discussion.

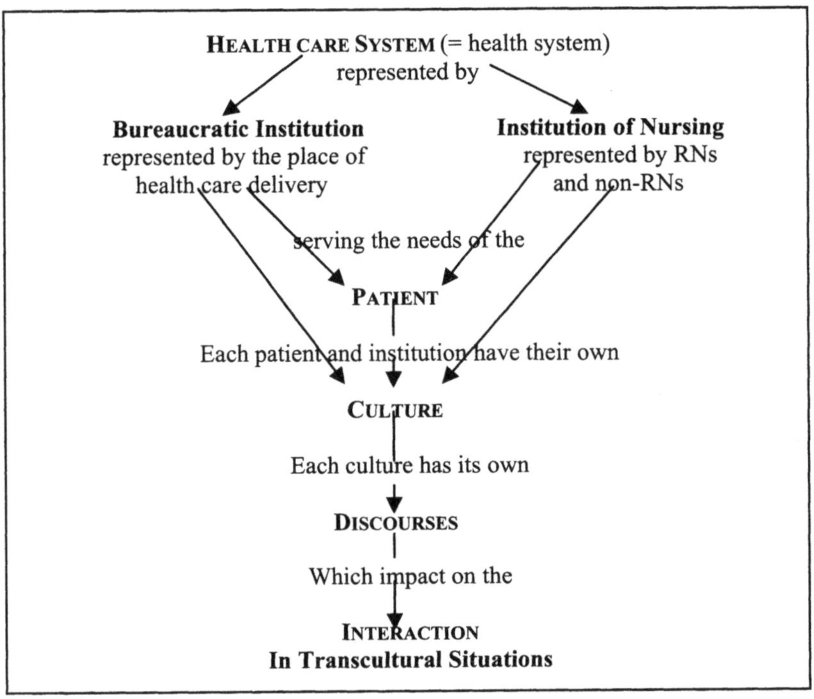

Figure 1. The cultures of different environments within the health care system.

2.2. The role of the expert nurse in the delivery of care

The situation where patients engage with the health care system can be challenging for both the individual patient and the nurse if an accurate nursing assessment is to be achieved and appropriate care delivered. It demands of the nurse a high level of expertise. This expertise is achieved not only by having a sound educational base, but also from gaining considerable experience within the practice setting. Benner (1984: 31-32) states that it is demonstrated by the nurse who has moved, in her professional practice, through stages from the novice practitioner where practice is rule-governed, to the expert nurse who no longer "relies on analytic principle (rule, guideline, maxim) [...]. The expert nurse, with an enormous background of experience, now has an intuitive grasp of each situation and zeroes in on the accurate region of the problem without wasteful consideration of a large range of unfruitful, alternative diagnoses and solutions". To deliver holistic care, considering the multidimensional needs of the patient, demands that her knowledge and experience refers not only to clinical tasks but also to the wider social and cultural world of the patient.

3. Cultures in contact: background to the research

As nursing care is dependent on the identification of goals which are determined in the health assessment of a patient, it is necessary that we clarify some of the issues which surround the concept of assessment.

3.1. Comparing nursing and other assessments

Nursing assessments are multi-dimensional in nature, addressing the total needs of the person: physical, social, emotional and spiritual. As such, this nursing activity has the potential to be different from other health-related assessments since it is comprehensive in nature with an emphasis on the totality of the individual's needs. It not only addresses the needs of the patient's physical domain, for example the maintenance of appropriate food intake or mobility, but also attends to other domains such as the psychosocial. Care is planned then according to the individual needs of each person.

Not every nursing assessment, however, is necessarily this comprehensive, nor is it the case that other health professionals, for example doctors, physiotherapists and occupational therapists, never perform comprehensive health assessments. Nevertheless this apparent generalisation is supported by other authors, for example Mishler (1984), Davis (1988), Fisher / Groce (1990), Fisher (1991), Fairclough (1992) and Faulkner (1992). Both Davis (1988) and Fisher (1991), for instance, found that doctors were far less inclined to address the psychosocial needs of patients than were nurses. The reason why it is important to draw attention to this issue is that patients have expectations of health professionals' behaviours. If, therefore, these expectations are not realised, then there is the potential for ambiguity in the professional relationship, whether the professional is a nurse, doctor or a member of an allied health group (as we shall see later). These behaviours, which contribute to the nature of the individual's identity, provide clues for the interlocutor who can then determine the strategies which will effect the successful negotiation of both nursing and interactional goals.

In comparing nursing assessments with other types of assessments, we should briefly consider the interactions which take place between patients and other health professionals. Because it has been difficult to locate discourse-based studies related to patients and allied health professionals, I discuss some of the studies of doctor-patient interactions. Consideration must be given however, to the differences between the practices of different health professionals. The point is made by Faulkner (1992: 14):

> Mr. West told his wife that everybody seemed to know his or her job. He then simplified matters enormously by telling his wife that "the doctor was wanting to make sure that he gave me the right treatment, the dietician, well she wanted to make sure that I get my food right". Mrs West then asked "Well what about the nurse – what did she want?" Mr West replied, "Oh she just looks after me, she needs to know what I want and how I feel". The simple

segregation is, of course far from the full reality of the team approach, but to Mr West each person had an allotted job [...].

3.2. Medicine

Because doctors and nurses both work in health-related situations one might expect that there would be similarities in their approaches to practice. However, partly because of the differing amounts of time spent by various practitioners with the individual patient (cf. Henzl 1989), there may, in fact, be considerable differences in their approaches. These differences may be related to the work of the nurse who is 'unable to get away' from the situation, a point made by Able-Boone (1989: 232) where she remarks that nurses must have "continuous responsibility for the infant's life". This situation contrasts with that of the doctor who is not with the patient continuously. It is to the nurse's observations that the doctor frequently refers for information about the patient's changing condition and needs. The amount of time spent with the patient contributes to the quality of the developing relationship and it is often the nurse from whom the patient first seeks help.

Davis (1988: 155) makes the point that in a culture where helplessness is not a desirable situation, asking for help carries face-threatening dimensions. When discussing the attitudes of doctors to patients who display varying degrees of helplessness, Davis (1988: 48) in her analysis of doctor-female patient interactions comments on the apparent 'niceness' of the General Practitioners (GPs). They were "unabashedly and unswervingly nice! They were friendly, interested, empathetic and quite obviously doing their best to provide patients with quality care". On closer examination of her data, however, she found that "it was precisely the intimate, pleasant quality of the medical encounter that made issues like power and control continuously seem like something else".

Within situations demonstrating varying degrees of need and helplessness, it is not surprising that a feature of the standard medical interview as described by Fairclough (1992:14) is the degree of interactional control by the doctor: "Doctors typically control the interaction [...]. It is the doctor who asks the question to which the patient responds and the doctor in turn accepts: a three part cycle, the topic of which is introduced by the doctor." Fairclough suggests that "the doctor is shifting and constraining topics in accordance with a pre-set agenda which the patient is not being allowed to disturb". Fairclough's observations echo those of C. Candlin, Coleman and Bruton (1983) when observing the interactions of dentists and patients, and also those of Fisher and Groce (1990: 241) who say that:

> it appears from these response patterns that doctors and patients share the perception of what kinds of information are more or less relevant for doctors. The participants do not, however, agree on what is appropriate for patients to talk about. Patients' accounting practices consistently move to broaden the medical discourse to include the social context of their lives as well as their assessment of health. Doctors' responses to their accounting practices consistently move to constrain their discourse and/or to legitimate the doctor's medical role.

3.3. The nursing assessment

Some nursing assessments are discourse-based addressing all the domains of health. And while there are many health-related topics, there may be no definitive order in which they are to be addressed. The order may relate to their importance at the time or simply woven into the 'flow' of conversation. Neither do all assessment topics necessarily need to be addressed. For example, the nurse might already be aware of, and possibly treating, a need in a specific domain. This might then not be raised in the discourse.

Other factors which may impact on the discourse include the environment in which the activity takes place. The influence of the surroundings is an observation made in personal practice experiences in both the hospital and community environment (for further discussion see S. Candlin 1995). Observations such as this support the argument put forward in the preceding discussion relating to cultural considerations and serve to emphasise the need for the nurse to enter the life world (LW) of the patient, making the LW pertinent to the nursing world (NW). Cazden (1970), when discussing the school situation, identifies the need for the teacher to consciously negotiate entry into the student's world. She argues that a child cannot enter the consciousness of the teacher unless the teacher has first entered the world of the child. A similar situation pertains to nurses and patients and can be captured in Figure 2 where we see that the worlds of the participating individuals overlap.

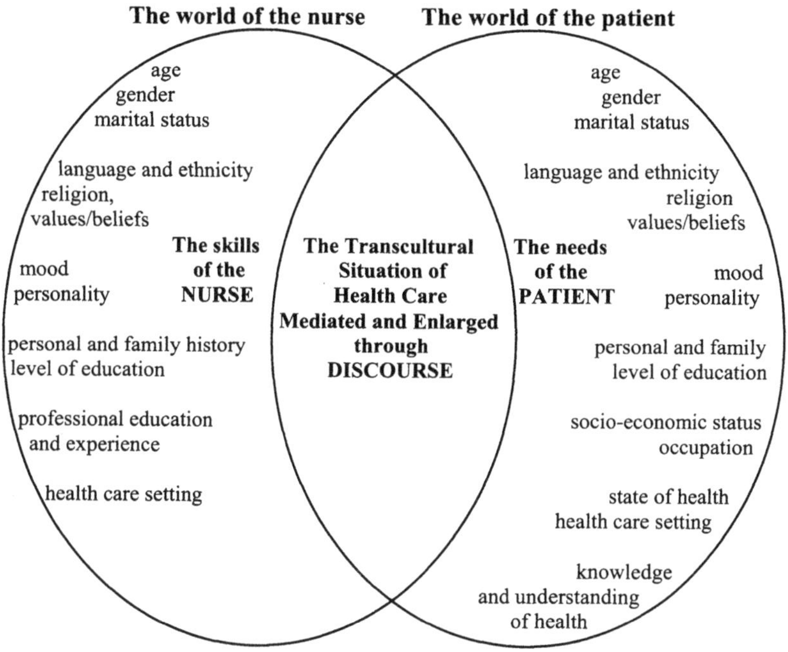

Figure 2. The transcultural health care situation mediated and enlarged through discourse (adapted from S. Candlin 1995).

Each world is dependent upon a number of variables (e.g. age, gender ethnicity, personality and the patient's state of health). These variables may need to be elicited by sensitive exploration of the patient's world. The further into the patient's world the nurse is able to enter, giving consideration to the different variables, the more the interlocutors will be able to create a shared 'space', and the more will the patient's needs be elicited and met. This transcultural space, demonstrated in the model, is mediated and enlarged by the competent use of discourse. The greater the space depends, therefore, on the skilful and strategic use of discourse and demonstrates the expertise of the nurse.

This expertise is reflected in, and may be measured by, the resulting identification and meeting of health needs. The situation that is presented in the model above implies that each participant can choose whether or not to tacitly invite the other into his/her world, and in turn choose whether or not to accept the tacit invitation – any 'shifting' patterns determining outcomes. The quality of the 'shift' determines the development of the relationship and the outcomes of the discourse.

The nurse-patient situation is different from many, in that to meet the patient's needs the nurse has a moral and legal duty to utilise particular professional skills. These skills are, I suggest, only truly effective if the variables of each world are considered. The nurse must identify and consider factors which can be used to empower the patient, thereby increasing capital (cf. Bourdieu 1991). She may, for example, elicit facts about the patient's health knowledge base, so that deficits can be appropriately addressed and existing knowledge exploited.

The demands on both interlocutors are considerable. While acknowledging and accommodating to individual variables, the person who enters into another world is stepping into an unfamiliar world which imposes constraints in a similar way to those imposed on members of ethnic groups, clubs and societies. The nurse who delivers care in a person's home enters an environment which represents the domain of another person. And while she is delivering a professional service, she is bound by the routines and expectations of the patient. Similarly the patient who is in a hospital or extended care facility, is not on 'home ground'. S/he faces an uncertain and unknown world, and having been removed by circumstances from the familiar world/culture, has had to enter another world/culture with its own values, beliefs, customs conventions, habits and practices that are the hallmark of another world (S. Candlin 1995). Not only is the physical location identified by its beliefs, expectations, rules and regulations that govern behaviours, but so too is the institution of nursing, and indeed all professional bodies. It is this complex and multi-cultural environment that the patient attempts to navigate if s/he is to make sense of this 'new' system.

From the outset, a patient might experience actual or perceived disadvantage in the relationship. The potential then for problems to arise in the developing relationship are always present. Without due recognition and understanding of this, it is possible that the purpose of nursing interventions will neither be understood nor acceptable to the patient or family, risking that the patient will not adhere to treatment. It is vital therefore that the activity is co-constructed by the nurse and patient so that differences can be understood, respected and accommodated, and particularly in the discoursal choices that each participant makes. These choices depend on making use of appropriate discoursal strategies in the context of the sensitivity and openness between the partners to the values and beliefs of both. The overall argument is supported by other authors and is relevant whether care is being delivered in the person's home or in a health care facility. When discussing the work of Blom and Gumperz (1972), Milroy (1986: 32-33) also emphasises

> the intimate manner in which choice of code is linked to an integrated system of local values and used to convey social meanings [...] linguistic choice takes place as a result of specifiable social and situational, constraints and incentives [...].

I suggest that the expert nurse recognises the social and situational constraints and chooses her discoursal strategies accordingly, since excellence in nursing care depends not only on sound nursing education and experience but also, as discussed above, on the sensitive discoursal skills of participants in the health care situation.

4. Research methodology

In the belief that there is benefit to be obtained from exploring further the discoursal strategies employed by expert nurses, I hypothesised that the expert nurse from her considerable experience and education is one whose communication and interpersonal skills have been finely honed. An observation of her strategies and the resulting outcomes might shed light on how successful interactions are conducted.

Data to explore how knowledge and understanding are constructed by nurses and patients are exemplified by the discourse of an experienced registered nurse (RN) and a patient in an assessment situation in the patient's home. This is compared, when appropriate, with the discourse of an untrained and less experienced assistant in nursing (AIN) in an extended care facility. It must be emphasised here that although AINs are not allowed to perform health assessments, it was agreed that they might participate in the study solely to observe communication strategies.

Following discussion with the related ethics committees, written informed consent was willingly given by 30 nurse–patient dyads to audio record interactions of assessment situations. A full explanation was given to each participant, and nobody was coerced into participating. The following discussion is illustrated with extracts from two dyads in the data corpus. To preserve confidentiality the names of people and places are fictitious. Cheryth (RN) is assessing the needs of Mrs. Y in her home, and Naomi (AIN) is talking with Mrs. G. in an extended care facility.

5. Discussion of the data

In Example 1, taken from the assessment of Mrs. Y, it is noticeable that the discourse is generally informal using the language of the LW (lines 1, 7 and 9) (cf. the work of Mischler 1984). Traces of formality and directness appear from time to time, seemingly when the nurse is requiring explicit information (e.g. lines 45-46 and 48). The formality, where the obvious agenda of the NW is seen, is demonstrated through the use of direct questions (e.g. lines 1-2 and 42). This strategy appears to gain information which could be seen as giving salience to the task-related goals of nursing, rather than the seeming interactional goals (e.g. lines 1 and 2). However the use of reference to the LW of Mrs. Y in lines 3-10, and the lexical items free of nursing 'jargon' (line 21, "Right and he thinks it's the shoulder" and 27-28, "Right the left one okay...") rather than a reference to 'the scapula' – which might be expected if the nurse was talking to a colleague, can be interpreted as an attempt to enter the world of the patient.

Example 1: Cheryth assessing Mrs. Y at home in the community

Cheryth: Now Mrs. Y can you let me
know what happened initially?

Mrs. Y: I was going to get some pot plants
from (?) it's a fern house my friend
is here for three weeks I was putting
them in the car this morning and I
just missed my footing and finished
up in the rock lilies and the azalea and
I've hurt the rock lilies but not the azalea
and I sat for a couple of minutes and then
called them out to help me in and then
(?) it's now x-rayed and the persons attending
me were extremely considerate to the pain
I had and I was asked to go back this
morning for an x-ray and said that I have
a broken shoulder possibly it's dislocated.
Am I talking loud enough?

Cheryth: Yes that's fine

Mrs. Y: And I see Doctor Z on Thursday
for C (?)

Cheryth: Right and he thinks it's the shoulder

Mrs. Y: Yes

Cheryth: Right

Mrs. Y: From what I gather it's a piece chipped off
this shoulder blade or shoulder bone
shoulder bone

Cheryth: Right the left one okay and how did you
go last night over the pain

Mrs. Y: Actually the pain wasn't as bad as I
expected they gave me a pethidine needle
and a lom something

Cheryth: Maxolon

Mrs. Y: And although I was waking up every
hour sort of thing I didn't have very much
discomfort I possibly leant on and wake up
woke myself up but I had the (?) so it's alright
What else do you want to know?

Cheryth: Right so they just put a sling on it on your arm to
support it and nothing else until you see Dr Z on
Thursday

Mrs. Y: Yes

Cheryth: Did he give any indication of what Dr Z might do?

Mrs. Y: He said I don't think there'll be any surgery but
he will assess it when he's read the report

Cheryth: Right and did he give some medication

46		for the pain
47	Mrs. Y:	Yes I had some panadeine for it
48	Cheryth:	Right and how often have you been taking those? […]

Throughout the interaction Cheryth appears to easily shift between the NW and the LW. This is particularly noticeable when she moves to the NW (line 252) from the Mrs. Y's LW. It is interesting that Mrs. Y, by attempting to joke (lines 249-251), is also able to make the LW part of the NW.

248	Cheryth:	Oh some of us have all the luck
249	Mrs. Y:	Everybody says that to me you know to lie down
250		on the beach and dig two holes you now (..) it's
251		terrible
252	Cheryth:	Just to get back to your medication do you are
253		you allergic to anything that you know of
254	Mrs. Y:	Foods but not medications that I know of
255	Cheryth:	Right but you are allergic to some foods are you

There is no sense in which Cheryth is seen simply to engage in social 'chit-chat' and 'passing the time of day'. Her discoursal choices, the questions (e.g. lines 1-2, 21, 27-28, 45-46) and topic choices (e.g. lines 2, 21, 27-28) are strategically selected with information garnered which is indicative of Mrs. Y's health needs: the diagnosis, x-ray and treatment of pain. Later there is reference to housework and what might in any other context be seen as 'idle talk' about domestic chores. Here the LW is very much part of the NW since an injury is likely to make it difficult to perform household work. Cheryth appears to make light of it in line 180 (below), but the following clause "that's good" indicates that she has considered and carefully acknowledged that the domestic arrangement accords with Mrs. Y's needs. Whether this interpretation is correct is one which only the participants can answer with certainty. At best it is an educated guess, albeit that of one who has worked in similar settings.

171	Mrs. Y:	Oh I don't like playing with the vacuum cleaner
172		that makes me tired
173	Cheryth:	Right makes you tired
174	Mrs. Y:	Makes me a little tired too
175	Cheryth:	Oh but do you normally do that do you normally
176		do the housework

177 Mrs. Y: No father usually vacs the floor for me
178 Cheryth: Right so he's pretty good
179 Mrs. Y: Oh he helps a lot yeah (?)
180 Cheryth: You've got him all organised ah that's good so
181 you usually share those sorts of things

The nursing assessment is seen to consider the social and emotional state of the patient since while the above exchange might appear to serve social goals, it acknowledges an area of need, but does so in such a manner that face is saved. Cheryth appears to lessen the threat to Mrs. Y's face in her admission of needing help by making light of the situation (line 180), but does not negate Mrs. Y's expressed need. Cheryth's goals are not only interactional. Before any physical task can be undertaken the nurse must elicit as much appropriate information as possible, and while 'moving the interaction along' the interlocutors are simultaneously engaging in 'nursing work'.

What is interesting about the discourse cited here is the ease with which both nurse and patient shift from the LW to the NW. Cheryth makes relevant the LW of Mrs. Y to the extent that the LW becomes the NW. This strategic intertextuality where Cheryth in line 252 refers back to an earlier text (lines 47-48) and blends LW with NW text is not a strategy which can be assumed, there being little sign of it in the following extract from the assessment of Mrs. B by Naomi. And yet this might have made earlier joking significant had Naomi been able to refer back to it and draw the LW into the NW.

Example 2: Naomi assessing Mrs. B in an extended care facility

225 Naomi: …you've got no problem with discharge or
226 bleeding have you energy level how's your
227 energy level
228 Mrs. B: nil
229 Naomi: nil (…..)
230 Mrs. B: I manage to wash meself
231 Naomi: Do you sleep well at night
232 Mrs. B: Oh with the help I take a very strong tablet
233 Naomi: Do you
234 Mrs. B: mm
235 Naomi: So you need help there now (……) how do you
236 class your health do you think it's bad or poor or
237 excellent
238 Mrs. B: Well I couldn't tell you but I'd say it was awful

Naomi: Poor all right
Mrs. B: I couldn't find the words to put in there
Naomi: No that's all right em (…) so you feel poor
Mrs. B: I can't find (…) I've said before I've told
you it's impossible for me to state because
I couldn't describe it only to say that (..)
I (..) feel you know like ….
Naomi: No well you feel well
Mrs. B: No I don't feel well
Naomi: No all right
Mrs. B: I get giddiness most of the time
Naomi: Illness I'll put illness there social activities
well you've got none have you
Mrs. B: No no
Naomi: No smoking
Mrs. B: No
Naomi: Nil (laughs**) alcohol
Mrs. B: No

Although earlier in the conversation there had been much joking and 'bantering' and, in the nursing sense, of apparently little consequence, we see Naomi posing direct questions from a proforma. This immediately aligns her with the institution and gives little control to Mrs. B who does not know what the topics are which must be addressed. Naomi has all the information: she calls the shots and controls the topic management with little opportunity for Mrs. B to initiate topic changes. Naomi is bound by the institutional agenda. As such Mrs. B has very little power – the relationship is asymmetrical and is reminiscent of the biomedical model where the institution is dominant. In contrast, by making little reference to a proforma, Cheryth hands much of the interactional control to Mrs. Y. She prefers to concentrate on the immediate and more urgent situation which is more significant and has more meaning to both Cheryth and Mrs. Y.

Cheryth is seen to be accommodating to Mrs. Y, a strategy proposed by Giles, Taylor and Bourhis (1973) where the speaker is prepared to 'move towards' the interlocutor discoursally. In this situation, the nurse, by using the language of the LW is, arguably, moving 'downwards' demonstrating a willingness to empathise with Mrs. Y. Whether the person moves 'upwards' (in an attempt to gain the approval of the other) or 'downwards', by acknowledging the individual social difference and making the move, the speaker can be seen to have made a strategic adjustment to allow the smooth flow of conversation. Important information might not have been elicited by a question/answer approach which demonstrates little move in the interaction.

But there is a further and equally significant issue which demands comment and relates to the manner in which information is elicited. Where Cheryth co-constructs knowledge and understanding with the patient, resulting in an assessment that is meaningful to Mrs. Y, there is little indication that Naomi's questions are meaningful to Mrs. B or that there is a deep understanding of the patient's needs (see lines 242-247). With her very minimal training and her lack of familiarity with the task, she has fewer members' resources to which Fairclough (1989) refers and from which she can draw, and displays little of the professional capital discussed by Bourdieu (1991) (see earlier discussion). Cheryth is aware that she must elicit considerable knowledge from the capital of Mrs. Y and make it significant to the NW. Only by co-constructing a mutual knowledge base, each drawing from and sharing in the capital of the other, can the participants develop a deeper understanding and make meaningful the health issues which are significant. Discoursally, by using the terminology of the LW and rejecting medical/nursing terminology, Cheryth demonstrates empathy with the patient, and by using similar terminology, she is further establishing cohesion in the discourse (Hoey 1991).

Nurse/patient interaction, as with other professional encounters, frequently involves the nurse in hearing relational narratives from patients. Cheryth, in the assessment task, conducts a narrative style interview and conforms to the two distinct stages proposed by Jordan and Little (2004). She encourages the story stage following the opening request, and follows this up with the stage of the weakly structured interview. The transformative task for the nurse is to make that relational narrative tractable in professional terms, in short to connect it to her professional knowledge and expertise. At the same time, however, there is a further transformative task which is to reformulate that expert interpretation in a form that is tractable to the patient. This is the essence of professional communication. It is co-constructed, it is transformative and it is continuously reformulated. The relational narrative of the patient may not, however, follow the traditional structures of canonical narrative, for example, the coda may precede the comment. In the case of Cheryth and Mrs. Y, the patient does follow the canonical form and the nurse is able to confirm and reformulate sections of the patient's story to make it tractable. Given the difficulties of the transformative process both ways, one facilitative procedure would be, as here, for the nurse and patient to co-construct the narrative, making minimal reformulation necessary. This is enabled by following the two stages posited by Jordan and Little. The assessment follows a series of story genres within the overall narrative until a comprehensive picture of the situation is drawn from which appropriate treatment can be planned. The strategies which the nurse utilises to achieve a successful outcome, I propose, is a hallmark of the expert nurse. Cheryth has not conformed to the structure of a proforma, but by using her extensive knowledge drawn from wide experience and her in-depth professional education and training, she has been able to home in on the immediate problems of the situation, loosely structuring the interaction and allowing the patient to establish what is of concern to her.

6. Conclusion

The importance of the patient's contribution to health care results not only in shifting power relationships between participants in the interaction, but also in the utilisation of the life world so that the nursing world becomes more meaningful to the patient. This facilitates the elicitation and utilisation of appropriate nursing information. While the data demonstrate that the process is not always easy to maintain, both the process and the resulting outcomes are found to be dependent on nursing expertise. Although there appears in Example 2 to be little movement of the patient into the world of the nurse, and indeed of the nurse into the world of the patient, in Example 1 – where the patient is on 'home ground' – the reverse is the case. The nurse, in the turn-taking and topic exchange, has listened to the patient's narrative and demonstrated a willingness to enter into the world and culture of the patient. But she has also drawn from the information to gain further knowledge which may be useful later. The transcultural world has been enlarged as the nurse has considered the variables that are part of the patient's culture. The discoursal strategies and nursing outcomes have been successful with quality nursing care being achieved.

Discourse analysts might, however, wish to address the validity of their interpretation of events, since, as Hak (1999) has indicated, it is not easy to interpret the behaviours of professionals who not only have their own unique body of knowledge, but where their behaviours and reasons for their discourse are frequently understood only by other professionals. It raises the question of the need for participants to reflect on the situation and to give confirmatory signals to the interpretation of the analysis. Such reflection and confirmation of the analyst's interpretation of data would give it richness and meaning and add to the body of knowledge of the professional workplace, at the same time giving deeper understanding of workplace practices to the discourse analyst.

It is important to consider also the ethics of data collection with participants understanding the intent of the study. The principles, for example, of beneficence and autonomy of the individual must be upheld. In a study involving the sensitive nature of health care, consideration must be given to the protection of the privacy and confidentiality of the participants and the facility, with the protocols of the latter understood. The discussion with participants of outcomes of studies should be considered, not only to ensure the accuracy of the interpretation by the analyst, but also to indicate acknowledgement of their contribution to the development of professional practices.

6.1. The way forward

The discussion in this chapter indicates and confirms the appropriate deployment of expertise and skills mix within the health care setting. But it also demonstrates the potential for impact on the preparation of individuals for practice. The data demonstrate that the quality and richness of care given by the expert nurse who is a highly trained, educated and experienced professional is, as would be expected, of high standard and quality. The process whereby this expertise is developed raises the question of the education of nurses. Of particular import is the value placed on communication as a fundamental and major component of both initial preparation programs and ongoing professional development. The strategies of the registered nurse demonstrate that not only does discourse contribute to excellence in health care, but when used sensitively, the therapeutic property of discourse is not only the vehicle of health care, but it *constitutes* that care in no small measure.

While the findings within the local situation are of interest, they are also of relevance and pertinent to the wider professional community. The population in western countries is ageing, bringing with it the potential for increasing demands on the health services. The professional nurse must be prepared adequately for these changes. This forward planning involves the planning and funding of education programs that are aimed at meeting the needs of contemporary society and enhancing the care of the individual.

References

Able-Boone, Harriet 1989. Parent-professional Communication Relative to Medical Care Decision Making for Seriously Ill New-borns. In von Raffler-Engel, Walburga (ed.) *Doctor Patient Interaction*. Amsterdam: Benjamins, 227-54.

Benner, Patricia 1984. *From Novice to Expert: Excellence and Power in Clinical Nursing Practice*. MenloPark: Addison Wesley.

Blom, Jan-Peter / Gumperz, John J. 1972. Social Meaning in Linguistic Structures: Code Switching in Norway. In Gumperz, John / Hymes, Dell (eds) *Directions in Sociolinguistics*. New York: Holt, Rinehart and Winston.

Bourdieu, Pierre 1991. *Language and Symbolic Power*. Cambridge: Polity Press.

Candlin, Christopher / Coleman, Hywel / Bruton, Clive 1983. Dentist-patient Communication: Communicating Complaint. In Wolfson, Nessa / Judd, Eliot (eds) *Sociolinguistics and Language Acquisition*. Rowley, Mass.: Newbury House, 56-81.

Candlin, Sally 1993. The Construction of Assessment in the Discourse of Older Patients. Paper presented at the *American Applied Linguistics Conference*. Atlanta, April 1993.

Candlin, Sally 1995. Transcultural Issues in Nurse–Patient Communication. *Geriaction* 13/7, 28-33.

Cazden, Courtney 1970. Children's Questions. Their Forms, Functions and Roles in Education. *Young Children*. 25/4, 202-20.

Davis, Kathy 1988. *Power Under the Microscope*. Dordrecht: Foris.

Fairclough, Norman 1989. *Language and Power*. London: Penguin.

Fairclough, Norman 1992. *Discourse and Social Change*. Cambridge: Polity Press.

Faulkner, Anne 1992. *Effective Interaction with Patients*. Edinburgh: Churchill Livingstone.

Fisher, Susan 1991. A Discourse of the Social: Medical Talk / Power Talk / Oppositional Talk? *Discourse and Society* 2/2, 257-83.

Fisher, Susan / Groce, Stephen, B. 1990. Accounting Practices in Medical Interviews. *Language in Society* 19, 225-50.

Giles, Howard / Taylor, Donald M. / Bourhis, Richard Y. 1973. Towards a Theory of Interpersonal Accommodation Through Speech: Some Canadian Data. *Language and Society* 2, 177-92.

Hak, Tony 1999. 'Text' and 'Con-text'. Talk bias in Studies of Health Care Work. In Sarangi, Srikant / Roberts, Celia (eds) *Talk, Work and Institutional Order. Discourse in Medical Mediation and Management Settings*. Berlin: Mouton de Gruyter, 427-51.

Helman, Cecil G. ^{2}1990. *Culture, Health and Illness*. Oxford: Butterworth/Heinemann.

Henzl, Vera M. 1989. Linguistic Means of Social Distancing in Physician-Patient Communication. In von Raffler-Engel, Walburga (ed.) *Doctor Patient Interaction*. Amsterdam: Benjamins.

Hoey, Michael 1991. *Patterns of Lexis in Text*. Oxford: Oxford University Press.

Jordan, Christopher / Little, Miles 2004. 'In This Scenario, I Do This, For These Reasons': Narrative, Genre and Ethical Reasoning in the Clinic. *Social Science and Medicine* 58, 1635-45.

Leininger, Madeleine 1985. Ethnography and Ethnonursing: Modes of Qualitative Data Analysis. In Leininger, Madeleine (ed.) *Qualitative Research Methods in Nursing*. Orlando, Fla: Grune.

Milroy, Leslie 1986. *Language and Social Networks*. Oxford: Basil Blackwell.

Mishler, Elliott 1984. *The Discourse of Medicine: Dialects of Medical Interviews*. Norwood, NJ: Ablex.

Roberts, Celia / Sarangi, Srikant 1995. 'But are they one of us?'. Managing and Evaluating Identities in the Work-related Contexts. *Multilingua* 14, 363-90.

Sarangi, Srikant 1996. Conflation of Institutional and Cultural Stereotyping in Asian Migrants' Discourse. *Discourse and Society* 7/3, 359-87.

Thompson, John B. 1990. *Ideology and Modern Culture.* Cambridge: Polity Press.

Maria Grazia Guido

The Discourse of Post-Traumatic Stress Disorder: Specialized-Genre Conventions vs. West African Refugees' Narrative Representations

1. Introduction

This chapter explores the ways in which past traumatic experiences of war and torture are first represented in the narratives of West African refugees and then reported and investigated in the specialized discourse of Psychiatry. More specifically, it analyzes the cognitive and discursive incongruities identified in the ways native trauma narratives come to be conventionally textualized into medical registers. This, it is argued, is mainly due to the fact that, so far, Western psychiatric enquiry has, with very few exceptions (cf. Devereux 1980), shown little concern for the consequences of prolonged and multiple war traumas in non-Western societies (cf. Summerfield 1999). Indeed, the possibility of different cultural representations of trauma does not fall within the biomedical parameters established in the *Diagnostic and Statistical Manual of Mental Disorders* (DSM-IV) issued by the American Psychiatric Association (APA 1994). On the one hand, such parameters determine the scientific terminology for the categorization and description of the psychiatric consequences of single-trauma exposure broadly labelled as Post-Traumatic Stress Disorder (PTSD), and thus fail to classify the complex post-traumatic syndromes associated with the victims of torture. Significantly, these syndromes have been only vaguely defined as Victimization Disorder, or Disorders of Extreme Stress Not Otherwise Specified (DESNOS) (cf. Herman 1992). On the other hand, the APA parameters have been developed to be specifically applicable to trauma impact on Western groups of people, such as the veterans of the Vietnam and Gulf wars living in North America (cf. Summerfield 1999). As a result, they have been found inadequate for the description of PTSD in non-Western cultures and, more specifically, insufficient as an instrument for the diagnostic assessment of PTSD in African populations (cf. Peltzer 1998) since they cannot represent any trauma category correlated to the effects of multiple-trauma exposure experienced, interpreted and recounted by refugees from African countries. The etiology associated with the trauma diagnostic constructs in African contexts can in fact encompass a multiplicity of factors which include natural/physical as well as supernatural/spiritual and even socio-political causes.

2. Rationale

On such contextual premises, the present study adopts a cognitive-functional approach (Sweetser 1990; Langacker 1991; Lakoff / Johnson 1999) to the analysis of the newly developed medical discourse of Transcultural Psychiatry. Its first aim is to investigate the extent to which the PTSD diagnostic parameters, such as those established by the APA/DSM-IV, fit not only the nosological concepts underlying the specialized lexical dimension of the conventional discourse of Psychiatry, but also the cognitive basis of its textual macro- and micro-structures (cf. van Dijk 1980; Gotti 2003). This would corroborate the hypothesis that psychiatric categories are encoded into generic conventions by Western psychiatrists so as to produce a discursive coherence reflecting a predetermined and homogeneous group of patients. Such a view inevitably gives rise to a 'category fallacy' (cf. Kleinman 1995) as soon as it comes to be challenged by different indigenous situated narratives whose deviating coherence reflects different knowledge systems (or 'schemata' – cf. Mandler 1984), symbols and expectations associated with traumatic experiences culturally embedded within contexts of violence and war.

This leads to the second aim of the present study, that is to illustrate how the labels conventionally attached to trauma disorders in Western Psychiatry do not encompass the mental imagery developed by West-African refugees in order to conceptualize, in their own metaphorical terms, the traumatic events experienced in situations of war. Such mental imagery crucially informs the refugees' native 'idioms of distress' (cf. Gibbs / O'Brien 1990) and trauma-narrative structures which are directly reflected in the English they use in narrating their experiences.

This chapter therefore investigates, through the implementation of a case study, how trauma stories narrated by West-African refugees, as well as their textualizations made by specialists according to the generic conventions of the Psychiatric Case Report, serve to clarify aspects of both life experiences and professional practices related to the problem of PTSD in non-Western cultures. The underlying research question is thus to find out whether the identification of divergent strategies of narrative representation of the PTSD may actually suggest alternative ways of understanding and, then, textualizing different sociocultural conceptualizations of the trauma experience.

3. Theoretical background

Central to this study is the notion of narrative coherence in both telling and interpreting traumatic experience. Indeed, even though non-Western trauma narratives report stories from another cultural world, these stories are normally understood by Western professionals with an exclusive reference to their own clinical-schema categories, and encoded according to the genre conventions of pre-established 'clinical plots' (cf. Eisenberg 1981; Adams Smith 1984; Mattingly 1998). At the basis of such established analytical procedure is Freud's (1920: 221) view that a clinician makes sense of the patient's associations, memories and dreams by imposing upon them a coherent interpretative pattern capable of filling the missing gaps. Sacks (1987) criticizes such patterns reflected in the textualization of psychiatric cases, as they conventionally thematize the pathology pattern rather than the human subject and his/her personal experience. He suggests, instead, a different transitivity pattern with a human subject shifting from the background position as a passive patient to the foreground position as an active agent in trauma narrative report. In describing the ways in which a staff of psychiatrists, specialized in the treatment of PTSD in US war veterans, related case histories to other staff members, Young (1995) notes how the semantic (transitive) and textual (rhetorical) organization of their clinical narrative reports remained in fact invariable. He concludes:

> in practice, the structure of these narratives exists prior to their content. [...] Even before the audience has heard all the details, they know, in a general way, what is coming next and how it all fits together. (Young 1995: 170).

In the case of non-Western PTSD reports, instead, native populations recount their stories according to *their own* sociocultural schemata and to the narrative types that their cultures make available. Linde (1993: 11), for instance, notes how life-story narratives about the self are not known in many native cultures where people have not conceptualized the subjective sense of having a private life story. Yet, life stories are considered as natural and even universal narrative forms to the point that they are adopted as coherent ethnographic frames for memory in Western anthropological and medical enquiry (cf. Kleinman 1995). By contrast, in non-Western cultures, narratives about physical or mental illness often serve to protect and pass on essential community values related more to social and political balance and welfare than to individual wellbeing. As such, they usually involve communal embodiment through collective and public involvement which is capable of conferring to a devastating trauma or illness story the quality of a shared and therapeutic 'fictional coherence' (cf. Mattingly 1998) which can help re-establish a culture-specific sense of order and ethics in the disrupted lives of people within an injured community.

4. Case study on transcultural psychiatry

4.1. Method and data analysis

The literature outlined so far constitutes the basis for a case study focused on the parallel analysis of two mini-corpora composed of:

1. 15 scientific articles in transcultural psychiatry regarding psychiatric case reports about the effects of war/torture-related trauma on non-Western populations (see Appendix);
2. some transcribed protocols of trauma stories narrated by seven West-African asylum seekers (from Sierra Leone, Nigeria, Liberia, Ghana) and collected, by means of semi-structured interviews, at a reception camp for asylum seekers and at a centre for refugee support.

The purpose of this investigation is to explore, by applying both qualitative and quantitative methods, four levels of deviation between clinical and native PTSD reports, which are: (a) epistemic vs. deontic modality; (b) transitivity vs. ergativity; (c) generic vs. ethnopoetic patterns; (d) technical lexis vs. native idioms of distress.

4.2. Discourse deviation at the level of modality

Qualitative register analysis of the scientific articles about PTSD case reports shows that all of them share the same tentative tone in interpreting post-trauma sequelae in non-Western contexts, due to the therapist's attempts to "construct coherent narrative out of symptoms and behaviours that make no sense" (Kirmayer 2000: 153). This can be explained by the fact that, unlike the unmarked structure of argumentation based on causal reasoning – and, thus, constructed on the primary 'embodied metaphor' of a 'journey' (Lakoff / Johnson 1999: 179) or a 'path' (Langacker 1991: 382) from an energy source (agent) causing an effect (goal) – traditional psychiatric argumentation entails a backward epistemic reasoning from the evidence of the effect to the inference of the cause (cf. Sweetser 1990: 57). This justifies its typical tentative tone conveyed by a frequent use of epistemic hedges (cf.

Salager-Meyer 1994; Skelton 1997) such as 'approximators' (Prince *et al.* 1982), consisting of quasi-negative expressions and adaptors of frequency which modulate statements as relatively true or false, as the following examples show:

(1) *Very little is known* about the consequences of trauma exposure in the survivors' lives.

(2) *Not all* refugee children, even those exposed to war, develop disorders and social impairment.

(3) The hallucinations are *most often* perceived in the individual's mother tongue.

By affecting the truth-conditions of the propositions, hedges determine vagueness of meanings, making them 'fuzzier' (Lakoff 1972) and, thus, conveying a sense of uncertainty. Often hedges function as 'shields' (Prince *et al.* 1982), mitigating the strength of the writer's claim and, thus, diminishing the therapist-writer's commitment to the truth value of the interpretative paths (s)he explores, as evinced by the frequent use of modal verbs, exemplified in the following extracts:

(4) The sensations provoked by an odor *may* trigger dysphoric associations (e.g. trauma associations and catastrophic cognitions) that *may* contribute to the production of panic.

(5) The concept of comorbidity *appears* to represent a less integrated approach, which *may* contain detrimental implications associated with refugee post-trauma.

By means of hedging, in sum, the writer advances possible interpretations of the non-Western trauma narratives and idioms of distress (s)he reports in order to make them coherently conform to pre-established interpretative frames in trauma psychiatry.

By contrast, the protocol analysis (Ericsson / Simon 1984) on the transcribed trauma narratives by West-African asylum seekers shows that the tone of such accounts is often assertive and marked by deontic modality of a high value (Halliday 1994: 357-358) signalling: (a) an obligation to act imposed upon the traumatized person by his/her own condition of sickness due to extreme events, and (b) his/her determination to perform the imposed actions in order to start a recovery process. In this sense, West-African trauma narratives turn the devastating effects of past traumatic events into present causal sources compelling future repairing actions. This deontic prompt to take action reveals how trauma, in West-African sociocultural schemata, cannot be directly traced back to individual experiences of grief, or personal painful memories, needing a therapeutic removal. On the contrary, it is experienced as a collective social distress marked by violent feelings of anger, hate and even revenge, often expressed through a process of metaphorical embodiment allowing a third-person detachment of the traumatized person from his/her personal shocking experience – as illustrated in the following transcription from a Liberian woman's account of her trauma-induced ghost possession:

(6) When the army attacked, my family and I make for escape to Ghana. So we're walking on a field and we're seeing this soldier behind a bush who's eating stolen food. He look us and quick my father hitted him with a machete unless he shoot us, and splitted his shoulder here down the trunk. So blood gush out the cut and he scream and die and we run for our lives. Now the spirit of this soldier had come inside my body 'cause he *must* gain revenge against my family and he *must* wake me up on every dawn and I shake for fear because he say he *should* split me in two if my family didn't obeyed him. I roll eyes and people say I speak with his voice and he say my family *must* bury him properly 'cause he's no guilty 'cause he was only eating, no attacking us.

This trauma narrative shows some features of West-African colloquial English such as the inaccurate use of prepositions, adverbs and, in particular, tenses, as evident from the application of the continuous aspect to verbs of perception ("we're seeing"), the incorrect formation of irregular verbs ("hitted", "splitted"), the double tense marking ("didn't obeyed"), and the inappropriate use of both past perfect ("his spirit had come") and basic infinitive forms ("he shoot", "blood gush", "he scream and die", etc.). Such tense indefiniteness, however, conveys the sense of a traumatic experience occurred in the past yet which still persists in the present of the speaker's world. The haunting memory of the soldier so brutally killed by her father compels the woman to undergo her trauma again on a different, trance-like level of public re-enactment. This consists in embodying the spirit of the soldier as an obligation to recover from her mind traumatic images and emotions associated with the savage murder of innocent people and to project them on to an external dimension of social recognition requiring moral reparation, which represents the first step towards individual and collective healing.

The intense degree of emotional involvement of the PTSD patients in the personal and social shock they undergo is often signalled in West-African English narrative by a decategorialization of phrasal constructions towards morphological structures that follow native strategies of minimal mental effort via minimal morphonemic differentiation (cf. Langacker 1977). These economical strategies are already grammaticalized in West-African indigenous languages (Fula, Igbo, Hausa, Mandinka), and then transferred to the typologically-different morphology of English (cf. Wise 1989; Elugbe / Omamor 1991) only to function as pragmatic markers iconically reproducing, by means of a reduced speech signal, the sense of perceptual immediacy of an action deontically prompted, in this case, by a situation of extreme distress. The following transcription from a man's trauma report in Sierra Leonean Krio English[1] illustrates these strategies:

(7) I was farming on the hill and I see the rebels se [that] were coming near our village foh kan kil mai traib [in order to kill my tribe]. Dehn bin *mek* mai pipul *foh khomoht* dehn hos dehn, ehn dehn *obubu* [*Igbo*: hasty moving] dehn na wan trit, ehn dehn bin tehl dehn se dehn *foh sidhon* na grohn. [They *obliged* my people to *come out* of their houses, they moved them rapidly to a street and told them that they *had to sit down* on the ground]. Afta, dehn bin se "go dohn" ehn dehn bin *mek* ohlman *foh ledhon* pan wan ston ehn dehn koht-koht dehn hed dhen. [After, they said "go down" and they *obliged* each of them to *lie down* on a stone and relentlessly cut their heads]. A noh *go* fohget. A *foh* go bak na Salone. Dehn *foh mohs* lib na wan ples. A *go* kil dehn ohl. [I *shall* never forget. I *must* go back to Sierra Leone. They *will most certainly* live in the same place. I *shall* kill them all].

In this report, the degree of the speaker's emotional involvement in his trauma memories increases as he switches from a detached use of Standard English to the more familiar Krio English, and even to his native Igbo when he introduces the typical pragmatic strategy of word

1 I wish to thank Professor Malcolm Awadajin Finney (California State University Long Beach) for his most helpful comments on the Krio and Pidgin English transcriptions reported in this chapter.

reduplication (*obubu*) to stress, by means of aural and articulatory iconicity, the sense of an immediate and uncontrollable action. This strategy is also transferred to the Krio reduplicative expression *koht-koht* (literally: *cut-cut*) reproducing the fierce beheading action. The speaker's emotional response to the tragic events he reports is especially signalled by his extensive use of Krio modal particles, such as *foh*, marking the sense of deontic obligation, *go*, entailing the speaker's commitment to a promise, and *mohs* (must), strengthening *foh* with an epistemic implication of certainty. Such modal particles, therefore, frame trauma narrative not as a sample of medical discourse, but as an essentially political one, where individual emotions are identified with social and moral obligations.

Most of these particles are here associated with decategorialized phrasal verbs resulting from a cliticization of the prepositional particle into a compact and reduced accentual unit – as in *khomoht* (come out), *sidhon* (sit down), and *ledhon* (lie down) – which forms a host+suffix construction of an agglutinative type. In trauma narrative, this particle suffixation also aims at reproducing the immediacy of a tragic action via aural and articulatory iconicity. This is particularly evident when a conceptual present simple is used to convey the sense of a past event that is still experientially actual and perceptually vivid in the narrator's mind. The immediacy of recall, in this case, requires a minimal mental effort which can automatically trigger the present-tense inflectional suffix '-s' directly attached to the phrasal-verb particles, as this extract from another trauma report in Krio/Standard English reveals:

(8) The soldiers drehb mai papa bifo wan hol. Mai papa *tinaps* ehn tis soldier shoots am ehn i *fohdohns* na hol, dehd dehd. [The soldiers drove my father before a hole. My father *stands up* and this soldier shoots him and he *falls down* into the hole, dead on the spot].

4.3. Discourse divergences at the level of transitivity

The specialized articles examined here conventionally textualize non-Western trauma reports by using passive or passive-like constructions characteristic of scientific text-types (cf. Gotti 2003: 96-99), which consist in defocusing the agent that would otherwise be the salient starting point of a natural transitive conceptualization of events, thereby conferring on the other secondary participant the starting-point status of theme. This means that in such passive constructions, Western categorizations of PTSD symptoms, diagnostic/interpretative criteria and treatment procedures are collocated in a thematic position within the structure of the sentence. Instead, non-Western PTSD-affected people, who represent the agentive experiencers (or 'sensers' – Halliday 1994: 117) of the traumatic and psychiatric processes, are either relegated to a rhematic background position as logical, psychological (and, indeed, actual) 'patients' (Halliday 1994: 108), or totally omitted, as the following examples show:

(9) Nausea and dizziness (*Theme: symptoms*) will tend *to be experienced* by many people (*Rheme: sensers*) during the traumatic event; the event will most likely *be strongly encoded* (*sensers omitted*) in memory, and the memory will *be readily recalled* (*sensers omitted*) upon exposure to odor and/or dizziness and/or nausea.

(10) Neurotransmitters and neuropeptides released during stress *may result in* [*passive-like causative structure, equivalent to* may be followed by] overconsolidation of memory traces, giving rise to intrusive memories of PTSD. Vivid re-experiencing and ordinary biographical memories of trauma *are represented* by separate memory systems so that sensory data, associated with an emotionally important event, *is stored* in memory without cortical processing. (*Sensers omitted*)

The description of trauma-inducing torture methods is also foregrounded as the thematic subject of sentence-structures:

(11) A particularly painful method of torture *is* [*intensive-identifying passive-like structure, equivalent to* is represented by + *-ing*-form (cf. Halliday 1994: 122-130)] to tie the wrists behind the back and then suspend the whole body weight by them. (*Sensers omitted*)

Notably, trauma-affected people are often described in conformity with the Western constructions of the non-Western mind as illogical and even 'primitive' (cf. Shore 1996: 54). This is evident in the way they are normally referred to in the examined articles by means of a patronizing tone, characterized by a reduction of their responsibility, agency, and even credibility, which is not only reflected in the sentence structure, but also in the use of adjectives and nouns (such as nerves, a Western idiom of distress implying personal and social culpability – cf. Kirmayer 2000: 159). These are some relevant examples:

(12) Upon encountering the stimulus, *there is no control of anxiety*, which may be *sufficient* to generate *even more anxiety* and an *increased* sympathetic outflow in the autonomic *nervous system*. (*Senser omitted*)

(13) It was found that disorders such as conduct disorder and major depression, were associated with *significant social impairment*. Other studies have shown *high rates of social impairment* to be associated with prolonged exposure to war, violence, separation and privation. (*Senser omitted*)

Unlike the transitivity patterns framing specialized case reports, the textualization of the traumatic events in West-African refugees' narratives follows, instead, native cause-effect conceptualizations. Typically, in refugees' native Niger-Congo languages, such event-conceptualizations in situations of emotional and physical stress occur according to ergative constructions (cf. Langacker 1991: 336), which are then transferred to the refugees' use of English. An ergative construction collocates the transitive object or 'medium' (Halliday 1994: 163) in a thematic position within the clause as if it were the actual energy-source of the action, thus running the transitive energy-flow directionality counter from a source-dynamic agent that causes a process directed to a patient/goal.

This means that, for instance, a sentence like "torture (*causal force: agent*) caused me (*affected entity: patient*) an unbearable pain (*effect: medium*)" may be rendered in West-African English varieties by an ergative form such as "an unbearable pain (*medium*) grabbed me (*patient*)", with the transitive object ('pain') placed in the thematic position of an animate subject, marked by components of volition and even force-dynamic motion (cf. Guido 2004). The implication is that trauma effects, like 'pain', come to be metaphorically experienced by West-African refugees as the actual animate source of their distress, thus removing the real physical and psychological causes initiating it (cf. Halliday 1994: 171), such as torturers and traumatic events. The role of the senser/experiencer, instead, is central in that it normally coincides with the first-person narrator. The following examples of ergative structures are found in the PTSD narratives of the refugees from Sierra Leone, Ghana and Liberia:

(14) [*Past-trauma narrative*] My skin (*energy source: medium*) ripped. My bones (*medium*) cracked and broke. An unbearable pain (*medium*) grabbed me (*patient*). [*Transitive equivalent:* The torturer (*omitted force-dynamic agent*) ripped my skin and broke my bones etc.]. (Liberian man)

(15) [*Present-recall narrative*] Heart (*medium*) rise up to the brain when it think the soldiers come on the camp and kill all people. [*Transitive equivalent:* The memory of the soldiers coming to the camp (*agent*) makes my heart rise up to the brain]. (Ghanaian woman).

(16) [*Present-recall narrative*] The mind (*medium*) think-think sickness and see fog and go out of place. [*Transitive equivalent*: The memory of the massacre (*omitted causal initiator*) makes my mind obsessed, etc.] (Sierra Leonean man)

In all these instances of narrative in West-African colloquial English, ergativity is justified by an 'emotional causation' (Lakoff / Johnson 1999: 221) metonymically representing an external (traumatic) cause in terms of the perceiver's emotional, embodied response to its effects. Consequently, in the textualization of first-person trauma experiences, the narrators' bodily reactions to them occupy the central, thematic role of the medium, as if such extreme reactions were the actual force-dynamic causes of trauma – here experientially represented by internal parts of the body (heart, mind, skin etc.) that arise ('rise up') or emerge ('go out') from a bodily 'container' (Lakoff / Johnson 1999: 213-214) which can rip or break. Such experiential metaphors would in fact prompt the narrators to acknowledge the inner fracture opened between themselves and their world.

4.4. Discourse deviation at the level of structure

The macro- and micro-moves that organize the specialized articles under analysis are the conventional ones characterizing scientific genres (cf. Bazerman 1988) and exemplified in the scientific abstract as 'purpose-method-results-conclusions' (cf. Salager-Meyer 1990). Such moves reflect the Western iconic conceptualization of a linear, progressive development of therapy over time (i.e., 'illness-treatment-healing'), as the following example illustrates:

(17) (*Purpose*) This paper will explore the usefulness of mainstream understandings of trauma work in the African context. (*Method*) This will be done by considering how the different conceptualizations of trauma relate to a research project undertaken with refugee women who were seen for rape trauma counseling. [...] (*Results*) Results show that many victims of sexual abuse experience post-traumatic stress reactions (PTSR). [...] (*Conclusions*) The approach directs our attention to the aftermaths of the events in which the subjective experiences of sexual assault are being re-elaborated.

These moves, however, may not correspond to non-Western conceptualizations of trauma distress and recovery. For instance, trauma stories narrated by West-African asylum seekers usually disrupt the Western conceptualization of a linear, cause-effect progression of time since they reproduce the schematic structure of actualized shocking memories within which past events and present recollections come to coincide. This particular narrative construction represents a native iconic and metaphorical mode of thought and action that is directly reflected in the 'ethnopoetic moves' (Hymes 2003: 98) of West-African oral narratives, emotionally organized according to a typical pattern of five and three verses (Guido 2005). The former five verses describe an outer social context, whereas the latter three verses introduce the narrator's inner mental state in response to it. The following two examples of trauma narratives are specifically patterned according to this ethnopoetic profile. The speakers' use of, respectively, Nigerian Pidgin and Sierra Leonean Krio Englishes makes their narrative reflect more closely their native structures:

(18) (A) *Verses 1-5: outer context. Nigerian Pidgin English transcript* [*Standard English translation*]

1. Das pipul dem bin don mek mi walk fo tri day dem, o, fo Niger border
   [Those people had made me walk for three days to the Niger border]
2. wie dem bin sell mi to won 'madam' and won car bin tek mi fo Al Zuwarah
   [where they sold me to a 'madam' and a car took me to Al Zuwarah]
3. wie won shack wit di sand-bed bin don lok mi and oda ten ten girl dem
   [where a shack with a sand-bed had locked me crammed with other ten girls]
4. wie di *oyibo* dem (*Yoruba*: white men) bin de kom evri de evri de
   [where the white men were coming every day, every day]
5. a remember di pain fo mai yansh and leg dem and di cut dem fo mai bodi
   [I remember the pain in my back and legs and the cuts in my body]

Verses 6-8: inner response

6. Wen di boat bin bring os fo Italy a bin mek mai pikin,
   [When the boat brought us to Italy I gave birth to my child]

7. but hie police dem bin spot os and dem bin pik os all.
   [but here the police found us and they took us all.]
8. Fo Nigeria a no get hope fo mari and fo mai pikin in future.
   [In Nigeria I have no hope for getting married and for my child's future.]

(19) (B) *Verses 1-5: outer context. Sierra Leonean Krio English transcript* [*Standard English translation*]

1. We dehn rebel dehn bin kam a bin de ple wit mai sista na do mai ples
   [When the rebels came I was playing with my sister outside my house]
2. ehn dehn kwik bin johs di nak-nak mi ed wit dehn rifle butt, ehn dehn bin pata mi
   [and they suddenly hit my head repeatedly with their rifle-butts and slapped me]
3. ehn dehn se if a noh bin kam wit dehn, dehn bin go mohs koht mi an wit dehn kohtlas
   [and they said that if I did not come with them, they would cut my hand with their machete]
4. ehn mai sista bin de krai-krai ehn dehn bin laf
   [and my sister started to cry incessantly and they laughed]
5. ehn wan rebel wit in kohtlas bin koht mai sista in fut ehn han ehn ed lehk wan banana tik.
   [and one rebel with his machete cut my sister's feet and hands and head like a banana tree.]

Verses 6-8: inner response

6. A bin du bohku at wok, dohti wok, foh rebel dehn,
   [I had done a lot of hard, dirty work for the rebels,]
7. a bin kil bohku pohsin dhen foh dehn, yehs.
   [I had killed a lot of persons for them, yes.]
8. A wan go foh pik dehn ehn dehn fambul ehn kil dehn lehk banana tik.
   [I want to go and pick them and their families and kill them like banana trees.]

As is evident from these two examples, embodied trauma schemata constitute the building blocks of ethnopoetic narrative. In both cases, specific link-words mark the ethnopoetic turning points that drive the story on, determining an alliterative pattern organizing the emotional construction of narration. In (A), for instance, verses 2-4 starting with *wie* ('where') stress the places of the narrator's agony (e.g., 'a car', 'a shack', 'a boat'), all of them thematized as force-dynamic medium in ergative constructions. Any description of herself undergoing rape and torture is instead avoided, except for a hint at abuse frequency (by reduplication: *evri de evri de* – 'every day every day') and consequences (pain on the back and legs and physical wounds). The woman's inner response to trauma in fact seems more focused on the sociocultural repercussions of rape, crushing her hopes for marriage and her illegitimate child's future back in Nigeria. Also in (B), the alliterative verses 2-5 starting with *ehn* ('and') and 6-8 with *a* ('I') speed the pace of a narrative focused on a ghastly escalation of violence. Yet, also in this case, the speaker is inwardly motivated by a feeling of social revenge for the family injury. Therefore, although in both cases reduplication emphasizes again the sense of obsessive thoughts (e.g., "mai sista bin de *krai-krai*" – 'my sister started to *cry and cry*'), psychiatric therapy should not be contemplated in the absence of a collective political action aimed at achieving community recovery by reconciliation.

4.5. Discourse deviation at the level of lexis

PTSD lexical items adopted in the specialized psychiatric articles are consistent with the APA categorizations and, as such, are conventionally assumed to be resistant to semantic/cognitive changes and meaning negotiations – which is typical of all technical words in specialized texts, according to a consolidated tenet in Western thought. The following are some examples:

(20) [*Specialized scientific text*] Dysregulation of the hypothalamic-pituitary-adrenal axis in patients with PTSD results in low urinary cortisol concentrations, raised concentrations of cerebrospinal fluid corticotrophin releasing factor, increased numbers of lymphocyte glucocorticoid receptor sites, and hypersuppression of cortisol with low dose dexamethasone.

(21) [*Specialized popular text*] After exposure to some traumatic event, one's initial response may include symptoms in the domains of physiology (e.g., rapid heart rate, body heat, sleep disturbance, appetite disturbance, nausea, shortness of breath, dizziness and palpitations, chocking sensation, chest tightness, shaking, sweating, chills/hot flashes and numbness/tingling).

In the case of transcultural psychiatry, however, technical lexis may need meaning negotiation so as to allow adaptation to different non-Western trauma categories. In fact, the idioms of distress used by the West-African refugees in their trauma narratives may totally diverge from the specialized APA definitions of post-traumatic stress disorders. This is so because West-African idioms are essentially of a metaphorical type, reflecting first-person trauma effects in terms of third-person concrete animate subjects affecting the patients, as the examples that follow reveal:

(22) When I escaped, I saw many bodies on the side of the road and I felt that the worms on them they started crawl up slow slow under my skin. I often feel the worms creep creep and make my blood to sleep. (Ghanaian woman)

(23) I suffer wind sickness, *fonyo kurango* we say (*Mandinka*), when I smell burning, like my village burning. Wind attacks my brain and rises. I hear wind inside my ears, like woo woo. It rise rise and press the eyes and I see black and my brain spin. (Sierra Leonean man)

These two trauma narratives perfectly convey, through the use of some features of West-African colloquial English varieties, the socioculturally-marked effects that an injured community can produce upon PTSD patients. In both cases, the strong physical reactions to extreme situations normally classified as loathing and panic attack are here embodied respectively by means of the native experiential metaphors of creeping worms (focused on the tactile iconicity of skin reactions) and wind sickness (focused on the aural iconicity of the inner perception of a high blood pressure). The metaphorical nature of such idioms makes them an integral part of the ethnopoetic pattern of West-African trauma narratives (cf. Kirmayer 2000).

5. Control study

A quantitative analysis was implemented as a control study, involving the same seven West-African refugees who supplied the trauma narratives. The purpose of this final check was to assess the possible sociocultural and schematic incongruities between the APA/DSM-IV parameters, reflected in the specialized PTSD lexicon, and the West-African idioms of distress identified in the asylum seekers' narratives. The adopted psychometric instruments were: (a) the *Harvard Trauma Questionnaire* (HTQ), asking about eight general categories of traumatic life events and providing four possible responses: (1) "no", (2) "heard about it", (3) "witnessed", (4) "experienced", and (b) the *Hopkins Symptom Checklist-25* (HSCL-25) determining PTSD criteria with a scale that include four categories of response, rated 1 to 4, respectively: (1) "not at all", (2) "a little", (3) "quite a bit", (4) "extremely". Table 1 reproduces the responses that the refugees (numbered [A] to [G]) supplied to the HTQ.

Refugees	[A]	[B]	[C]	[D]	[E]	[F]	[G]
[a] Material deprivation	4	4	4	4	4	4	4
[b] War-like conditions	4	4	4	2	4	4	4
[c] Bodily injury	3	4	4	4	4	3	3
[d] Forced confinement and coercion	4	3	3	4	3	2	2
[e] Forced to harm others	4	3	4	1	2	3	3
[f] Disappearance, death, or injury of loved ones	4	4	4	2	4	4	2
[g] Witnessed violence to others	4	4	4	4	4	4	4
[h] Brain injury	3	3	2	2	3	2	3
Average Total	*3,75*	*3,62*	*3,62*	*2,87*	*3,50*	*3,25*	*3,12*

Table 1. Refugees' responses to the HTQ.

The high rates of first-person involvement in traumatic events emerging from Table 1 clearly reveals the refugees' deep awareness of having undergone extreme experiences whose physical and psychological effects are assumed to be tremendously serious, but also quite easily identifiable by means of well-tested diagnostic criteria. To verify this assumption, the same refugees were asked to provide responses to an adapted version of the HSCL-25 that specifically focused on PTSD symptoms. Their responses are reproduced in Table 2. Correlational analysis carried out on the average responses to the two scales shows a lack of correlation (Pearson correlation = .003; $p \approx 1$). This would confirm that the impact of trauma such as that experienced by this group of West-African refugees is so experientially and metaphorically complex that Western assessment instruments, like the HSCL-25, cannot be adequate to represent it. From their responses to this scale, these refugees do not appear to be extremely affected by the extreme trauma situations they asserted to have undergone by responding to the HTQ. Indeed, it emerges that many typical trauma symptoms in the list have "not at all" been experienced, or just "a little", although in their narratives they clearly described, in culturally-marked metaphorical ways, many of such PTSD symptoms. This incongruity, therefore, indicates the need to develop new culturally and linguistically sensitive instruments for assessing and then reporting in new clinical terms trauma effects as they are represented in the West-African discourse of PTSD.

Refugees	[A]	[B]	[C]	[D]	[E]	[F]	[G]
[a] Dizziness	1	3	1	1	3	1	2
[b] Palpitations	2	1	1	2	3	1	2
[c] Nausea	1	2	2	2	2	2	2
[d] Panic attacks	1	1	2	2	4	2	4
[e] Flashbacks	4	3	4	2	3	4	4
[f] Shaking	1	1	1	1	4	2	3
[g] Blurry vision	2	4	1	1	3	1	3
[h] Nightmares	3	3	2	3	3	3	3
[i] Social isolation	2	2	3	3	1	1	1
[j] Suicidal ideation	1	2	1	1	1	1	1
Average Total	*1,80*	*2,20*	*1,80*	*1,80*	*2,70*	*1,80*	*2,50*

Table 2. Refugees' responses to the HSCL-25.

6. Conclusions

This chapter has discussed the ways in which Western medical professionals and researchers reconstruct PTSD experiences through established patterns of psychiatric cases that are coherent only to solution-oriented templates of clinical reasoning, directly reflected in the conventional structure of medical genres. Yet, it has been argued that such structures actually ignore the original cultural, social and political contexts of non-Western populations for whom the traumatic experience of physical and psychological violence is often perceived principally as a collective shock, rather than as a private abuse. The chapter has therefore explored some parallel constructions in both PTSD case reports and refugees' trauma narratives, by focusing on the cognitive and structural deviations at the levels of modality, transitivity, textuality, and lexis. The discourse analysis has been carried out through the implementation of a case study on transcultural psychiatry applied to the PTSD experience of a group of West-African refugees. The outcome of analysis clearly reveals a deep interpretative gap between the original trauma accounts by the West-African subjects and their clinical textualizations into psychiatric registers. To fill such a gap, a specialized mediation is thus urgently needed to negotiate between the non-Western narrators' sociocultural schemata which construct reality by organizing traumatic experience into native forms of discourse, and the Western mental-health professionals' interpretation of such native narrative constructions according to conventional PTSD clinical schemata.

References

Adams Smith, Diana 1984. Medical Discourse: Aspects of Author's Comment. *English for Special Purposes* 3, 25-36.

APA (American Psychiatric Association) [4]1994. *Diagnostic and Statistical Manual of Mental Disorders*. Washington, DC: American Psychiatric Press.

Bazerman, Charles 1988. *Shaping Written Knowledge: The Genre and Activity of the Experimental Article in Science*. Madison: University of Wisconsin Press.

Devereux, Georges 1980. *Normal and Abnormal: Basic Problems of Ethnopsychiatry*. Chicago: University of Chicago Press.

van Dijk, Teun A. 1980. *Macrostructures: An Interdisciplinary Study of Global Structures in Discourse, Interaction, and Cognition*. Hillsdale, NJ: Erlbaum.

Eisenberg, Leon 1981. The Physician as Interpreter: Ascribing Meaning to the Illness Experience. *Comprehensive Psychiatry* 22, 239-248.

Elugbe, Ben / Omamor, Augusta 1991. *Nigerian Pidgin*. Ibadan: Heinemann.

Ericsson, Anders / Simon, Herbert A. 1984 *Protocol Analysis: Verbal Reports as Data*. Cambridge, MA: The MIT Press.

Freud, Sigmund 1920. *A General Introduction to Psychoanalysis*. New York: Boni and Liveright.

Gibbs, Raymond / O'Brien, Jennifer 1990. Idioms and Mental Imagery: The Metaphorical Motivation for Idiomatic Meaning. *Cognition* 36, 35-68.

Gotti, Maurizio 2003. *Specialized Discourse: Linguistic Features and Changing Conventions*. Bern: Peter Lang.

Guido, Maria Grazia 2004. Cross-cultural Miscommunication in Welfare Officers' Interrogations. In Candlin, Christopher N. / Gotti, Maurizio (eds) *Intercultural Aspects of Specialized Communication*. Bern: Peter Lang, 127-145.

Guido, Maria Grazia 2005. Context Misconstructions in Professional Entextualizations of 'Asylum' Discourse. In Cortese, Giuseppina / Duszak, Anna (eds) *Identity, Community, Discourse: English in Intercultural Settings*. Bern: Peter Lang, 183-207.

Halliday, M.A.K. 1994. *An Introduction to Functional Grammar*. London: Arnold.

Herman, Judith Lewis 1992. Complex PSTD: A Syndrome in Survivors of Prolonged and Repeated Trauma. *Journal of Traumatic Stress* 5, 377-391.

Hymes, Dell 2003. *Now I Know Only So Far: Essays in Ethnopoetics*. Lincoln: University of Nebraska Press.

Kirmayer, Laurence J. 2000. Broken Narratives: Clinical Encounters and the Poetics of Illness Experience. In Mattingly, Cheryl / Garro, Linda C. (eds) *Narrative and the Cultural Construction of Illness and Healing*. Berkeley: University of California Press, 153-180.

Kleinman, Arthur 1995. *Writing at the Margin: Discourse Between Anthropology and Medicine*. Berkeley: University of California Press.

Lakoff, George 1972. Hedges: A Study in Meaning Criteria and the Logic of Fuzzy Concepts. *Journal of Philosophical Logic* 2, 458-508.

Lakoff, George / Johnson, Mark 1999. *Philosophy in the Flesh: The Embodied Mind and its Challenge to Western Thought*. New York: Basic Books.

Langacker, Ronald W. 1977. Syntactic Reanalysis, in Li, Charles N. (ed.) *Mechanisms of Syntactic Change*. Austin: University of Texas Press, 57-139.

Langacker, Ronald W. 1991. *Foundations of Cognitive Grammar. Volume II: Descriptive Application*. Stanford: Stanford University Press.

Linde, Charlotte 1993. *Life Stories: The Creation of Coherence*. Oxford: Oxford University Press.

Mandler, Jean M. 1984. *Stories, Scripts and Scenes: Aspects of Schema Theory*. Hillsdale, N.J.: Erlbaum.

Mattingly, Cheryl 1998. *Healing Dramas and Clinical Plots: The Narrative Structure of Experience*. Cambridge: Cambridge University Press.

Peltzer, Karl 1998. Ethnocultural Construction of Post-traumatic Stress Symptoms in African Contexts. *Journal of Psychology in Africa* 8, 17-30.

Prince, Ellen / Bosk, Charles / Frader, Joel 1982. On Hedging in Physician-Physician Discourse. In di Pietro, Robert J. (ed.) *Linguistics and the Professions*. Norwood, NJ: Ablex, 83-97.

Sacks, Oliver 1987. *The Man Who Mistook His Wife for a Hat and Other Clinical Tales*. New York: Perennial Library.

Salager-Meyer, Francoise 1990. Discoursal Movements in Medical English Abstracts and their Linguistic Exponents: A Genre Analysis Study. *Interface* 4, 107-124.

Salager-Meyer, Francoise 1994. Hedges and Textual Communicative Function in Medical English Written Discourse. *English for Specific Purposes* 13, 149-170.

Shore, Brad 1996. *Culture in Mind: Cognition, Culture, and the Problem of Meaning*. New York: Oxford University Press.

Skelton, John R. 1997. The Representation of Truth in Academic Medical Writing. *Applied Linguistics* 18, 121-140.

Summerfield, Derek 1999. A Critique of Seven Assumptions Behind Psychological Trauma Programmes in War-affected Areas. *Social Science and Medicine* 48, 1449-1462.

Sweetser, Eve, E. 1990. *From Etymology to Pragmatics: Metaphorical and Cultural Aspects of Semantic Structure*. Cambridge: Cambridge University Press.

Wise, Akintola 1989. *Krio of Sierra Leone*. Madison: University of Wisconsin Press.
Young, Allan 1995. *The Harmony of Illness*. Princeton, N.J.: Princeton University Press.

Appendix

PTSD articles examined for the comparative analysis.

Boehnlein, J.K. / Kinzie, J.D. 1995. Refugee Trauma. *Transcultural Psychiatric Research Review* 32, 223-52.
Bolton, P. 2001. Local Perceptions of the Mental Health Effects of the Rwandan Genocide. *Journal of Nervous and Mental Disease* 189, 243-8.
Carlson, E. / Rosser-Hoggan, R. 1994. Cross-cultural Responses to Trauma: A Study of Traumatic Experiences and Post-traumatic Symptoms in Cambodian Refugees. *Journal of Traumatic Stress* 7, 43-58.
Falsetti, S. / Resnick, H. 1997. Frequency and Severity of Panic Attack Symptoms in a Treatment-seeking Sample of Trauma Victims. *Journal of Traumatic Stress* 10: 683-9.
Fox, S. H. 2003. The Mandinka Nosological System in the Context of Post-Traumatic Syndromes. *Transcultural Psychiatry* 40, 460-87.
Hinton, D. / Pich, V. / Chhean, D. / Pollack, M. 2004. Olfactory-Triggered Panic Attacks Among Khmer Refugees: A Contextual Approach. *Transcultural Psychiatry* 41, 155-99.
Hodes, M. 2002. Three Key Issues for Young Refugees' Mental Health. *Transcultural Psychiatry* 39, 196-213.
Kinzie, D. / Boehnlein, A.K. 1993. Psychotherapy of the Victims of Massive Violence: Countertransference and Ethical Issues. *American Journal of Psychotherapy* 47, 90-103.

Medical Foundation 1999. Reported Patterns of Human Rights Abuse and Torture. UK Medical Foundation for Care of Victims by Torture.

Mezey, G. / Robbins, I. 2001. Usefulness and Validity of Post-traumatic Stress Disorder as a Psychiatric Category. *BMJournal* 323, 561-3.

van Ommeren, M. / Sharma, B. / Sharma, G.K. / Komproe, I. / Cardena, E. / de Jong, J.T. 2002. The Relationship Between Somatic and PTSD Symptoms among Bhutanese Refugee Torture Survivors: Examination of Comorbidity with Anxiety and Depression. *Journal of Traumatic Stress* 15, 415-21.

Rousseau, C. 1995. Mental Health of Refugee Children. *Transcultural Psychiatric Research Review* 32, 299-331.

Silove, D. 1999. The Psychosocial Effects of Torture, Mass Human Rights Violation and Refugee Trauma: Toward an Integrated Conceptual Framework. *Journal of Nervous and Mental Disease* 187, 200-7.

Sinnerbrink, I. / Field, A. / Steel, Z. / Manicavasagar, V. 1997. Compounding of Premigration Trauma and Postmigration Stress in Asylum Seekers. *The Journal of Psychology* 131, 463-70.

Tang, S.S. / Fox, S.H. 2001. Traumatic Experiences and the Mental Health of Senegalese Refugees. *Journal of Nervous and Mental Disease* 189, 507-12.

RICK IEDEMA*

(Post-)bureaucratizing Medicine: Health Reform and the Reconfiguration of Contemporary Clinical Work

1. Introduction

The twentieth century confirmed medicine as one of the few privileged professions in western industrialized nations, thanks to the support it was able to muster from the State (Rose 1994). While predictions about its future are inevitably precarious, it appears from developments over the last two to three decades that medicine may not be able to maintain the levels of support, protection and privilege that characterized its relationship to the State during the previous century. A number of developments can be isolated as playing a particularly central role in this shift in medicine's power.

The developments I have in mind here flow forth from various governmental initiatives that have begun to crowd into medical-clinical space in order to render medicine accountable to stakeholders other than doctors. The first of these initiatives was introduced in a number of industrialized countries and centred on transmuting existing classifications of medical work into costing mechanisms, such as Disease Related Groupers and casemix,[1] both of which sought to impose resource calculations on types of medical practices, such as hip replacements, stent surgery and appendicectomy. In some countries, such as the U.K. and Australia, clinicians were exhorted to involve themselves as 'clinician-managers' in spreading acceptance of

* University of New South Wales, Australia.

1 Disease Related Groupers (DRGs) are classifications of diseases. Casemix provides a DRG map of health organizations, such that we know what disease types these organizations (can) handle.

these calculations and in promoting the implications of the resulting resource usage (wastage?) data to their frontline staff, in the expectation that this would lead to self-induced rationing.

A second initiative centred on the integration of scientific evidence into bureaucratic regulations, such as guidelines and protocols governing the use of drugs and other resources. At the heart of this contingent of initiatives was the drive towards clinical work systematization, in the hope that individuals' medical autonomy be balanced against organizational accountability, and unnecessary or counter-productive variation in practice be minimized. This initiative sought to base medical practice on scientific evidence whose 'gold standard' status was guaranteed by a resource-intensive form of population-based experimentation called 'randomized control clinical trial' or RCT. In recent years, this drive towards evidence-based practice has been given renewed impetus by being made one of the cornerstones of 'clinical governance', or the expectation that clinicians do not just do their work well, but that they also produce the means (data) through which to improve what it is they do, and base their practices on established (preferably RCT-generated) evidence.

This rhetoric of practice improvement has recently intensified following publications revealing the epidemiology of medical error across nations' health care systems and the recurrent practice problems of substandard services, in addition to reports about rogue professionals whose inappropriate practices went unchecked by their medical authorities. These revelations have served to tighten the link between what clinicians do, the data that they produce about what they do, their enactment and measurement of practice improvement, and their accountability to agencies that straddle medical and State authorities and that are given increasing power to scrutinize and intervene in how medical clinicians do their work. This accountability to non-medical stakeholders is given additional moral weight by aligning the intent behind governmental policies with the interests of patients, carers and consumers generally. The significance of this is that the point of gravity of medical legitimation has begun to shift back to the State, undoing some of the gains medicine began to accrue over a hundred years ago.

The thesis just outlined about the delegitimation of medicine remains a topic of much debate among scholars of health and illness

(Williams / Calnan 1996; Armstrong 2005; Stevenson / Scambler 2005). These scholars' disagreements notwithstanding, it is surprising that few of the arguments raised by these commentators address the issues raised in the previous paragraphs, and centre almost exclusively on how medicine is enacted in the domains of primary care or general practice, how medicine is represented in the public media, how the general public's perceptions of medicine are changing (or not), and the extent to which medicine is appropriating or being displaced by non-western medical approaches to healing. While each of these factors is important, it would appear to this author that the current bureaucratic-scientific redefinition of medicine lends credibility to the view that doctoring is taking place in an increasingly crowded space, and that its practices of legitimation are becoming increasingly publicly played out and contested.

Against this background, the present chapter develops the argument that the shift towards knowledge economies in many western nation states appears to have the attendant effect of involving medicine in micro-managerial practices that undermine medicine's organizational autonomy, put limits on its resource expenditures, and complicate its definitions of patient treatment in specific and health care more generally. The chapter mobilizes evidence from two recent studies carried out in New South Wales (Australia), the first of which centred on the analysis of written reports about clinical errors or 'critical incidents', and the second of which focused on clinicians acting on these incident reports to do what is called root cause analysis (RCA) in order to discover the logics of practice that set clinicians up for making those errors, and to change those systems such that similar errors no longer occur. The remainder of the chapter is structured as follows. The next section is divided into four sub-sections, the first two focusing on critical incidence reporting (CIR) and the other two on RCA. These sub-sections include a brief background to contextualize CIR and RCA and to explain their rising significance in contemporary health care organizations, and an analytical sub-section that presents data examples and an outline of their main discursive features. The chapter then moves to a discussion that summarizes the contours of the argument, which leads into a conclusion about the importance of accounting for how post-industrialization and the intensification of knowledge practices and relationships affect modern medicine as a result of its participation in self-reflexive techniques such as CIR and RCA.

2. Critical Incident Reporting and Root Cause Analysis

This section focuses on two interventions promoted across the western world to rationalize medical work. In essence both 'post hoc' approaches to medical process analysis, CIR and RCA, are promoted as central to contemporary quality and safety initiatives in health care, and have in some jurisdictions become mandatory (as of 2005 in New South Wales, Australia). Complementing a priori ways of mapping out the contours of clinical work such as guidelines, protocols and pathways, CIR and RCA are nevertheless often deployed to address particularly 'problematic' domains of health care; that is, domains that are not necessarily routinizable in advance (Lillrank / Liukko 2004). The uncertainty about what is right and wrong in these domains, on top of the uncertainties about how to enact these new kinds of work, increase the emotional burden of contemporary clinical work. Before elaborating this issue in the discussion section below, I will provide a discourse analytical account of CIR and RCA, using selected empirical examples. I will address CIR first, as the lodging of an incident report provides the trigger for an RCA, provided the incident is considered serious enough to deserve an RCA investigation (e.g. involving a death or near-death) but does not concern a criminal matter that goes to the Coroner.

2.1. Critical Incident Reporting: Background

CIR was developed to understand the errors and mishaps surrounding fighter pilots during World War II (Flanagan 1954). These studies led to considerable cockpit and instrument panel redesign on the one hand, and to specifications governing the appropriate conducts of fighter crews on the other hand. As Runciman and Moller (2001: 35) explain, the technique led not just to "setting criteria for selection, training, performance and motivation of personnel, but also for improved job design, operating procedures and equipment". Early examples of the use of CIR in health care are described in publications by Safren and Sanazaro and colleagues (Safren / Chapanis 1960; Sanazaro / Williamson 1970), whose introduction of CIR into anaesthesia constituted the first public acknowledgement by medical professionals of the occurrence of iatrogenic injury in hospitals.

The technical orientation of CIR notwithstanding, this practice of recording 'what happened' and 'what I did' puts an affective dimension in play by requiring clinicians to record their (inter)personal experiences of an error. As the examples below will bear out, this means that writing about the specifics of an event is hardly ever a neutral affair, particularly in circumstances where people's life was at risk. Thus, the writings that clinicians produce when reporting mishaps are therefore not necessarily 'bureaucratic', and not infrequently resemble 'narratives' (Iedema *et al.* 2006). Research has shown that narratives have a number of characteristic features. One is the way that narratives are 'staged'. Their staging is most typically characterized by the presence of a complicating event: 'but all of a sudden …'. Another typical feature is 'evaluative assessment' by the author, focusing on how serious the disruption of the usual was experienced to be. This narrative feature seeks to engender sympathy on the part of the reader for the protagonists of the story and enhances the reader's interest in the events described (Rothery / Stenglin 1997). In sum, the peculiarity of the discursive resources deployed in narratives is that they weave representations about 'what happened' seamlessly into expressions about 'how it felt' and 'how the event was resolved' (Labov / Waletzki 1967; Mitchell 1981; Plum 1988).

Thus, in describing the details of the mishaps they witnessed or perpetrated, clinicians weave together 'factual' events with personal experiences, interested positionings and moral feelings in complex ways. In earlier work, I argued that this interweaving ensnares clinicians not just in reconciling views on 'what went wrong', 'who was responsible', 'how did it feel' and 'how much do I need to reveal', but also in translating these 'molecular' issues into implications for their 'systems of practice' – a move mandated by the broader health-organizational agenda of governance, practice improvement, work systems redesign, and clinical quality and safety (Iedema *et al.* 2006). This argument went on to say that in making their moral, personal and political sentiments 'public' to their superiors in the organizational and health departmental hierarchy, clinical professionals 'risk' re-orienting away from the values and norms that define their professional peer relationships, to ones that favour their health organization, or at least, the organization of their health services. Narratives are hypothesized to operate as the means of change here thanks to their affective pull, inducing clinicians to fold this public and systems-oriented self-scrutiny 'into their soul' (Rose 1999). Put in more theoretical terms, CIR is a narrative technique through which affectivity, identity, practice reflexivity and organizational strategy are made to converge.

2.2. Critical Incident Reporting: Analysis

In this section, I will present two critical incident report examples. The first example comes from the area of retrieval medicine; that is, that domain of medicine that is involved with flying doctors, nurses and other specialist clinicians to distant accident sites to provide emergency care. This first report describes how a medical team at a rural hospital failed to provide care as advised by the retrieval team to a patient they were scheduled to collect for treatment in one of the better-resourced metropolitan hospitals.

2.2.1. Critical Incident Report #1

> *Story*
> Patient with suspected acute abdomen at referral hospital. Complicated by multi-system organ failure. Intubated at time of initial contact. Mode of ventilation, fluid resuscitation extent of monitoring and blood investigations were inappropriate as not complete.
> Advised to do ventilatory changes, and changes in monitoring, insertion of nasogastric tube and other medications. Nothing done despite one hour till retrieval team arrived at referral hospital.

Outcome
Prolongation of organ dysfunction, metabolic acidosis and need to increase FiO_2.

Steps taken or treatment required
Sedate, optimise ventilation, N/G tube, external and central access, repeat ABG.

Was this incident preventable?
Yes. Medical staff present were capable of following retrieval team phone advice but chose not to.

The 'story' part of this report (a required 'field' on the critical incident report form) begins with setting the scene ("Patient with suspected [disease]"), before presenting the source of the disruption of usuality: "Mode of ventilation, fluid resuscitation extent of monitoring and blood investigations were inappropriate as not complete." What follows this is a negative assessment of the work done by staff in the rural hospital: "Advised to do ventilatory changes, and changes in monitoring, insertion of nasogastric tube and other medications. Nothing done despite one hour till retrieval team arrived at referral hospital." Despite the retrieval team having requested specific action be taken, nothing was done. In this case, then, the disruption of usuality centres on what specific people did not do, and on the consequences of their inaction ("Prolongation of …"). The report finishes with steps that needed to be taken on the part of the retrieval team to rectify the situation and salvage the patient ("Sedate, optimise ventilation, N/G tube, external and central access, repeat ABG").

As this analysis demonstrates, the incident report is a device through which technical issues and interpersonal sentiments become interwoven. The fact that the rural hospital's staff did not follow the retrieval team's orders produced what the latter saw as an incident worthy of being reported to their management. Moreover, the report leaves no doubt that due to the rural's team failure to do what was requested, the patient was unnecessarily put at risk. This failure to follow advice incurs a negative assessment of the rural team's clinical competence. In stark contrast to conventional ways of silencing these tensions, failures and emotions, the power of this bureaucratic-administrative device is that it creates a public space (the critical incident report) where technical judgments, clinical activities and interpersonal relationships are not just played off against one another, but also made to resolve into some kind organizational action ('what action was taken?').

The resolution of critical incidents may remain a within-department affair, but it may also necessitate involvement of clinicians from around the organization to investigate what happened and produce recommendations for change and learning. While in fact a report produced for the local health authority rather than for a clinical department or hospital, the incident report reproduced below is an example of such a case.

2.2.2. Critical Incident Report #2

Synopsis
Patient admitted following MBA had a respiratory arrest following large doses of narcotics administered to control severe pain.

Description of incident
MBA trauma patient admitted via helicopter retrieval with multiple fractures experiencing severe pain.
30 mgs morphine and 100mgs ketamine were administered by ambulance and retrieval team between 1800 and 2000, and 65mgs morphine administered for pain relief in emergency department between 2015 and 2240.
Patient transferred to theatre for emergency surgery.
Experienced a respiratory arrest in anaesthetic bay pre anaesthetic.
Narcosis successfully managed by anaesthetist. Patient required Naloxone infusion and monitoring in HDU overnight.
Nil permanent injury.

Action taken
• Advised A/Director Emergency Department
Suggested response for use by department or minister in media or other public comment.
Nil Response required.
Further planned action: eg. Root Cause Analysis, public response, contact with other agencies, staff debrief.
• RCA.
• Discuss with patient on [date].

This report is slightly different from the one seen above, because it is a summary about an incident produced from an internal CIR, hence its rather 'telegrammatic' style. Leaving the 'Synopsis' aside for now, this report too starts out with setting the scene: "MBA trauma patient admitted via helicopter retrieval with multiple fractures experiencing severe pain." It then describes the disruption of usuality, but does so in a rather technicalized way, leaving the seriousness of the error of over-prescribing implicit:

> 30 mgs morphine and 100mgs ketamine were administered by ambulance and retrieval team between 1800 and 2000, and 65mgs morphine administered for pain relief in emergency department between 2015 and 2240. Patient transferred to theatre for emergency surgery. Experienced a respiratory arrest in anaesthetic bay pre anaesthetic.

This higher level report, then, has reduced the interpersonal impulse that generally informs narrative down to a single expression in the Synopsis (in italics): "Patient admitted following MBA had a respiratory arrest following *large* doses of narcotics administered to control severe pain." While this second report has been shown to harbour the staging of a narrative, its interpersonal impact is further absorbed by the final recommendation to conduct RCA investigation. That is, any negative judgments about particular staff's activities have by this stage been transformed into a very specific kind of bureaucratic action ("Advised Director ED [...] RCA, Discuss with patient on [date]").

As its section 'Further planned action' indicates, this incident was considered critical enough to order an RCA investigation. I will turn to an analysis of the transcript of one of the RCA meetings that addressed this incident after providing some historical and procedural background.

2.3. Root Cause Analysis: Background

The technique of applying RCA to the investigation of clinical errors originated in 1997 following new hospital accreditation standards set by the US Joint Commission on Health Care Safety (Wald / Shojania 2001). Following that, the US National Centre for Patient Safety of the Department of Veterans Health Affairs (VA) piloted RCA at four of its hospitals in 1999, and accomplished a full roll-out in 2000 (GAO 2004). The VA models of RCA and RCA training to induct hospital clinicians into enacting the technique were adopted (Bagian

2001; Bagian *et al.* 2002) by NSW Health in 2002 and by the NHS in 2005. NSW Health has now trained over 2500 people and has also produced a second-tier training scheme called RCA Train the Trainer, with the aim of further expanding the network of certified RCA investigators in the NSW Health workforce.

Importantly, RCA and CIR are inter-dependent techniques. In a number of jurisdictions, incident reporting has begun to shift from a local paper-based practice used to alert local units and departments to mishaps, to becoming an inter-departmental reporting system that connects clinicians via a centralized server to a wider range of actors. In this virtual environment, clinicians' choices about whether and how to investigate their and their colleagues' errors are attracting increasing levels of scrutiny. The move from reporting errors to investigating errors, then, is one that is becoming not just increasingly 'tightly coupled' (Weick 1995) but also visible for an increasing number of stakeholders. This means, in turn, that the enactments and outcomes of such error investigations also gain in public attention and importance.

Root cause analysis is currently promoted as the technique par excellence for ensuring appropriate analysis of what went wrong. 'Appropriate' here means, among other things, that the volunteer clinicians who populate RCA teams home in on systems of practice, not individuals' actions. Our research has shown that this rule is difficult to follow in practice for a number of reasons. Before turning to these problem issues, let us consider the way that RCA has been defined as an investigative technique. The unique thing about this practice is that RCA is to be conducted by the clinical colleagues of those who were involved in the error, without sharing relationships that may become the basis for a conflict of interest. Once enrolled as team members, RCA team members do interviews with relevant personnel about the incident, so they can begin to articulate the causalities that they see as having contributed to the incident, and formulate conclusions and recommendations targeting systems and practice redesign.

The practice of investigating the details of colleagues' clinical work engages RCA team members in not just a micro-sociology of others' medical processes, but also in a reflexivity of clinical practices more generally. As earlier research showed, team members explore and articulate 'what happened' by drawing parallels with the clinical processes that they are familiar with. This dual focus implies, we argue elsewhere (Iedema *et al.* 2006; Iedema *et al.* submitted), that RCA intensifies the reflexivity which is already increasingly expected from medical-clinical professionals regarding how they interact with patients (Armstrong 2002), by broadening it to cover the *full* range of clinical practices. In extending clinicians' critical attention from the patient encounter to the whole of clinical-medical practice, RCA could be argued to complete "the rotation of the prism of illness to focus on the doctor" (Armstrong 2002: 185).

The details of RCA as technical procedure are as follows. RCAs are set in motion when a critical incident report is lodged about a mishap that is severe enough to necessitate an RCA (usually involving a patient death). The quality coordinator or quality manager of the hospital convenes a working party or RCA team by inviting appropriate (clinical or administrative) staff to participate in the investigation. This team has three meetings. In between these meetings, the team conducts interviews with the clinicians who were involved in the adverse event, it does targeted research into the clinical domain in question to understand the dynamics of the relevant disease(s) and treatment(s) and the organizational aspects of care, and it formulates causal relationships conjectured to underlie the incident. At the last meeting, the team prepares a report that outlines the main 'systems' causes behind the adverse event (Reason 1997), as well as recommendations to prevent future failures.

Below we will consider some selected extracts from an RCA meeting. As these extracts demonstrate, RCA's objective of clarifying the systems causes behind clinical failure involves clinicians in delicate discussions. Investigating errors in which one's colleagues were involved is a difficult process, even in organizations where trust levels are high. We know from other research that discussions of clinical practices among departmental colleagues *before* errors have occurred are fraught with difficulty (Iedema / Scheeres 2003), so it is not surprising that the examination of failure by a team of clinicians[2]

2 In what follows we will use the term 'clinicians' to describe RCA team members for brevity's sake, but we should emphasize that many people

from different departments might give rise to anxiety and defensiveness.

2.4. Root Cause Analysis: Some empirical data

The morphine overdose incident, of which we saw the report above, was deemed to require further investigation due to its potentially serious consequences for the patient (the patient had to be resuscitated). The investigation was structured according to the RCA technique described in the previous section. The data reproduced below are from a transcript made from a recording of the first RCA meeting organized by the team.[3]

The analysis of the transcript focuses on the new kind of work that comes into play for clinicians in doing these investigations. Rather than just being about a technical enquiry into a failure of clinical procedure, RCA involves clinicians in scrutinizing each others' approaches to their work, and this, in turn, involves them in interviewing colleagues, witnesses, and potentially patients. This kind of scrutiny, as I argue elsewhere, has profound emotional implications for all the individuals involved (Iedema *et al.* in press). When we consider how the RCA team confronts these challenges, it becomes evident that they too are torn between the technical and rational objectives inscribed into the RCA process, and the inevitable emotional cost of this kind of 'immaterial' work (Iedema *et al.* 2005).

This contradiction is clearly manifest in the meetings we tape-recorded, in so far that team members move back and forth between technical and interpersonal or relational concerns. In the following turns (313 and 368[4]), the chair of the RCA team meeting explains the team's technical brief.

---

participating in RCA teams in our study were in fact clinician-managers as well as non-clinical managers.

3 We attended five RCA meetings in total of which two were tape-recorded and transcribed.

4 These numbers represent 'turn numbers' as they appear in the original manuscript.

313 Yeah. RCA's can't look at a group of problems, they're only designed to look specifically at one incident. If we've got a group of them then we do – have a different process for doing that. So, we've got the process for checking – who, where, when, you know, do they have an armband … followed every case … got to try and remember … [?] … I've just written on the side here, "Do they check all that against the original …".

368 Yeah, because I was thinking … you'll probably want to know the usual sort of thing that … the usual processes, don't you? And then specifically what happened on that day to sort of have a comparison of, "Well, is that what they normally do?" Or it's, you know, what fell outside that, that may have contributed to this or is it just extremely lucky that 99% of the patients get to x-ray from ED and get the right x-ray?

Shortly after, the meeting moves towards considering the effect that the investigation will have on the interviewees ("so they don't freak out" at turn 469).

469 Now, what I'll do – I've already spoken to [name]. We need to sort of speak to [name], if you wouldn't mind doing that [name] to say that, "There's an RCA going on", dah, dah, dah, dah, that someone will be contacting him shortly to find out, you know, who the nurses are, the nurses will be interviewed, so they don't freak out.

A little later, the discussion turns towards team members' 'interviewing style', to make sure interviewees are not 'put on the backfoot'. The chair also explains what happens with the data that is collected and the procedures that are in place to make sure that confidentiality of the interviewees is preserved (at turn 491).

491 So, in the group of questions, it'll say, "Take the chronology along with you so you can sort of, you know, go through it all". You'll have a list of questions, the interviewing style or whatever, helps you to … you know, how to phrase so you're not putting people on the back foot and making them comfortable. They need to know that, when you finish … when you're finished with the interviews and you've collected all the information, that all the [?] completely destroyed and remains anonymous – which becomes a bit of a problem sometimes when you're trying to convince the department heads about how you arrived at your conclusion, so that's another story. Now, in terms of the next meeting … now, does a week … a week long enough for everyone to do their…to conduct those interviews? It's usually about a week, but I'll give you an opportunity to say no. Does next … next Wednesday or Thursday? [?] available?

The emotional work that needs to be done to ensure the cooperation and trust on the part of the interviewees is not the only concern the RCA team has, however. While it is in the interviewees' interest to have all the interview transcripts and information destroyed, this procedure in fact makes it more difficult for the RCA team to convince those who have to manage their recommendations into existence: unit and department heads, clinician-managers, and others with clinical responsibility for the processes that the RCA team feels need to be redesigned.

The RCA team is therefore caught in a bind. To make sure frontline clinicians will provide the necessary information about 'what happened' for the RCA team to deduce causes behind what happened and recommend clinical process changes, the team needs to destroy evidence, maintain secrecy and respect people's need for confidentiality. On the other hand, and in contrast with this, once the team issues its recommendations for change, those responsible for carrying out the changes will want to know the data and reasoning upon which the recommendations are based. While in the first case the RCA team faces the challenge of acting like confidants and creating spaces of personal trust, in the second case the team is faced with having to morph into an organizational change authority that can mount convincing grounds for legitimizing its recommendations. Both positions are demanding; not so much because of technical-clinical reasons, but because of the very different kinds of immaterial labour that are at the heart of the RCA team's hybrid or 'boundary-riding' position.

3. Discussion: Re-knowledging medicine

The analyses above have aimed to provide support for the thesis that contemporary clinical work in many post-industrial nation states is becoming increasingly immaterial; that is, increasingly oriented towards communicating, producing and sharing information, and working out, maintaining and fixing organizational relationships. CIR and RCA play a complementary role in this: while CIR involves clinicians in narrativizing errors of care, thereby reconfiguring local experiences and personal judgments into organizational concerns (Iedema *et al.* 2006), RCA involves clinicians in enacting new kinds of face-to-face relationships across disciplines, units and departments in ad hoc and temporary ways, requiring extraordinary emotional and relational skills.

Above, the point was made that CIR and RCA are post hoc devices for making visible the logics of clinical practice: only when a clinical process fails do clinicians become involved in scrutinizing the organizational dimensions of their work. This needs to be seen in the context of the fact that for some time now there has been a push for clinicians to engage in a priori mappings of their practices using the principles of the critical pathway (Campbell *et al.* 1998). However, the obstacles that clinicians confront in making their work explicit are numerous. Their university training notwithstanding, once in the hospital clinicians generally have (or make?) little time for negotiating the general principles that inform what they do. Moreover, clinicians are not trained to negotiate such principles, and they therefore tend to lack the necessary discourse for articulating them. Additionally, turning people's understandings of their own work processes into comprehensive descriptions of what goes on is less easy than might be assumed, because their understandings are to a large extent tacit. Complicit with this is the lack of comprehensive clinical documentation in many hospitals. Under-documentation in hospital care is a problem of long-standing (Codman 1917; Berg 2003) but it does render local disagreements about and discontinuities affecting clinical decisions invisible, thereby to some extent staving off inter-departmental and inter-specialty conflict over differences in clinical approaches and methods. This lack of data however makes it difficult for clinicians to develop meta-discursive insight into their own work, preventing them from being able to redesign it.

Given the problems that exist around the prospective mapping of clinical processes, CIR and RCA have the added advantage of embodying moral legitimacy: something went wrong and that something needs to be fixed. If prospective approaches to rationalizing medical work come up against differences in opinion leading to a lack in work systematization, retrospective approaches come up against that and more: as demonstrated above, CIR and RCA are methods that implicate clinicians in immaterial labour in ways that go well beyond sorting out differences in opinion about whether to prescribe a nebulizer or an inhaler for asthma patients, for example. CIR relies on clinicians turning personally-held values and norms regarding their clinical work into organizational change narratives, some of which (as did the one about the morphine overdose) produce investigations and recommendations that can have serious implications for how people do their work. For its part, RCA involves clinicians in a contradictory role, part of which centres on engendering trust with those from whom the team needs information, and another part of which centres on creating legitimacy and authority around RCA recommendations.

In both instances, what we are witnessing is what Munro (2003) has called the 'withdrawal of management'. Instead of managers eliciting information from frontline staff and making strategic decisions about details of the work, both CIR and RCA create spaces where personal concerns, emotions and judgments are connected to organizational processes, procedures and designs. Seen in these terms, CIR and RCA provide important examples of how new kinds of work are beginning to reconfigure work in general and health care practices in particular: as complementary techniques, they herald a new stance on how relationships between clinicians, professions, units, managements and policy makers are arbitrated.

Finally, this analysis suggests that CIR and RCA are what we may call *post-bureaucratic* devices (Iedema 2003). The notion of post-bureaucracy refers to a shift in organizations from pre-determined task and rank specifications towards ones that are emergent and responsive to changing requirements and local exigencies of work (Heckscher 1994). To remain responsive to these dynamics and exigencies, employees are increasingly obliged to communicate and share information about what they do with each other: their work involves not just doing what they do, but talking and writing about what they do. This communication work has been labeled 'immaterial labour' (Hardt / Negri 2004) and has been defined as encompassing not just problem solving, analytical tasks and intellectual work, but also negotiating emotions and judgments. As the data analysed above reveals, CIR and RCA put this immaterial labour centre stage in ways that are highly complementary, with team members being expected now to move seamlessly between writing about and collectively enacting emotional matters, normative judgments and technical expertises.

4. Conclusion: Post-bureaucratizing medicine

This chapter has described and presented an analysis of two new initiatives in hospital care: CIR and RCA. These initiatives emerged from increasing public concern about and say in the efficacy of medical work, and the perceived need for greater public accountability about what goes on in medicine. With other initiatives, such as critical pathways and clinical guidelines having achieved only a precarious relevance for medical practitioners (Woolf *et al.* 1999; Shojania / Grimshaw 2005), CIR and RCA appear to be having a greater impact on the way that doctors do and design their work. Both devices are being rolled out across a number of post-industrial jurisdictions, backed up with responsibilities and accountabilities that are increasingly enshrined in law and policy. It appears that from now on, doctors have increasingly limited scope to ignore the organizational, communicative and patient outcomes dimensions of their work, and are expected to conduct their written and face-to-face communications in increasingly public forums. Central here is the post-bureaucratic ethos that requires staff to communicate about the knowledge basis of their practices and to openly evaluate its evidence and principles.

In sum, the practice of clinicians reframing their norms and experiences in the form of the organizational incident report, and the practice of clinicians interviewing each other about mishaps together represent a broadening and intensifying of communication about medical work *as work*. This communication work constitutes a closer inspection of medical work not just by doctors, but is also by stakeholders from outside of medicine: nurses, allied health staff, managers, policy makers, and, last but not least, the public (consumers of health care services). The shift that is identified here is towards an inspectorial ethos: events that in the past would have been discussed in closed, 'paper-less' settings (Bosk 2003) are now reported through the organization (albeit still in restricted ways!),[5] and this affects how clinicians structure and perform their professional identities, their support networks and their disciplinary methods. In not being able to deny the moral authority of bureaucratic-managerial devices such as CIR and RCA due to their roots in practice improvement and patient-centredness, medicine is pushed towards more public forms of accountability compared to the ones into which it has thus far inducted its students and juniors. Instead of continuing to centre itself on medical-scientific knowledge, personal clinical experience and closed peer assessment, then, medicine can be argued to have begun to occupy a new social-organizational space where its claims to authority, expertise and legitimacy are articulated in ways that are increasingly measurable, verifiable and challengeable.

References

Armstrong, David 2002. *A New History of Identity: A Sociology of Medical Knowledge.* Basingstoke: Palgrave.

Armstrong, David 2005. The Myth of Concordance: Response to Stevenson and Scambler. *Health: An Interdisciplinary Journal for the Social Study of Health, Illness and Medicine* 9/1, 23-7.

Bagian, James P. 2001. Patient Safety – The VA's Experience. *Michigan Health & Hospitals* 37/4, 62-3.

Bagian, James P. / Gosbee, John. / Lee, Caryl Z. / Williams, Linda / McKnight, Scott D. / Mannos, Dea M. 2002. The Veterans Affairs Root Cause Analysis in Action. *Joint Commission Journal on Quality Improvement* 28/10, 531-45.

5 Anecdotal evidence has it that critical incident reporting is much less effective and more political than its proponents claim: CIR 'captures' only those errors that clinicians cannot not report (because they are so serious), those that are not really serious enough to report, those that they have to report due to 'uncooperative' witnesses, and those that they think may yield political or personal advantage.

Berg, Marc 2003. *Health Information Management.* London: Routledge.

Bosk, Charles 2003. *Forgive and Remember: Managing Medical Failure.* Chicago: University of Chicago Press.

Campbell, Harry / Hotchkiss, Rona / Bradshaw, Nicola / Porteous, Mary 1998. Integrated Care Pathways. *British Medical Journal* 316, 133-7.

Codman, Ernest 1917. Case-Records and Their Value. *Bulletin of the American College of Surgeons* 3/1, 24-7.

Flanagan, John 1954. The Critical Incident Technique. *Psychological Bulletin* 51, 327-58.

GAO (US Government Accountability Office) 2004. *VA Patient Safety Program: A Cultural Perspective of Four Medical Facilities.* Report to the Secretary of Veterans Affairs, Washington: United States Government Accountability Office.

Hardt, Michael / Negri, Antonio 2004. *Multitude: War and Democracy in the Age of Empire.* New York: The Penguin Press.

Heckscher, Charles 1994. Defining the Post-bureaucratic Type. In Heckscher, Charles / Donnellon, Anne (eds) *The Post-bureaucratic Organization.* Thousand Oaks: Sage, 14-62.

Iedema, Rick 2003. *Discourses of Post-Bureaucratic Organization.* Amsterdam: Benjamins.

Iedema, Rick / Flabouris, Arthas / Grant, Susan / Jorm, Christine M. 2006. Narrativizing Errors of Care: Critical Incident Reporting in Clinical Practice. *Social Science & Medicine* 62, 134-44.

Iedema, Rick / Jorm, Christine M. / Braithwaite, Jeffrey / Travaglia, Jo / Lum, Martin under review. Root Cause Analysis: Confronting the Disjunction between Formal Rules and Situated Clinical Activity. *Social Science & Medicine.*

Iedema, Rick / Jorm, Christine M. / Long, Debbi / Braithwaite, Jeffrey / Travaglia, Jo / Westbrook, Mary 2006. Turning the Medical Gaze in upon Itself: Root Cause Analysis and the Investigation of Clinical Error. *Social Science & Medicine* 62/7, 1605-15.

Iedema, Rick / Rhodes, Carl / Scheeres, Hermine 2005. Presencing Identity: Organizational Change and Immaterial Labour. *Journal of Organizational Change Management* 18/4, 327-37.

Iedema, Rick / Scheeres, Hermine 2003. From Doing Work to Talking Work: Renegotiating Knowing, Doing and Identity. *Applied Linguistics* 24/3, 316-37.

Labov, William / Waletzki, J. 1967. Narrative Analysis: Oral Versions of Oral Experience. In Helm, June (ed.) *Essays in the Verbal and Visual Arts, American Ethnological Society, Proceedings of the Spring Meeting.* Washington DC: University of Washington Press, 12-44.

Lillrank, Paul / Liukko, Matti 2004. Standard, Routine and Non-routine Processes in Health Care. *International Journal of Health Care Quality Assurance* 17/1, 39-46.

Mitchell, William J.T. 1981. *On Narrative.* Chicago: University of Chicago Press.

Munro, Rolland 2003. Disorganization. In Westwood, Robert / Clegg Stewart (eds) *Debating Organization: Point-Counter-point in Organization Studies*. Oxford: Blackwell, 283-97.

Plum, Gunther 1988. Textual and Contextual Conditioning in Spoken English: A Genre-Based Approach, Sydney: University of Sydney.

Reason, James T. 1997. *Managing the Risks of Organizational Accidents.* Aldershot: Ashgate.

Rose, Nikolas 1994. Medicine, History and the Present. In. Jones, Colin / Porter, Roy (eds) *Reassessing Foucault: Power, Medicine, and the Body*. London: Routledge, 48-72.

Rose, Nikolas 1999. *Powers of Freedom: Reframing Political Thought.* Cambridge: Cambridge University Press.

Rothery, Joan / Stenglin, Maree 1997. Exploring Experience Through Story. In Christie, Frances / Martin, Jim (eds) *Genre and Institutions: Social Processes in the Workplace and School.* London: Cassell, 231-63.

Runciman, William B. / Moller, Jerry 2001. *Iatrogenic Injury in Australia*. Canberra: Australian Patient Safety Foundation.

Safren, M.A. / Chapanis, A. 1960. A Critical Incident Study of Hospital Medication Errors. *Hospitals* 34, 32-66.

Sanazaro, P.J. / Williamson, J.W. 1970. Physician Performance and its Effects on Patients: Classification Based on Reports by Internists, Surgeons, Paediatricians and Obstetricians. *Medical Care* 8, 299-308.

Shojania, Kaveh / Grimshaw, Jeremy 2005. Evidence-based Quality Improvement: The State of the Science. *Health Affairs* 24/1, 138-51.

Stevenson, Fiona / Scambler, Graham 2005. Rejoinder to 'The Myth of Concordance': A Response to Armstrong. *Health: An Interdisciplinary Journal for the Social Study of Health, Illness and Medicine* 9/1, 39-40.

Wald, H. / Shojania, Kaveh 2001. Root Cause Analysis. In Shojania, Kaveh / Duncan, Bradford / McDonald, Kathryn / Wachter. Robert / Markowitz, Amy (eds) *Making Health Care Safer: A Critical Analysis of Patient Safety Practices.* Evidence Report / Technology Assessment: Number 43. Rockville, MD.: Agency for Healthcare Research and Quality.

Weick, Karl 1995. *Sense-making in Organisations.* London: Sage.

Williams, Simon J. / Calnan, Michael 1996. The 'Limits' of Medicalization? Modern Medicine and the Lay Populace in 'Late' Modernity. *Social Science and Medicine* 42/12, 1609-20.

Woolf, Steven / Grol, Richard / Hutchinson, Allen / Eccles, Martin / Grimshaw, Jeremy 1999. Potential Benefits, Limitations and Harms of Clinical Guidelines. *British Medical Journal* 318/20 February, 527-30.

FLORIAN MENZ / JOHANNA LALOUSCHEK

"I just can't tell you how much it hurts." Gender-relevant Differences in the Description of Chest Pain

1. Introduction

Chest pain can be caused by many different diseases, ranging from trivial muscle pain to life-threatening disorders like acute myocardial infarction (Hofgren *et al.* 1994). If chest pain is due to coronary heart disease, a prompt diagnosis is important to survival and quality of life. Since laboratory investigations like EKG or blood tests are only of limited value to confirm or exclude a coronary cause of chest pain, the clinical history remains an important diagnostic tool (Fruergaard *et al.* 1996, Douglas / Ginsburg 1996). Medical studies show that there exist gender differences in diagnosis and therapy of coronary heart disease with a strong bias. Coronary heart disease is less well diagnosed with women than with men. This means that although sometimes women suffer from coronary heart disease, it is not diagnosed as such. This may have severe influence on survival and/or death rate (Tobin *et al.* 1987, Steingart *et al.* 1991, Ayanian / Epstein 1991, Silbergleit / McNamara 1995, Schulman *et al.* 1999). An improvement of the clinical history is therefore desirable. Up to now, only a few medical studies have investigated cause- and gender-specific differences in the description of chest pain and found only slight differences in the symptoms (Hofgren *et al.* 1994, Penque *et al.* 1998, Meischke / Larsen / Eisenberg 1998, Goldberg *et al.* 1998, Milner *et al.* 1999). These slight differences do not sufficiently explain the gender differences regarding diagnostic and therapeutic measures in patients with chest pain. Linguistic analysis, however, has indicated that gender-specific differences in language behaviour exist in many situations of social relevance, especially in institutional contexts where laypeople are confronted with experts, as is the case in doctor-patient interaction (Hein *et al.* 1984, West 1984, Tannen 1993, Crawford 1995, Kotthoff / Wodak 1997, Wodak 1997, Talbot 1998, Goddard / Patterson 2000). Therefore, the aim of this prospective transdisciplinary cardiologic-linguistic study of patients admitted to a cardiological department was to assess whether 1) cause-specific differences exist in the symptoms reported, 2) gender-specific differences exist in the symptoms reported (cardiologic investigation), 3) the description of chest pain differs between causes of chest pain, and 4) the description of chest pain differs between female and male patients (linguistic analysis). In this chapter I will concentrate on the last hypothesis.

2. Literature review

Since the 1970s, communication between doctors and patients has been established as a major research area within discourse analysis, both internationally and in the German speaking world (Becker-Mrotzek 1992), focusing primarily on the institutional conditions (Hein *et al.* 1984, Lalouschek / Menz / Wodak 1990, Menz 1991b). Numerous volumes summarise the state of linguistic research in this field (e.g. Atkinson / Heath 1981, Ehlich *et al.* 1989, Corney 1991, Löning / Rehbein 1993, Todd 1993, Redder / Wiese 1994, Morris 1995, Sarangi / Roberts 1999).

The scope of medical talk can be categorised as transforming personal 'narratives' into a scheme in order to find a diagnosis, an interactive task that has to be performed by both patient and physician (Mishler 1984). In this respect the medical interview can be seen as a decision making process (Rehbein 1993). To gain this goal, physicians tend to interrupt patients' narratives, to ask questions with narrow focus and to talk more than patients themselves (Hein *et al.* 1984, Frankel 1990, Menz 1991b), sometimes even with problematic results (Cicourel 1985, Menz 1991a). On the other hand, patients' questions are frequently ignored (Lalouschek / Menz / Wodak 1990). Moreover, as in most institutional settings, several studies have shown strong gender and class related differences within doctor-patient communication as well (Fisher / Todd 1983, West 1984, 1990, Hein 1985, Hein *et al.* 1984), Similar results have also been established in the medical literature (Richards *et al.* 2000). Despite the extensive and abundant discourse analytic literature on doctor-patient communication, specific studies on the descriptions of pain are scarce.

As Ehlich (1985) has pointed out, three types of pain expression can systematically be distinguished: a) weeping, crying, whining, b) interjections of pain (archetypically for English: *ouch!* and German: *au!*), and c) descriptions of pain. Only the latter are of interest in the context of this chapter. The problem with pain descriptions is that our everyday language is not particularly rich in expressions of the symbolic field, in contrast to visual and acoustic phenomena, where the linguistic typology is rather distinctive. This scarcity of direct linguistic expressions urges interactants to make use of indirect forms such as metaphoric or figurative descriptions (Baumgartinger *et al.* 2002). Moreover, Kütemeyer (2002) presents some facts which show that metaphorical expressions of pain are only used by patients with psycho-somatically induced pain, thus differing significantly from patients with clearly organically diagnosed pain causes.

Heath's (1989) study reveals that both expression of pain and description of pain hamper, even exclude, each other mutually in the medical setting. The medical diagnosis is dependent on an exact description of pain; the expression of immediate pain is of little help for the diagnostic process, it is actually even obstructive in a way that other witnesses have to be relied on in cases where the patient him/herself is not able to give 'objective' descriptions (Heath 1989: 114). The emotional stress of physicians in cases of severe pain has been elaborated on by Ehlich (1993: 90).

3. Data description and design of the study

Due to the scarcity of work on pain description, our study had primarily an explorative character which favoured an open focus (Miles / Huberman 1996). Therefore, for the sampling of the data, an important precondition lay in the consideration to find a setting which, on the one side, was close to naturally occurring interactions between patients and physicians, and, on the other side, was not severely influenced by the institutional constraints of the hospital. For this reason, we decided not to take medical interviews as a data basis but to conduct specific interviews which took the criteria mentioned above into account. In these semi-standardised interviews, the topics, but not their exact order, were fixed in advance. Thus, the interviewer had the chance to stimulate a conversation as close as possible to naturally occurring interaction, pursuing the goal of giving the patients the opportunity to describe and talk[1] about their chest pain as spontaneously and completely as possible in order to attain a comprehensive overview of different pain descriptions. These phases with open focus were supplemented by a number of questions primarily oriented towards the medical differential diagnosis with its specific, rather narrow focus. The length of the interviews ranged from 15 to 50 minutes.

The data were gathered during an eight-month period between February and September 2000 in the intern ward of a major hospital in Vienna. Included were patients who were admitted because of chest pain at the 2nd medical department. Chest pain had to be the main symptom leading to admission. Additional symptoms could, but did not need to be, present. Chest pain was defined as pain located between the throat (*jugulum*) and the stomach (*epigastrium*). Within 48 hours after hospital admission, the patients were asked to take part in the study. After having obtained informed consent, all included patients were interviewed by the same investigator, a medical student completing her thesis. The medical therapy was documented, and the patients were categorised according to the primary cause of their chest pain. The interviews were de-personalised and made available for transcription and linguistic analysis.

1 For narration cf. Gülich / Quasthoff (1985).

All in all, 102 interviews were tape-recorded and subjected to a quantitative medical analysis (Vodopiutz *et al.* 2002). Out of these 102 interviews, 24 were selected for a deeper discourse analytic examination. The selection criteria were gender (female/male), cause (coronary/ non coronary), and age (<56, 56-69, >70 years). As can be seen in Table 1, with one exception, each cell was filled with at least two cases.

	Code number of female patients	*Code number of male patients*
coronary cause <56 years	039, 092	085, 078
coronary cause 56-69 years	062, 058, 059	094, 080
coronary cause > 70 years	071, 095	027, 053
non-coronary cause <56 years	054, 074	028, 056
non-coronary cause 56-69 years	057, 060	077, 065
non-coronary cause > 70 years	029, 055	091

Table 1. Data distribution according to gender, cause, and age.

4. Some results

The qualitative linguistic analysis of the 24 interviews showed strong gender differences in two directions: on a more global level of self-presentation (4.1 and 4.2) and on a more local level of pain description (4.3 and 4.4), which in the following sections will be described and illustrated by some excerpts of the transcripts.

4.1. Focus: cause of pain vs experiencing of illness

The interviews with the patients took place at a semi-standardised level with the discourse analytic goal of gathering comprehensive and spontaneous descriptions of pain. For this reason, an introduction as open as possible was chosen, which allowed the patients to set their own foci rather effectively, by making relevant specific themes and interactional goals. All in all, five general foci were found:

- Self-presentation as being well informed
- Psycho-social strain
- Illness as a threat to life and fear
- Downgrading or upgrading of illness
- Cooperativity or passivity (together with delegation of illness to the medical institution).

Table 2 shows the tendencies found in focus-setting of the interviews.

Code	*Gender*	*Age*	*Focus*
027	m	75a	being informed / self-presentation
053	m	75a	being informed / self-presentation
085	m	46a	being informed
077	m	59a	being informed
080	m	64a	being informed
094	m	61a	illness being something special
095	f	73a	illness being something special
056	m	41a	illness as threat/clarification of pain cause
078	m	47a	illness as threat/clarification of pain cause
074	f	33a	illness as threat/clarification of pain cause
057	f	58a	illness as threat/clarification of pain cause
039	f	52a	downgrading
058	f	62a	downgrading / delegation to institution
060	f	64a	co-operation / delegation
055	f	76a	passivity/ delegation
071	f	70a	rejection of illness
059	f	66a	stressing of seriousness
028	m	54a	stressing of seriousness
054	f	36a	psycho-social strain
092	f	57a	psycho-social strain
062	f	60a	psycho-social strain
029	f	76a	psycho-social strain

Table 2. Gender and global focus of the interview.

The category of the concentration on specific foci showed gender-specific differences. The main interest of men seems to be to know about the cause of their pain on a very somatic level and to present themselves as being well informed about illness, medication and/or therapeutic measures. Women, on the other hand, focused on the psycho-social strain caused by the illness: increasing dependence on others, concern about family and relatives, limitations in daily life, fear and anxiety because of physical problems and handicaps.

4.2. Self-presentation: pain managing vs pain enduring

An additional gender difference was found in the self-presentation of 'pain management'.

			Self-presentation	
Code	*Gender*	*Age*	*Pain enduring*	*Pain managing*
074	w	33a	+	
054	w	36a		
039	w	52a	+	
092	w	57a	+	
057	w	58a	+	
062	w	60a		
058	w	62a	+	
060	w	64a	+	
059	w	66a		
071	w	70a	+	
095	w	73a		
029	w	76a	+	
055	w	76a	+	
056	m	41a		
085	m	46a		+
078	m	47a		+
028	m	54a		
077	m	59a		+
094	m	61a	+	
080	m	64a		+
065	m	69a		
091	m	72a		
053	m	75a		
027	m	75a		+

Table 3. 'Pain management' and gender.

Female patients tended towards an emotional self-description and presented themselves as prevailingly pain enduring: they accepted their suffering passively, did not frequently care about former pain attacks, and would not have been admitted to hospital if they had not been sent by relatives. Furthermore, they did not show interest in the clarification of the pain causes and delegated their pain treatment to the expert system. The self-presentation by the patients, however, did not necessarily coincide with actual information or co-operation, i.e. although women did not interactionally present themselves as co-operative, they may well have been co-operative during their stay in hospital. This type of self-description, however, implies a certain degradation of the individual pain experience. One of the consequences may well be that the pain is not taken seriously by the physicians either. Some illustrative examples are the following:[2]

(1) 055WLW (w, 76a, Ucardncu)
173 I: KENNen Sie so einen SCHMERZ von: IRGENDwas ANderem?
P: EIgentli[ch nicht.
I: [NEIN. GANZ neu AUFgetretn? (-) mhm\/
P: (---) WISSnS *ich BIN EIne die SOGT wos aLLEIne KOMMT muss aLLEIne verGEHN.*
I: aha\/
P: jo? (--) drum (.) BIN i zu kan OAZT <<GONGen> lachend>

(1a) 055WLW (f, 76a, Ucardncu)
I: Have you ever experienced such a pain from somewhere else?
P: rather [not
I: [no. occurred for the first time? – hm\/
P: --- you know, *I'm among the ones who say: what appears by itself that has to disappear by itself as well*
I: aha\/
P: yeah – therefore I haven't gone to the <<doctor's> laughing>

(2) 058 KAW (w, 62a, Ucoron)
168 P: JA/ aber ich bin SO: wie ich schon SAgte ein: M:ENSCH der wos hoit .hh (--) *WEMMa a BIßi einen SCHMERZ hat, SO denkt ma „naja es WIRD schon wieder AUFhörn .hh und wenn es dann AUFhört dann: (---) verGEß ich das halt wieder. nicht*?
I: mhm\/ (-)
P: SO: in der HÜBSCH in dem SINN: NED? wenn (-)
I: ja'
P: *MANche LAUfn halt GLEICH zum Arzt* oba ich BIN: (--) lieber SO:
.hhh daß ich NICHT GLEICH geh. ned?

2 The relevant parts are highlighted by italics.

(2a) 058KAW (f, 62a, Ucoron)
P: yes, but as already said, I'm among the people who – when one has a little bit of pain – who think "well, it will stop again .hh and *when it then actually stops then --- well then I forget about it again, don't I*
I: hm\/
P: so, in that way, you see
I: Yes
P: *Others may run to the doctor's at once, but I myself .hh don't go immediately.*

(3) 057FCW (w, 58a, Uspondyl)
310 I: und WANN hat DAS beGONNen? (---)
P: no ich DENke so DONNersTAG A:bend ja:
I: der KRAMPF auch? das KLEIne:? (--) das SCHWACHe auch?
P: ah des SCHWACHE: (-) .hh na UNgefähr ACHT TAge so was. ACHT ZEHN TAge: (-) MÜßT man sagn;
I: ACHT zehn TAge. (---)
P: das WEIß ich WIRKlich NICHT mehr. *weil ich HAB des am ANfang, .hh GAR nicht ah: beACHtet*

(3a) 057FCW (f, 58a, Uspondyl)
I: and when did it start? ---
P: well I think around Thursday evening, yeah
I: the cramp as well? The little one, the twinge as well?
P: uh the twinge - .hh no about 8 days or something like that. Eight to ten days one would have to say
I: eight to ten days ---
P: That I really don't know anymore. *Because in the beginning I really didn't pay attention to it*

Male patients presented themselves as well informed about their illness(es), as actively pain-managing, as co-operative, and as interested in the detection and diagnosis of the pain causes. In addition, male patients observed their pain extensively, took it seriously and stressed the importance of treating it. With regard to the medical diagnosis, this strategy of self-presentation facilitates the interactive reconstruction of the development of the pain and the disease in general. As this kind of self-presentation as well informed and actively pain-managing seems to relate with a high degree of self-observation and upgrading of one's own pain (cf. 4.3), this strategy of self-presentation might effect the assessment of relevance on the part of the physicians. Preliminary results of a matched guise test with physicians point in this direction but have to be further validated.

(4) 085SKM (m, 46a, Ucoron)
223 I: Also Sie ham nicht gedacht, das ist das Herz ist
P: *I hobs sofort gwusst.*
I: Ham Sies gwusst,
P: I hobs glei gwusst (---) Weil i hob um ein Uhr die ersten Schmerzen gspürt
I: mhm\/
P: do bin i aufgstandn und i hob in die letzten drei vier Wochn ghobt (.) ah (-) ah na a Knattern (xxx) dass wonn i so woch worn bin hob i so richtig gspürt wies wies wies orbeit, oisi i i [wor i hob scho
I: [mhm\/
P: gwusst dass i geh soi und (--) jetz so zu spät ned

(4a) 085SKM (m, 46a, Ucoron)
I: Well, you didn't think it was your heart
P: *I knew it instantly*
I: You knew it
P: I knew it at once --- because I felt the first pains at one o'clock.
I: hm\/
P: I got up and the last three four weeks I've had a, well, some rattling (XXX) that when I woke up, I really felt how it worked, well, I I [was I
I: [hm\/
P: I knew I had to go and – well

4.3. Experiencing of pain: foregrounding vs backgrounding

A strong connection between the global orientation and focusing is to be found with the self-evaluation of the patients' own pain. Men stressed the distinctiveness, the particularity, and the importance of taking their illness seriously. This was categorised as foregrounding.

(5) 027VPM (m, 75a, Ucoron)
041 P: dann *hab ich eben meinen Arzt gesprochen*, praktisch, no aber nachdem des halbwegs abgeklUngen is durch stoarke AntibiOtika, so wie [sie, hh(-)
I: [ja-
P: sag mer, *des kummt mer spanisch vor*, net woar,(.) der koide Schweiß, des kann do nit mitn (-)hh mitn (.) mit die Bronchien ztuan ham, wos=wos *wos ma da umadum ah lie:st im Laufe der vielen [Ja:hre*,
I: [ja-
P: sogt ma einfach, des is a Herzinfa:rkt, (.) net woar, aber natürlich *a*

Herzinfarkt, h müßte aber dann dAuernd ,(.)h ah dA sein, und ni:cht, net woar, sag mer h (.) einma:l (.) sog mer, einma:l (.) h fünf Minuten kummen und und=und wieder verge::hn, net? No, *da hamma EKG gemocht*, des hat nix zeigt, net woar, s nächste Mal hob i h(.) bin i wieder zu ihm, hob (i) gsagt, Sie:, jetz is: h heart net a:uf, hat er wieder an EKG gemocht,

(5a) 027VPM (m, 75a, Ucoron)

P: Then *I talked to my doctor*, practically, well but having eased by heavy antibiotics
I: yes
P: let's say, *that's Greek to me*, isn't it . the cold sweat, it can't have to do with the bronchial tubes anyway, *what one is reading around in the course of many [years.*
I: [yes
P: One simply says it's a heart attack, all right?, but of course, *a heart attack, .h it would have to be there uhm continuously* and not, let's say, once, let's say come once . .h for five minutes and then disappear again, right?. Well, *we've made an EKG*, it didn't show anything, right? Next time I went to him again, I said: Doctor, it is, it doesn't stop, he made an EKG again

In the above excerpt, by using the pronoun *we,* the patient reduces the institutionally motivated hierarchy between himself and the physician, i.e. the difference between experts and lay-people, which is further strengthened by his remarks on symptoms of myocardial infarction. He presents himself as well informed, as a person who takes his illness seriously.

Women, on the other hand, tended to play down their suffering from pain, described it as not serious and underestimated it.

(6) 039BRW (w, 52a, Ucoron)

038 I: Und wo genau war der Schmerz?
P: Do.
I: Do.
P: Do. Es woa ned, *es woa zum Aushoidn oba es woa hoit unangenehm irgendwie.*

(6a) 039BRW (f, 52a, Ucoron)

I: And where exactly did you feel the pain?
P: Here
I: here
P: Here. It wasn't, *it was endurable, it was just unpleasant somehow*

In the following excerpt, the backgrounding of relevance is created by the repeated use of the (Austrian German) discourse particle *halt*, which can only approximately be translated by 'in a way', 'somehow':

(7) 058KAW (w, 62a, Ucoron)
064 P: WIE wenn das SO (--) geDRÜCKT wird.
I: mhm\/ (-) mhm\/
P: SO: hab ICH das GeFÜHL daß das SO (---)
I: mhm\/ (-)
P: und das HAB ich *halt* so'(-) SO' ZWIschndurch halt. WIE geSAGT WENN ich MEHR (-) A:rbeit MACHe so. bißl
<...>
P: WENN=s SO: (-) WAR, DAß ma MANCHmal (-) MEHR oder ÖFTers, .hh ah so geDRÜCKT hat DANN: (---) BIN ich *halt* zu der: (--) ja HAUSärztin geGANgen und (-) beim LETZtn Mal: HAT sie ebm *halt* DANN mi:chs: zum INternist geSCHICKT, so: RADfahrn und SOLche SACHN

(7a) 058KAW (f, 62a, Ucoron, lines 38ff)
P: as if it were pressed somehow
I: hm\/ - hm\/
P: well I've the feeling that well
I: hm\/
P: Well, and that I've so, so now and then somehow. As I said when I work more, little bit
<...>
P: If it was the way that – sometimes – more or more often .hh I felt the pressure then --- well then I went to my family doctor and – the last time, well then she sent me to the internist, kind of bicycling and such things

4.4. Pain description: concrete vs diffuse

Some of the most evident gender-specific differences could be found on the level of pain description. In the interviews an enormous band-width of pain description could be found which we allocated on a scale of concreteness. The main allocation parameter was, first, the presence or absence of a description of symptoms and, secondly, the richness of description. To take the description of symptoms as a parameter of differentiation is reasonable, as this is in accordance with the expectations of the interviewing physicians. On this basis we distinguished among three types of pain description:

- *Very concrete*: patients gave long and detailed descriptions of the pain symptoms;
- *Concrete:* patients gave shorter symptomatic descriptions of pain and changed the topic rapidly towards general pain experience;
- *Diffuse:* patients gave no symptomatic pain descriptions and made meta-communicative comments on the impossibility of pain description.

The evaluation showed that, with one exception, all 'very concrete' pain descriptions were produced by men, whereas, with one exception, all 'diffuse' pain descriptions were produced by women (Table 4).

Code	*Gender*	*Age*	*chest pain for the first time*	*Cause of pain / diagnosis*	*Pain description*
054	f	36a	No	psychogenic cause	very concrete
085	m	46a	Yes	coronary cause	very concrete
028	m	54a	No	musculoskeletal cause	very concrete
077	m	59a	Yes	Gastrointestinal	very concrete
094	m	61a	Yes	coronary cause	very concrete
080	m	64a	No	coronary cause	very concrete
027	m	75a	No	coronary cause	very concrete
053	m	75a	No	coronary cause	very concrete
039	f	52a	Yes	coronary cause	concrete
057	f	58a	Yes	musculoskeletal	concrete
062	f	60a	No	coronary cause	concrete
060	f	64a	No	cardiac non-coronary	concrete
056	m	41a	Yes	pulmonary cause	concrete
078	m	47a	No	coronary cause	concrete
074	f	33a	Yes	cardiac non-coronary	diffuse
092	f	57a	No	coronary cause	diffuse
058	f	62a	No	coronary cause	diffuse
059	f	66a	No	coronary cause	diffuse
071	f	70a	No	coronary cause	diffuse
095	f	73a	No	coronary cause	diffuse
029	f	76a	No	gastroesophageal	diffuse
055	f	76a	No	cardiac non-coronary	diffuse
065	m	69a	No	pulmonary cause	diffuse

Table 4. Pain description and gender.

The only woman with very concrete symptomatic description was very young and desperately tried to avoid to be diagnosed as psychogenic. Therefore she definitely wanted a 'somatic' diagnosis. The only man with diffuse descriptions of pain did not co-operate in the interview and consequently produced only diffuse and vague pain descriptions. With only one exception, all very concrete pain descriptions are produced by men. Not only is the description detailed in the way they refer to the symptoms, but also with regard to the onset, the intensity and the duration of pain. The following example may illustrate this:

(8) 027VPM (m, 75a, Ucoron)
09 I: was hat's mit den Schmerzen auf sich, (.) wie is das-
P: jaha(.) das setzt plötzlich ein (.) Druck hier(-) h im im Brustbereich, im oberen Brustbereich e:in, (--) h der ein kleines bIßchen so: zu Atemno:t(-)
I: ja,
P: ah (.) fü:hrt, (-)h und außerde:m h ah=ah=m kalten Schweißaus ausbruch verursacht. h und ein gewisses Angstgefühl. Net? (-) Und dos(.) ah sagmer bewegt mich dann sofort ah=ah so mich hInzulEgn,
I: ja,
P: ja, und (.) h und nach tIefen ah A:temzü:gen, ja, sag mer h (.) hat des ph sag mer meinetwegen nach (.) fünf, sechs oder zehn Minuten aufgehört-
I: ja-
P: es war alles wieder norma:l. (-) (net),(.) so.

(8a) 027VPM (m, 75a, Ucoron)
I: What about this pain, (.) what is it like?
P: we:ll (.) it starts suddenly (.) pressure here (-) .h in the chest area, upper chest area, (--) h which leads a little bit to dispnoea [difficulty in breathing]
I: Yes
P: and besides that er er causes cold sweating .h and a certain feeling of anxiety, doesn't it? (-) and this, let's say makes me immediately lie down this way
I: yes
P: yes, and (.) after some deep er breaths, well, let's say, .h (.) after five, six or ten minutes, if you like this has stopped-
I: yes
P: everything was back to normal

Frequently, very concrete pain descriptions go hand in hand with focusing on the clarification of pain cause and a preference of presenting oneself as well informed. This high degree of self-observation seems to be stronger in men than in women. Typically male patients are able to reconstruct the onset of the pain attack very exactly:

(9) 094VLM (m, 61a, Ucoron)
040 I: WIE WA:R das mit dem SCHMERZ? (--)
P: BeGONNEN? (-) EI:gentlich (-) VÖLLIG überRA:SCHEND?
I: JA:?
P: IN der NA:CHT von SONNtag (.) auf MO:Ntag. (--) WIE: GESAGT (--) ZEI:Tpunkt (-) ZIRKA (-) EI:N Uhr ZWANZIG (.) FRÜH:? (-) MIT (-) PLÖTZlich AUFtretenden (-) KA:LTEN SCHWEI:ßausbrüchen? (--) KOPFschmerzen. (-) ERBRECHEN (-) DURCHFALL. (-) SCHWINDELGEFÜHL (-) und einen DRU:CK in der (--) BRU:ST der (--) der RICHtig zum ANGSTGEFÜHL (-) WURDE!

(9a) 094VLM (m, 61a, Ucoron)
I: What was it like with the pain?
P: started – actually – completely surprisingly
I: Yes?
P: In the night of Sunday (.) till Monday – as I said – point of time – around – one twenty . in the morning – with suddenly appearing cold sweating, head ache – vomiting – diarrhoea – dizzy feeling – and pressure in the chest which turned into a real feeling of anxiety

Except for one male patient, only women produced diffuse pain descriptions in the sense of our categorisation, i.e. with little or no description of symptoms, but a long dwelling upon detailed descriptions of pain experience. Patients who give diffuse descriptions of pain frequently use vagueness markers such as expressions of doubt and uncertainty, relativising particles, hesitations, and also show efforts in re-formulating their answers to the question of the quality of pain (see examples 10-11).

Frequently not only is the description of pain diffuse, but also the whole experience of pain is characterised as virtually indescribable, incomparable and/or peculiar:

(10) 057FCW (w, 58a, Uspondyl)
310 I: und WANN hat DAS beGONNen? (---)
P: no ich DENke so DONNersTAG A:bend ja:
I: der KRAMPF auch? das KLEIne:? (--) das SCHWACHe auch?

P: ah des SCHWACHE: (-) .hh na UNgefähr ACHT TAge so was.
ACHT ZEHN TAge: (-) MÜßT man sagn;
I: ACHT zehn TAge. (---)
P: das WEIß ich WIRKlich NICHT mehr. weil ich HAB des am
ANfang, .hh GAR nicht ah: beACHtet

(10a) 057FCW (f, 58a, Uspondyl, lines 310ff)
I: and when did it start? ---
P: ,well I think around Thursday evening, yeah
I: the cramp as well? The little one, the twinge as well?
P: uh the twinge - .hh no about 8 days or something like that. Eight ten
days one would have to say
I: eight ten days ---
P: That I really don't know anymore. Because in the beginning I really
didn't pay attention to it

(11) 045 P: Es ist NET ein KRAMPF - (.) kann man das aber eigentlich AUCH
ned sagen. (--)
I: Ist das INNEN? (-)
P: Is INNEN. (-)
I: Is innen. (--) mhm:\/ (-) U:ND (-) es tut WE:H. (--)
P: Es tut WE:H. (---)
I: WIE:: tut=s WE:H? (--)
P: Wie SOLL ich Ihnen das erKLÄREN? (--) Das KANN man gar ned
SA:GEN wie das WEH tut. (-) DAS: (-) das: KOMMT (--) tut so weh;
DAS: (---) da (-) das: ZIEHT sich so ZUSAMMEN und tut WE:H. (-)
Aber ich KANN Ihnen das: (-) gar ned SAGEN (--) WIE: es: weh tut.
(-) Es TUT halt WE:H. (-)
I: mhm\/. (--) STICHT das oder BRE:NNT das:?
P: NEI:N. (---) Nur SCHME:RZEN. (--)
I: DRÜCKN (.) AUCH nicht? (-)
P: Nein.

(11a) 057FCW (f, 58a, Uspondyl, lines 45ff)
P: it's not a cramp - . one couldn't actually say that –
I: Is it inside?
P: it's inside
I: It's inside. .. hm\/ - AND – it hurts –
P: it hurts ---
I: How does it hurt? --
P: How shall I explain that to you - - you can't even say HOW much
it hurts. – it – it comes – hurts so much, this --- this here is contracting
and hurting. – But I can't really describe to you the WAY it hurts. –
it just hurts. –
I: hm\/. – is it piercing or burning?
P: No just pangs

I: pressing pain, neither?
P: No.

The patient in the last excerpt very briefly localises the pain ("das zieht sich so zusammen und tut weh"/ "this here is contracting and hurting"), and then moves over to the actual indescribability of the emotions and sensations. Specifying questions do not add to a more detailed description either.

5. Conclusions

Medical investigations have shown that coronary heart disease is under-diagnosed and under-treated in women. A purely medical approach does not seem to explain this phenomenon. The results of the linguistic analysis, however, might give an explanation. They are in accordance with other findings in the linguistic literature on gender-specific differences in language behaviour in many situations of social relevance (cf. Sections 1 and 2). Historically, coronary heart disease developed as a disease predominantly occurring in male patients and was described and treated mostly by male physicians. Regarding chest pain description, male language behaviour seems to match physicians' expectations better than female language behaviour. Clear descriptions of symptoms with exact chronological data appear to be considered more relevant, whereas female self-presentation as pain enduring combined with less concrete pain descriptions seems to make it more difficult for physicians to reconstruct pain development. As the self-presentation as pain enduring (cf. Section 4.2) implies a certain deprecation of the importance of one's own pain, this may be one reason why descriptions of pain by women may be assessed as less relevant and why women with coronary causes of chest pain are less well diagnosed and less extensively treated than men. Furthermore, it has been shown that in the evaluation of chest pain the physician's diagnostic approach can be profoundly affected by the patient's presentation style. These findings were recently substantiated by a study showing that the race and sex of a patient independently influence how physicians manage chest pain (Richards *et al.* 2000). Therefore, training in gender-specific language attitudes and preferences in order to get satisfactory results when taking the clinical history might well be suitable for the education of physicians and healthcare professionals in general and especially for those working in emergency rooms.

However, there are a few limitations to be considered. First, as doctor-patient interaction is highly language-sensitive, it is clear that our results are limited to the German-speaking population (and probably even to the ones using the Austrian variant of German), although gender-related differences sound plausible for other (Western) language communities as well (Schulman *et al.* 1999). Regarding socioeconomic status, there might also be some restrictions on the validity of our study.

The following conclusions for clinical routine can be drawn from our study: when taking the clinical history of patients with chest pain, especially in female patients, pain description should be supported by enhancing the patients' ability to describe the kind and course of the symptoms. If patients play down their symptoms, physicians should encourage them to take their disease seriously. If patients describe their pain only diffusely, physicians should help them to more concretely describe their pain and make them aware of the fact that, in such a setting, patients rather than physicians are experts for describing their pain.

References

Atkinson, Paul / Heath, Christian 1981. *Medical Work: Realities and Routine.* Westmead, Farnborough, Hants: Gower.

Ayanian, J.Z. / Epstein, A.M. 1991. Differences in the Use of Procedures between Women and Men Hospitalized for Coronary Heart Disease. *New England Journal of Medicine* 325, 221-225.

Baumgartinger, Barbara / Sator, Marlene / Binder, Ernst C. / Pobaschnig, Gerd 2002. Metapherngebrauch bei der Beschreibung von Brustschmerzen. *Wiener Linguistische Gazette 70,* 45-69.

Becker-Mrotzek, Michael 1992. Kommunikation und Sprache in Institutionen. Teil III. Arbeiten zur Kommunikation in medizinischen Institutionen. *Deutsche Sprache* 20, 336-369.

Cicourel, Aaron 1985. Doctor-Patient-Disourse. In van Dijk, Teun (ed.) *Handbook of Discourse analysis.* Vol. 4. London: Academic Press, 193-202.

Corney, Roslyn H. (ed.) 1991: Developing Communication and Counselling Skills in Medicine. London: Tavistock / Routledge.

Crawford, Mary 1995. *Talking Difference: On Gender and Language.* London: Sage.

Douglas, P.S. / Ginsburg, G.S. 1996. The Evaluation of Chest Pain in Women. *New England Journal of Medicine* 334, 1311-1315.

Ehlich, Konrad 1985. The Language of Pain. *Theoretical Medicine* 6/2, 177-187.

Ehlich, Konrad 1993. Sprachliche Prozeduren in der Arzt-Patient-Kommunikation. In P. Löning / J. Rehbein (eds) *Arzt-Patienten-Kommunikation. Analysen zu interdisziplinären Problemen des medizinischen Diskurses.* Berlin: de Gruyter, 67-90.

Ehlich, Konrad / Koerfer, Armin / Redder, Angelika / Weingarten, Rüdiger (eds) 1989. *Medizinische und therapeutische Kommunikation.* Opladen: Westdeutscher.

Fisher, Sue / Todd, Alexandra D. (eds) 1983. *The Social Organization of Doctor-Patient Communication.* Washington, DC: Center for Applied Linguistics.

Frankel, Richard 1990. Talking in Interviews: A Dispreference for Patient-Initiated Questions in Physician-Patient-Communication. In G. Psathas (ed.) *Interaction Competence.* Washington, DC: UPA, 231-262.

Fruergaard, P. / Launbjerg, J. / Hesse, B. / Jorgensen, F. / Petri, A. / Eikenm, P. / Aggestrup, S. / Elsborg, L. / Mellemgaard, K. 1996. The Diagnoses of Patients Admitted with Acute Chest Pain but without Myocardial Infarction. *European Heart Journal* 17, 1028-1034.

Goddard, Angela / Patterson, L. Mean 2000. *Language and Gender.* London: Routledge.

Goldberg, R. / O'Donnell, C. / Yarzebski, J. / Bigelow, C. / Savageau, J. / Gore, J.M. 1998. Sex Differences in Symptom Presentation

Associated with Acute Myocardial Infarction: A Population-based Perspective. *American Heart Journal* 136, 189-194.

Gülich, Elisabeth / Quasthoff, Uta 1985. Narrative Analysis. In T. van Dijk (ed.) *Handbook of Discourse Analysis*. Vol. 2. London: Academic Press, 169-197.

Heath, Christian 1989. Pain Talk. The Expression of Suffering in the Medical Consultation. *Social Psychology Quarterly* 52, 113-25.

Hein, Norbert 1985. *Gespräche beim praktischen Arzt.* Wien: Univ. Wien (unpublished M.A. thesis).

Hein, Norbert. / Hoffmann-Richter, Ulrike / Lalouschek, Johanna / Nowak, Peter / Wodak, Ruth 1984. Kommunikation zwischen Arzt und Patient. *Wiener Linguistische Gazette, Supplement 4.*

Hofgren, C. / Karlson, B.W. / Gaston-Jonsosson, F. / Herlitz, J. 1994. Word Descriptors in Suspected Acute Myocardial Infarction: A Comparison between Patients with and without Confirmed Myocardial Infarction. *Heart and Lung* 23, 397-403.

Kotthoff, Helga / Wodak, Ruth (eds) 1997. *Communicating Gender in Context.* Amsterdam: Benajmins.

Kütemeyer, Mechthild 2002. Metaphorik in der Schmerzbeschreibung. In Brünner, Gisela / Gülich, Elisabeth (eds) *Sprechen über Krankheiten.* Bielefeld: Aisthesis.

Lalouschek, Johanna / Menz, Florian / Wodak, Ruth 1990. *Alltag in der Ambulanz. Gespräche zwischen Ärzten, Schwestern und Patienten*. Tübingen: Narr.

Löning, Petra / Rehbein, Jochen (eds) 1993. *Arzt-Patienten-Kommunikation. Analysen zu interdisziplinären Problemen des medizinischen Diskurses*. Berlin: de Gruyter.

Meischke, H. / Larsen, M.P. / Eisenberg, M.S. 1998. Gender Differences in Reported Symptoms for Acute Myocardial Infarction: Impact on Prehospital Delay Time Interval. *American Journal of Emergency Medicine* 16, 363-369.

Menz, Florian 1991a. "Zucker! Des Hams ma gar net gsagt!" Zur Kommunikation zwischen Arzt und Patient im Krankenhaus. In H. Tüchler / D. Lutz (eds) *Lebensqualität und Krankheit. Auf dem Weg zu einem medizinischen Kriterium Lebensqualität.* Köln: Deutscher Ärzteverlag, 33-43.

Menz, Florian 1991b. *Der geheime Dialog. Medizinische Ausbildung und institutionalisierte Verschleierungen in der Arzt-Patient-*

Kommunikation. Eine diskursanalytische Studie. Bern: Peter Lang.
Miles, Mathew B. / Huberman, A. Michael 1996. *Qualitative Data Analysis: An Expanded Sourcebook*. Thousand Oaks, Cal: Sage.
Milner, K.A. / Funk, M. / Richards, S. / Wilmes, R.M. / Vaccarino, V. / Krumholz, H.M. 1999. Gender Differences in Syptom Presentation Associated with Coronary Heart Disease. *American Journal of Cardiology* 84, 396-401.
Mishler, Elliot 1984. *The Discourse of Medicine: Dialectics of Medical Interviews*. Norwood, NJ: Ablex.
Morris, G.H. (ed.) 1995. The Talk of the Clinic: Explorations in the Analysis of Medical and Therapeutic Discourse. Hillsdale, NJ: Erlbaum.
Penque, S. / Halm, M. / Smith, M. / Deutsch, J. / Van Roekel, M. / McLaughlin, L. / Dzubay, S. / Doll, N. / Beahrs, M. 1998. Women and Coronary Disease: Relationship between Descriptors of Signs and Symptoms and Diagnostic and Treatment Course. *American Journal of Critical Care* 7, 175-182.
Redder, Angelika / Wiese, Ingrid (eds) 1994. *Medizinische Kommunikation – Erfahrungen in Ost und West*. Opladen: Westdeutscher.
Rehbein, Jochen 1993. Ärztliches Fragen. In Löning, Petra / Rehbein, Jochen (eds) *Arzt-Patienten-Gespräche. Analysen zu interdisziplinären Problemen des medizinischen Diskurses*. Berlin: de Gruyter, 311-364.
Richards, H. / McConnachie, A. / Morrison, C. / Murray, K. / Watt, G. 2000. Social and Gender Variation in the Prevalence, Presentation and General Practitioner Provisional Diagnosis of Chest Pain. *Journal of Epidemiological Community Health* 54, 714-9.
Sarangi, Srikant / Roberts, Celia (eds) 1999. *Talk, Work, and Institutional Order. Discourse in Medical, Mediation and Management Settings*. Berlin: de Gruyter.
Schulman, K.A. / Berlin, J.A. / Harless, W. *et al.* 1999. The Effect of Race and Sex on Physicians' Recommendations for Cardiac Catheterization. *New England Journal of Medicine* 340, 618-24.
Silbergleit, R. / McNamara, R.M. 1995. Effect of Gender on the Emergency Department Evaluation of Patients with Chest Pain. *Academic Emergency Medicine* 2, 115-121.

Steingart, R.M. / Packer, M. / Hamm, P. / Coglianese, M.E. / Gersh, B. / Geltman, E.M. / Sollano, J. / Katz, S. / Moyé, L. / Basta, L.L. / Lewis, S.J. *et al.* 1991. For the Survival and Ventricular Enlargement Investigators. Sex differences in the Management of Coronary Artery Disease. *New England Journal of Medicine* 325, 226-230.

Talbot, M. M. 1998. *Language and Gender. An Introduction.* Cambridge: Polity Press.

Tannen, Deborah (ed.) 1993. *Gender and Conversational Interaction.* New York: Oxford University Press.

Tobin, J.N. / Wassertheil-Smoller, S. / Wexler, J.P. / Steingart, R.M. / Budner, N. / Lense, L. / Wachspress, J. 1987. Sex Bias in Considering Coronary Bypass Surgery. *Annals of Internal Medicine* 107, 19-25.

Todd, A.D. (ed.) 1993. *The Social Organization of Doctor–Patient Communication*. Norwood, NJ: Ablex.

Vodopiutz, Jiulia / Stöllberger, Claudia / Menz, Florian / Lalouschek, Johanna 2002. Chest Pain in Hospitalized Patients: Cause- and Gender-specific Differences? *Journal of Women's Health and Gender-Based Medicine* 11/8, 1-9.

West, Candace 1984. *Routine Complications. Troubles with Talk between Doctors and Patients.* Bloomington: Indiana University Press.

West, Candace 1990. Not just 'Doctor's Orders': Directive-response Sequences in Patients' Visits to Women and Men Physicians, *Discourse & Society* 1/1, 83-112.

Wodak, Ruth (ed.) 1997. *Gender and Discourse*. London: Sage.

BRANCA TELLES RIBEIRO / DIANA DE SOUZA PINTO

The Psychiatric Interview: An Insider's Perspective

"The patient will narrate the illness. Try to listen to what he/she is saying."
(Dr. Cardoso)

1. Introduction

This is an excerpt from a psychiatric interview. While eliciting information, the doctor often has to shift gears so as to adjust to the patient's implied requests, complaints, and needs. Shifting alignments also allows for bits of a story to unfold:[1]

Doctor:	but I want to know one thing- [acc]
Patient:	of the crisis, the crisis, the crisis, the crisis, the crisis, the crisis, the crisis, the crisis, the crisis, the crisis.
Doctor:	but ah Irene-
Patient:	I heard my father tell me.
Doctor:	mmm.
Patient:	do whatever you feel like doing. I threw everything on | the floor.
Doctor:	| I see.
Patient:	I left on my tiptoes, quite well dressed. (pause)
Doctor:	smartly dressed? (pause)
Patient:	I- I am short. no I can't look too good, | I can only look nice.=
Doctor:	| no? =you can only look nice?
Patient:	because short women, it's awful to be short, y'know?
Doctor:	oh, really? (laughs)
Patient:	five feet one, doctor...

1 See transcription conventions in the appendix.

Doctor:	that's not tall enough to look good?
Patient:	only in high heels. I won't wear high heels anymore, not even if they pay me to.
Doctor:	really?
Patient:	( ) very high heels.
Doctor:	but let's get back to the crisis, you threw things on the floor (pause) then what?

In a psychiatric interview, participants often talk at cross-purposes. Topics are brought up by the doctor in a disjointed way, frequently interrupting the ongoing conversation. The patient may bring up idiosyncratic topics and get progressively 'off the track'. In this case, the interviewer is expected to get back on topic, and lead the patient into less digression. With all its complexities, the psychiatric interview defines an interactional process where each encounter is singular and where communication may be facilitated or inhibited. The crux of the matter is the psychiatrist's competence and style of interviewing (Shea 1998).

This chapter focuses on the art and tension of interviewing – specifically in the psychiatric setting. It discusses how one doctor's professional and personal alignments in the interview situation help create moments of quasi-conversation between him and the patient. We will also examine the tensions the doctor experiences between institutional and professional demands on the one hand, and his own preference for a more open approach to patients and interviewing, on the other hand. Though the medical inquiry – the institutional context – prevails, talk shifts between institutional and personal framings (Ribeiro / Hoyle 2002). Shifts to a personal frame not only establish rapport but also provide relevant information about the patient's illness and discomfort. Personal alignments seem to provide a space for the patient and the doctor to speak in their own terms. This discussion is a reflection on the psychiatric interview and addresses issues raised by Cicourel (1992) on the interpenetration of professional and personal communicative contexts. It also points to doing research with participants in a more integrated way (Sarangi / Roberts 1999).

2. Background to this study

The data presented here derives from an ongoing research project developed at the Institute of Psychiatry of the Federal University of Rio de Janeiro.[2] The Institute is considered one of the model hospital schools for the study of mental health in Brazil. Its work policy is grounded on interdisciplinary and cross-disciplinary research, learning, and clinical assistance. Admittance to psychiatric wards, Day Hospital (providing daily activities regarding re-insertion in the family and at the work place), and Outpatient Clinic are some of the institutional resources available to patients. As a state hospital, the Institute serves the working, lower middle classes as well as homeless patients. The focus of the research project is the analysis of psychotic discourse. We observe, tape, transcribe and analyze talk and interaction among psychiatric patients, doctors and patients, patients and mental health care providers, patients and researchers in varied contexts, such as conversations among patients in the wards, staff meeting, and rounds. The project enables sociolinguists to work together with psychiatrists, psychoanalysts, psychologists, and speech pathologists.

The psychiatrist discussed in this study – Dr. Cardozo – has been a consultant to the project for the past ten years and has participated in several psychiatric interviews which were video and audio-taped. He is also a successful neuropsychiatrist (with a large private clinic) whose research interests focus on the investigation of Attention Deficit Disorder. He is a Professor of Psychiatry at a prestigious Brazilian public institution where he is the coordinator and teacher of interns in Clinical Psychiatry. Finally, it is worth mentioning that Dr. Cardozo has been an English/Portuguese interpreter and has attended a graduate course on Discourse Analysis in the Clinic, which attests to his awareness of the close relationship between Discourse and Psychiatry.

The patients are Brazilian women diagnosed with bipolar disorder which is characterized by altering phases of mania, or great

2 Grants from CNPq – the Brazilian National Research Council – and FAPERJ – the Rio de Janeiro State Research Foundation – sponsors of the project.

euphoria, and phases of severe depression. Each patient had been hospitalized for a week.[3] The videotaped interviews, granted while the patients were in a manic episode, were conducted at the Institute of Psychiatry of the Federal University of Rio de Janeiro.

Our research methodology derives from qualitative analysis as developed in Interactional Sociolinguistics. Based on an interactional approach for the analysis of talk (Goffman 1981; Gumperz 1982, 1992; Tannen 1984, 1993), we investigate how discourse is jointly constructed by the participants in face-to-face interactions. Specifically, we inquire what sorts of alignments and relationships are established through talk and how these are negotiated in interaction.

Speakers and hearers enact social and discursive roles that are constantly changing; these are changes in alignments or footings (Goffman 1981), which may occur linguistically, paralinguistically and non-verbally. These shifts allow participants to change the frame of the interaction, and provide a definition for what is going on (Tannen 1984). Given the sociological and linguistic nature of the frame, Gumperz suggests that interactants use *contextualization cues* (linguistic, paralinguistic and non-verbal devices) to "signal and interpret what the activity is, how semantic content is to be understood and how each sentence relates to what precedes or follows" (1982: 131). Lexical choices, overlaps, lengthened vowels and posture are some of the features that altogether contribute to contextualize and recontextualize frames. More specifically, one would ask "How do frames shape the ongoing discourse?" and "What do frames indicate about the way we communicate with one another?". As a "bracketing device of a higher phase or episode of interaction" (Goffman 1981: 128), framing captures participants' ever-changing alignments to each other and to what is being communicated. It captures participants' definitions (and on-going redefinitions) of a social situation, that is what they believe they are doing (what speech act they are producing

---

3 We are indebted to the doctor and the patients for their time and availability. All names have been changed to protect confidentiality. The participants are Brazilian, and the interviews were conducted in Brazilian Portuguese. The excerpts were translated by the authors with the purpose of preserving the functional meaning of what participants were communicating to each other at a given context. Thus these excerpts do not capture a word-by-word translation.

or what activity they are performing) and in what way their words and gestures are to be understood. Such signaling among interactants is necessary, because intersubjectivity is not pre-ordained but is, rather, achieved. Frame analysis captures a speaker's relation to his or her own previous or upcoming utterance, a speaker's relation to an audience, an interlocutor's relation to a speaker, and a speaker's relation to nontextual aspects of the self (Ribeiro / Hoyle 2002). This analysis is particularly interesting to use in describing the shifts that take place in the interview situation.

The psychiatric interview is an institutional encounter where social and professional identities are negotiated. As an institutional discursive practice (Drew / Heritage 1992), there is a (clinical) task that needs to be fulfilled through talk-in-interaction. The doctor is the official representative who follows an institutional agenda: he/she gathers patients' information, reaches a diagnosis and establishes a course of action (Ribeiro / Pinto 2005). Nevertheless, most often than not, patients have different expectations towards this encounter. He/she sees it as an opportunity to introduce personal narratives unrelated to their illnesses. Being positioned as a listener, the doctor is then faced with the complex duty of balancing his assigned institutional role and the moment-to-moment interactional demands from the patient.

In this chapter, our discussion focuses first on excerpts from psychiatric interviews performed by the same clinical psychiatrist. In these interviews, Dr. Cardozo positions himself both as a listener (as in a conversation) and as an inquirer (as interviewer); shifts between these two types of alignment are viewed as crucial. While the interviewer seeks information to get a better understanding, the conversational listener sustains the development of narratives. Second, the discussion describes research interviews conducted by one of the authors with the psychiatrist about his professional and institutional alignments in the interview situation. As mentioned previously, this psychiatrist has participated in several psychiatric interviews that constitute the database of our research project (Pinto 2000; Pinto / Ribeiro / Lopes Dantas 2005; Ribeiro 2000; Ribeiro 2002). As a result, we decided to probe further into how this clinician portrayed himself and his practice by interviewing him. In a set of two long interviews (one hour each), Dr. Cardozo gives voice to the underlying tension of balancing institutional demands, professional positioning, as well as conversational frames that seem to be at the heart of psychiatric clinical practice as he sees it.

3. The standard psychiatric interview: instructions on how to listen

Psychiatrists in a teaching institution share a common complaint: the fact that the standard medical interview – the doctor/patient interview – serves as a model for structuring the psychiatric interview. From the institutional perspective, the medical interview aims at gathering patients' information to reach a diagnosis and establish a course of action for proper treatment. An agenda should be followed to address and assess topics related to why the patient has been hospitalized, the history of the illness, its previous episodes, among other clinical concerns.

Unlike other medical specialties, such as oncology, heart disease, diabetes, among others, Psychiatry does not have any specific diagnostic laboratory exams available; thus, this field of medicine relies solely on the expert's interpretive practices of the patient/client symptoms (Sullivan 1970) which are evaluated in psychiatric interviews. Therefore, these two encounters are of different natures: the medical encounter is a search for clinical information, whereas the psychiatric interview is an assessment of thought, language, and communication disorders as well as other behavioral disorders.[4] Despite these differences, the medical model still prevails in the psychiatric setting. Its general plan for the construction of the interview can be captured by looking at the institutional framings of the interview, where the doctor requests information or clarification, and introduces and closes topics from the institutional agenda (cf. Excerpt 1).

---

4 Disturbances in the use of language are displayed in most of psychiatric conditions, such as mania, severe depression, organic disorders, and schizophrenia.

1 Patient: I'm pretty good in everything. [pause] ( ) I I when I left home to school [pause] at ahm ( ) have you ever heard of the town of (Ararupinho- Ararupinho)?
2 Doctor: no.
3 Patient: where Caetano Veloso- the songs of Caetano Veloso,[5] Caetano Veloso speaks of: (Ararupinho.)
4 Doctor: no, no I don't know- I don't remember.
5 Patient: the Apolo, [pause] when you hear a song from- uhm Caetano Veloso, one that speaks of (Ararupinho), the Apolo [pause], where I studied. [pause]
6 Doctor: oh, so you were going to tell me about the crisis, how was this crisis?
7 Patient: the crisis, [pause] the crisis, the first crisis was a rape, see?
8 Doctor: mmm mmm.
9 Patient: this rape [pause], I:: what did I do my God [pause] I got really upset at everything.
10 Doctor: were you agitated? you got agitated?
11 Patient: I stripped off the clothes of a doctor who looked after me in Salvador.
12 Doctor: oh, really? [laughs]
13 Patient: I left him naked, with ( ) in his hands
14 Doctor: and were you aggressive with people?
15 Patient: no, I wasn't.
16 Doctor: and tell me something, did you use to hear voices at the time?
17 Patient: I never heard voices.

Excerpt 1.

In turns (1-3-5), the patient frames interaction as conversation. Initially, she brings in personal topics by introducing references to her native town (Ararupinho – turns 1 and 3) and to her school (turn 5). She asks the doctor a question to establish a common ground ("have you heard of ...?"); by bringing up a well known Brazilian singer – Caetano Veloso. The doctor, however, minimally sustains this frame: he does not provide any back channeling signal nor expands the topic, despite the pauses the patient has provided in turn 5. He eventually interrupts (turn 6), sticking to his professional ground and moves back to the institutional agenda by introducing topics: the crisis, the history of her illness (turn 10), her affective behavior (turn 14), and her perception of reality (turn 16). He asks direct yes/no questions on different topics related to her illness (agitation, aggressivity, hearing

---

5 A famous and popular Brazilian composer and singer, born in Bahia, a northeast state of the country, where the patient was also born.

voices). These questions constitute the standard psychiatric examination as prescribed by the biological approach.

Following the clinical interview structure, the psychiatric interview is thus framed as an *inquiry* and not a conversation. It sets an agenda for how the psychiatrist is expected (and trained) to listen to the patient's information. There is a set of topics to inquire about, pre-determined as a format for recording medical data (identifying data, chief complaint, present illness, past history, family history, and so on). There are also specific ways of requesting and responding to information. An inquiry establishes the inquirer as a predisposed listener: he/she asks questions and listens for responses.

4. Personal alignments in the interview situation

There are, however, different understandings of how the encounter could proceed. Let us now examine how the doctor views his role as interviewer:

> I let the encounter flow as close to a conversation as possible, as the traditional agenda disturbs me. I always greet the patient informally, thus creating an opening for the interview in a more personal way. I never start out the interview with the section 'identifying data' – (patient's name, age, occupation). This information I obtain in the development of the interview. I try to investigate issues through conversation and I accept a more personal relationship. Sometimes I even talk about personal issues of my own. I find this makes the patient more comfortable.

A conversation on a nonclinical/medical topic is what we see in the following excerpt:

1 Patient: that ANIMAL, where's that animal? where is he?
2 Doctor: animal, Zeca? [a famous Brazilian soccer player of the 90's often referred to in the media as 'animal']
3 Patient: yeah.
4 Doctor: he's around, making trouble, had a problem somewhere, he hit someone.=
5 Patient: =he hit someone?

6 Doctor: yeah. he crashed his car and all. |no he didn't hit [someone], he crashed.
7 Patient: |but he's okay? but he's okay? he's very crazy.
8 Doctor: you like Zeca?
9 Patient: I'm crazy about him.
10 Doctor: you're crazy about him?
11 Patient: so what? I'm drawn to him, I go deep, see, when you're drawn to someone, you do it, right?
12 Doctor: oh yeah.
13 Patient: yeah.
14 Doctor: you go deep.

Excerpt 2.

Both participants are fully engaged in talk. Turns latch (4 and 5) and overlap (6 and 7), with each participant repeating the other's prior information (turns 4 and 5, 9 and 10, 11 and 14) attesting to a conversation with a high involvement style (Tannen 1984, 1989). The inquiry has changed to a conversational frame where the patient brings up referents and the doctor takes a secondary position. In these moments, the patient takes an active role: she brings up topics unrelated to her mental problem and to the clinical setting – a famous Brazilian soccer player Zeca about whom she asks a series of questions (turns 1 and 5); she presents challenges (turn 11), provides explanations (turn 9) and evaluations (turn 7 "he's very crazy"). This conversation provides a frame for the patient to narrate brief segments of her (life) story (Ribeiro 2000).

5. The active listener

As narratives unfold, Dr. Cardozo is an active listener. He frequently probes into topics brought up by the patient ("who is this guy you talk so much about?", "you like him a lot, right?", "and why do you also like Eric?"). His contributions ratify personal topics. He also contributes to a playful alignment, as in the following excerpt taken from the same interview that originated Excerpt 1:

1	Doctor:	but I want to know one thing- [acc]
2	Patient:	of the crisis, the crisis, the crisis, the crisis, the crisis, the crisis, the crisis, the crisis, the crisis, the crisis.
3	Doctor:	but ah Irene-
4	Patient:	I heard my father tell me.
5	Doctor:	mmm.
6	Patient:	do whatever you feel like doing. I threw everything on | the floor.
7	Doctor:	| I see.
8	Patient:	I left on my tiptoes, quite well dressed. (pause)
9	Doctor:	smartly dressed? (pause)
10	Patient:	I- I am short. no I can't look too good, | I can only look nice.
11	Doctor:	| no? you can only look nice?
12	Patient:	because short women, it's awful to be short, y'know?
13	Doctor:	oh, really? (laughs)
14	Patient:	five feet one, doctor ...
15	Doctor:	that's not tall enough to look good?
16	Patient:	only in high heels. I won't wear high heels anymore, not even if they pay me to.
17	Doctor:	really?
18	Patient:	( ) very high heels.
19	Doctor:	but let's get back to the crisis, you threw things on the floor (pause) then what?

Excerpt 3.

This is a different interaction from the standard inquiry. First we see the patient completing the doctor's statement and predicting what he would say (turns 1 and 2). This joint construction also conveys a criticism implied in the many repetitions of 'the crisis', a topic the doctor had requested information about twice before. His next turn attests to his lack of comfort: he uses a discourse marker to introduce contrastive information ("but"), then he follows with an attention device ("ah"), and addresses the patient by name ("Irene"), all of this to preface a statement that the patient interrupts, returning to a previous narrative that had been left unconcluded ("I heard my father tell me"). As she starts telling her story (turns 4, 6, 8), the doctor ratifies (turns 5 and 7) and then joins in and participates by requesting her to expand the topic (turn 9). His supportive and evaluative request triggers a pause and a reframing from the patient (turn 10).

The next nine turns are constructed within a personal frame proposed by the patient and co-sustained by the doctor. Here the yes/no questions (turns 11, 13, 15 and 17) – quite typical in doctor/patients interviews – are employed to request confirmations on a personal topic that is not related to the institutional task of the interview. It is a conversation about height and looking good, the sort of intimate conversation women might have. Finally, in turn (19) the doctor shifts back to the institutional frame of the inquiry, prefaced by the discursive marker *but*.

The reframings we see here are typical of interactions with this doctor. Instead of rocking the boat of the interview, they actually work to make the interview more conversational and therefore more personal, where participants often display more involvement.

6. The insider's perspective

Framing captures a composite of projected selves or multiple alignments that one brings to an interaction. Among the relatively stable social and cultural traits that a participant has (education, social class, language background, ethnicity, gender, etc.), there are those that would be most salient in a given interaction. Goffman alerts us to look at the enactment of social traits in interaction: "note that it is not the attributes of social structure that are here considered, such as age and sex, but rather the value placed on these attributes as they are acknowledged in the situation current and at hand" (1979: 62). Thus, in the psychiatric encounter, one must take into consideration the knowledge participants have and share in the encounter, the social and conversational attributes that surface in that encounter (which are enacted face to face), and the effect these attributes have on the interactant(s). The set of attributes one enacts in a given interaction is also related to one's projected expectations about the encounter.

We will now discuss three key issues concerning expectations as they came up in the research interviews with Dr. Cardozo. Each relates to the analysis just presented: the doctor's different alignments to self, to other (in this case, the patient), and to the institutional discourse.

7. Traditional definitions: who is this person? who is this doctor?

A key issue in these interviews relates to how one defines 'the other' in the interview situation. The field of psychiatry creates a reflection on who we are and who the other is. Taking an interactional approach to the doctor/patient encounter, Dr. Cardozo says that "how one defines the other entails how one defines the encounter". Thus, if the doctor has a more traditional view of psychiatry (i.e., more rigid, where categories are more clear-cut, with set boundaries between 'normality' and 'abnormality', etc.), this view will define a distant relationship between the participants in the interview situation:

> When one defines the other as different, as crazy – then there will be very little [possibility] of intersection [of contact with you] – because that one is crazy and you are normal. So the dialogic situation will be completely different because 'it's a madman that I am examining'. Then I am really investigating, it's almost an investigation. Because there's no possibility of meaningful contact.

The traditional assumptions are still in place at this medical school where the culture defines a psychiatrist as a professional who, in Dr. Cardozo's words, "deals with crazy people". Here "craziness means very different." Separation and distance from the other do not stop there. They extend to the profession as well. Psychiatrists are also viewed as 'very different' by their peers (and lay people in general, well portrayed in the arts). Most of all, the profession is poorly evaluated in the medical field:

> when I decided to become a psychiatrist, I told a professor of semiology who really liked me. He was so frustrated. Psychiatry is not really considered medicine, it's not well regarded. [...] So within the field, I chose to practice a type of psychiatry closer to the traditional medical model, the field of

> neuropsychiatry, following the biological model, [a path] which is better evaluated. I chose what was best regarded in a nonprestigious field.

Dr. Cardozo's comments are particularly interesting when one considers how much attention he gives to the patient. He points out this paradox of being attentive to the relationship ("Patients liked me. My approach was different. Things happened in a different way.") while having chosen a biological rather than a psychological path:

> In my case, given the concerns I have, it would have been natural to bend more towards psychotherapy than pharmacology, to be more interested in neurosis than organic illnesses such as ADD or dementia.

And yet, it is indeed this paradox which makes Dr. Cardozo an interesting doctor. While taking a critical stand on the traditional discourse of medicine, he sought today's most prestigious domain within psychiatry. And in his medical practice, he adopted a model provided by his semiology professor:

> And he would tell us "the patient will tell you the diagnosis. He/she will tell you". I remember him saying that "the patient will narrate the illness. Try to listen to what he is saying". And this came from a traditional doctor, who viewed psychiatry poorly, a clinician. But he would say this: "listen to how the patient will tell you his own diagnosis".

This doctor also showed how communication would happen beyond words, demonstrating "a gentle way of approaching the patients, having a true fondness for them". From this discussion we see that the institutional discourse (of the school, the professors, the peers) clearly discriminates among more and less distinguished fields of knowledge and clinical practice, where psychiatry seems to rank at the lower end of the scale. However, ways of being as a professional and caring for the patient seem to cut across different medical domains, whether prestigious or not.

8. On clinical practice and the interview situation

Psychiatry is driven by diagnostic procedures. The doctor must investigate each one of the symptoms and search for a standard definition. Such guidelines are problematic and this doctor voices strong criticism openly:

> To teach psychiatry, based on the model of classic psychopathology favors the medical model of identifying symptoms in an external body to reach a diagnosis. It does not favor interaction. And that may be the reason why one teaches a type of anamnesis which is really pretty bad. Because it's pretty bad. Most of them are pretty bad.

However, one can interpret symptoms without having to perform a standard interview. An 'assessment' opens the possibility for a variety of discourse types, and professional conversation may take different shapes. Dr. Cardozo states that psychiatric interviewing could change:

> It could be a technique related to the sort of person we are interviewing; so which questions to ask would be related to what type of person he is. This technique would derive from the relationship one establishes with the person. This would be a crucial change – instead of searching for a diagnosis, one would search to establish a relationship and then understanding who the patient is. It would derive from the situation. That's an art. The psychiatric interview as it is performed today derives from the German model – from extracting information in psychopathology. It's a technical training. And we go on teaching this investigators model.

So this doctor views the possibility of a significant change in the interview situation. The nature of the conversation may shift and contribute to a different relationship and different understandings, as he adds:

> The way to interview could change greatly. One reason for change is to modify people's views about the psychiatrist. People don't like having to see a psychiatrist, they feel bad, they don't know what type of question we're going to ask, if we are evaluating, then what's the diagnosis? [...] Another reason for change is therapeutic. If the patient participates, gets involved or engaged in her treatment, then the treatment will be easier and more effective. She has to

> be aware of the causes for her troubles. It's the difference between 'adherence' and 'compliance' with a treatment.[6]

This reflection points out how much the interview format is geared towards the institutional discourse (the medical school, the diagnosis, etc.). A change as proposed by this doctor would entail a paradigm shift. It would place the patient at the center, the patient as a person, and consequently affect mental health care providers at large.

9. On language and ways of interviewing

Now, even if we keep this asymmetrical model, there are ways of improving talk and interaction. The techniques could differ but share similar goals such as reaching across to the patient, asking sensible questions, listening for understanding. In his classes, this doctor emphasizes that:

> In psychiatry there are no complementary exams; everything will depend on what the patient tells you. [...] If you find yourselves in a good dialogic situation, you'll get to find out more than through a question/answer process. So you must improve this dialog. And this can be done without changing the model of searching for symptoms to arrive at a diagnosis.

While he adds that patients are unsatisfied with the interview as an inquiry, he also says that most professionals are not aware of the inadequacies of the present model and that this situation is often true in the field of medicine as a whole.

Turning specifically to the interview situation, he describes some required conversational skills:

---

6 The doctor goes on to point out that adherence means being involved and actively participating in the treatment, while compliance relates to merely going along with the treatment prescribed. In this case, patients often stop taking care of themselves at some point, especially taking the prescribed medication.

> There are situations where one must cut, where one won't allow for that branch of the tree to blossom. You must cut there to look for other things. But I think this is done in an inappropriate way. For example, if I must attend to ten patients between 2 and 5, I must divide my time accordingly. But the way we interrupt to check things up we don't really understand the patient's anxiety in bringing up certain topics. At that moment in the interview, a given topic may be crucial to understanding certain issues. So I think conversational skills are crucial. I can even interrupt a patient, for example, a patient with manic disorder, who starts to speak tangentially or indicates intense flight of ideas. While I would like to discuss a specific issue, I will need to interrupt several times. But just like with a tree, I will need to learn where to cut. I can't just cut anywhere. I will have to know where to do it, how often, under what circumstances.

Thus, attending to different needs requires expertise and care. While being aware of the patient's suffering (anxiety) and to institutional constraints, one must also work to understand why certain issues come up or may be troublesome. In doing all this social and clinical work, one is also attentive to meandering topics or excessive details, which may result in a digressive interview. Shea (1998) points out that a true wandering interview is the joint creation of both the patient and the clinician. Such co-construction is well described out by Dr. Cardozo as he reports on the communicative skills of medical students:

> The problem lies in how they got the story, the questions they asked, what they heard the patient saying. In reporting actual words, one wonders if they got this right, as no one really speaks like this. So I often ask them "maybe it was the way you asked about the story that led to this?" or I tell them "your doubts may be related to the way you framed the question" or "did the person understand what you were asking?". Frequently I myself feel that the patient has not understood what I was saying. I tell them: "this is a little tricky, a little complicated." They say "I got it" but I have the feeling that they did not. I always try to spell out the question, but I still get the feeling that it didn't make sense.

Where does this feeling come from? In interpreting a response, one stumbles upon contextualization cues (Gumperz 1982, 1992) that may signal embarrassment, discomfort, concern, or uncertainty. These cues may be verbal or nonverbal (such as a change in pitch, a longer pause, a sigh, or a change in gaze), and they work indirectly. Dr. Cardozo is not only attuned to capturing implicit meaning. He also criticizes the present institutional model, where students are taught to actually "report on [the patient's] actual words".[7] Anyone involved in this exercise knows how impossible this task is. Tannen (1989) even proposes changing the linguistic term 'reported speech' to 'constructed dialog', which asserts the speaker's creative authoring of someone else's words and indicates its dialogical nature.

The above thematic discussion and vignettes highlight some clear positions that Dr. Cardozo takes regarding the psychiatric patient, the psychiatrist, and the interview situation, as well as the professional and institutional discourses. Critical viewpoints come up as well as some of the difficulties associated with this profession.

10. Conclusion

In this chapter, we first discussed a series of segments from different psychiatric interviews performed by the same doctor. We pointed out that, while the institutional frame of the inquiry (where doctors request information or clarification and introduce and close topics related to mental illness) prevails, both the doctor and the patient also construct talk within personal framings. These frames are mostly proposed by the patient and the doctor goes along. When this happens, there are changes in pace (faster talk), rhythm (more overlap, more latching), laughter and smiles. Responses tend to provide more details, leading to bits and pieces of stories. The local context thus changes to foster an interaction that is quasi-conversational rather than strictly interviewing.

In the discussion that followed, we see how this doctor's professional and institutional beliefs match his actions in the interview situation. While performing as a role model for his students – the neuropsychiatrist at the Institute – he advocates proximity (the patient is different but not *that different*) and a more flexible posture (he openly criticizes the traditional approach). The patient is actually

7 It is worth adding that this professor has recently been awarded a prize as the best medical school professor in psychiatry at a prestigious university in Rio de Janeiro (based on a poll conducted with all last year medical residents).

someone one can relate to. As an example, the doctor brings up stories about a gentle and caring clinician, a major influence in his professional life. It is thus no surprise that Dr. Cardozo can often align himself in the interview situation as someone the patient can trust and confide in – someone the patient may even disclose secrets to. The art of interviewing, as pointed out by Shea (1998), rests upon the competence of the expert and his/her style of successfully engaging the patient. In several excerpts, this doctor's interviewing style is shown to create involvement and a feeling of rapport (Tannen 1989).

There is, however, also a tension between the doctor's beliefs (being more flexible) and the mind set of some of his students:

> Psychiatry is learning to cope with what is different, with not having a mind set. A lot will depend on the system of personal beliefs. I teach students that, and some understand where I am coming from, while others think that's silly talk, psychiatrists' talk.

Thus, the psychiatrist faces prejudice too. In being evaluated as 'different', the doctor indicates how the institutional discourse (the discourse of clinicians, students, valued texts and associations) points at difference regarding *both participants* in the interview situation: the psychiatrist and the patient.

Tension also occurs relating to the present teaching model, which is oriented towards diagnosis and psychopathology. While performing his institutional roles as a professor, he must teach medical students the standard and traditional way of interviewing, following a strict institutional agenda which hardly ever leaves room for personal topics. Yet he remains critical of it, as "it does not favor interaction", rather it favors an investigation, and adds "this may be the very reason why one performs a bad anamnesis". This critical position calls for a radical shift in the interview situation: a change to focus on the doctor/patient relationship. While some professionals and researchers involved in the field of psychiatry work for this transformation to take place, institutional constraints which shape the discourse of medicine (Mishler 1984) make professors conform to the present situation. However, slight changes do take place. Making such adjustments so as to progressively focus on the interaction is an art (Shea 1998). Dr.

Cardozo works his way to teach and improve the conversation even within the traditional interview inquiry and agenda.

Appendix: Transcription conventions[8]

.	sentence-final falling intonation
?	sentence final rising and fall intonation (BP question pattern)
,	phrase-final intonation (indicating more talk to come)
-	glottal stop or abrupt cutting off of sound
(pause)	noticeable break in rhythm with no speech length of time was not assigned
:	lengthened sound (extra colons indicate greater lengthening)
CAPS	very emphatic stress, loudness or shouting
[acc]	spoken quickly, appears over the line
( )	transcription impossible
(words)	uncertain transcription
[words]	in the original Brazilian Portuguese utterance
=	two utterances linked by = indicate no break in flow of talk
|	overlapping speech: two people talking at the same time

References

Cicourel, Aaron 1992. The Interpenetration of Communicative Contexts: Examples from Medical Encounters. In Duranti / Goodwin (eds), 293-309.

Drew, Paul / Heritage, John 1992. Analyzing Talk at Work: An Introduction. In Drew, Paul / Heritage, John (eds) *Talk at Work. Interaction in Institutional Settings*. Cambridge: Cambridge University Press, 3-65.

Duranti, Alessandro / Goodwin, Charles (eds) 1992. *Rethinking Context*. Cambridge: Cambridge University Press.

8 Most of these conventions are based on Tannen (1984).

Goffman, Erving [1972] 1979. The Neglected Situation. In Giglioli, Pier Paolo (ed.) *Language and Social Context*. New York: Penguin. 61-6.

Goffman, Erving 1981. Footing. In Goffman, Erving *Forms of Talk*. Philadelphia: University of Pennsylvania Press, 124-59.

Gumperz, John 1982. *Discourse Strategies*. Cambridge: Cambridge University Press.

Gumperz, John 1992. Contextualization and Understanding. In Duranti / Goodwin (eds), 229-52.

Mishler, Eliot 1984. *The Discourse of Medicine*. Norwood, N.J.: Ablex.

Pinto, Diana de Souza 2000. *A Construção da Referência no Discurso de uma Paciente Psiquiátrica: análise lingüística para distúrbios de pensamento, fala e comunicação*. Ph.D dissertation, Instituto de Psiquiatria da Universidade Federal do Rio de Janeiro.

Pinto, Diana / Ribeiro, Branca Telles / Lopes Dantas, Maria Tereza 2005. 'Let the heart speak out' – Interviewing Practices by Psychiatrists from Two Different Traditions. *Journal of Communication & Medicine* 2/2, 177-88.

Ribeiro, Branca Telles 2000. Listening to Narratives in Psychiatric Interviews. In Coulthard, Malcom. / Cotterill, Janet / Rock, Frances (eds) *Dialogue Analysis VII: Working with Dialogue*. Tübingen: Niemeyer, 283-92.

Ribeiro, Branca Telles 2002. Erotic Discourse Strategies in Powerless Women: Analyzing Psychiatric Interview. In Litosseliti, Lia / Sunderland, John (eds) *Gender Identity and Discourse Analysis*. Amsterdam: Routledge, 193-219.

Ribeiro, Branca Telles / Hoyle, Susan 2002. Frame Analysis. In Verschueren, Jef (ed.) *Handbook of Pragmatics*. Amsterdam: Benjamins, 1-20.

Ribeiro, Branca Telles / Pinto, Diana de Souza 2005. Medical Discourse, Psychiatric Interview. In Brown, Keith (ed.) *Encyclopedia of Language and Linguistics*. 2nd edition. Oxford: Elsevier, vol 7, 1-7.

Sarangi, Srikant / Roberts, Celia 1999. The Dynamics of Interactional and Institutional Orders in Work related Settings. In Sarangi,

Srikant / Roberts, Celia (eds) *Talk, Work and Institutional Order*. New York: Mouton, 1-57.

Shea, Shawn Christopher 1998. *Psychiatric Interviewing. The Art of Understanding*. Philadelphia: Saunders.

Sullivan, Harry Stack 1970. *The Psychiatric Interview*. New York: Norton.

Tannen, Deborah 1984. *Conversational Style*. Norwood, NJ: Ablex.

Tannen, Deborah 1989. *Talking Voices*. Cambridge: Cambridge University Press.

Tannen, Deborah 1993. *Framing in Discourse*. New York: Oxford University Press.

CELIA ROBERTS

Continuities and Discontinuities in Doctor–Patient Consultations in a Multilingual Society

1. Introduction

Consultations between doctors and patients, like many other workplace encounters, are positioned by contradictory pressures. On the one hand, they are part of the growing instabilities of all organisations in late modernity resulting from globalisation. And on the other, they are still subject to the same influences and requirements of more traditional medical practices. So, for example, there are anxieties about de-professionalisation as earlier assumptions about medical authority begin to melt down in new less stable ways of working. However, the textbooks on doctor–patient communication are still organised around twentieth century notions of communication and 'patient-centeredness' as if roles, power relations and identities were not changing.

An important part of the instabilities in health, as in other areas of public life, is the increasing diversity of cities throughout the world, as a result of globalisation. This chapter will examine the impact of this 'superdiversity' on doctor–patient consultations in British cities. In particular, it will look at some of the continuities and discontinuities in the detail of day-to-day talk between family doctors from a range of ethnic and linguistic backgrounds and patients for whom English is not their expert language.

2. The discourses of change in contemporary health care practice

The changing landscape and 'emerging discontinuities' (Hoff *et al.* 2004) of health care produce new discourses for health professionals which require them to be and act in new ways. Increasingly, workplaces are implicated in a 'new work order' (Gee / Hull / Lankshear 1996; du Gay 1996) where surveillance and measurement produce discourses of accountability and where individual professional autonomy gives way to team working (Iedema / Scheeres 2003). In medical settings, doctors are becoming business managers; the organising and managing of resources are pushed down to surgery level as hierarchies are flattened and professionals take on wider organisational responsibilities. At the same time they are more constrained by discourses of accountability, including targets and protocols. This new work order has led to concerns of de-professionalisation (Dent 2002; Halford / Leonard 1999) or at least the formation of new kinds of professionalism. One aspect of this is the 'backstage' work (Barton 2004) where doctors increasingly communicate in multidisciplinary teams where their insider professional knowledge has to be translated into talk which healthcare workers and other staff can make sense of. Another aspect is the impact of technology and specifically the computer as a third presence in the consultation.

The widely-researched encounters between doctors and patients have not focussed on these discursive issues and have tended to look at the consultation as a bounded encounter, relatively unaffected by the discursive changes of these new times (but see Wodak 1997; Iedema *et al.* 2004). Similarly, the 'superdiversity' arising from globalisation and the movement of workers and refugees throughout the world has not been dealt with systematically in either the general literature on communications in healthcare or in the discourse analysis of doctor–patient consultations. Either diversity is not addressed at all, or tends to be dealt with in essentialist or functional ways. Most of the medical studies of minority ethnic groups discuss communication in terms of the health beliefs of specific groups on the assumption that they are homogenous entities and that these beliefs are transmitted wholesale into the consultation (but see Ahmad 1993 for a critique). Alternatively, diversity is dealt with in a functional way in terms of the need for interpreters and how they are used (Smaje 1995). However, the reality of such cities as London is that patients do not come from a small number of well-established ethnic and minority linguistic groups whose health beliefs can be readily summarised and for whom interpreters are easily available. In London over 300 languages are spoken (Baker / Eversely 2000) and each year the ethnic landscape changes as new workers, refugees and asylum seekers enter the city.

3. Some of the continuities in doctor–patient consultations

Despite the discursive and professional changes of late modernity suggested above, much of what happens in the consultation is continuous with the past. Conversation and discourse analysis of doctor–patient communication over the last 30 years or so has repeatedly shown asymmetrical power relations (West 1984; Fisher / Todd 1983; Freeman / Heller 1987; Ainsworth-Vaughn 2003), with patients' voices muted by the medical 'voice' (Mishler 1984). And conversation analysts have charted patterned phases in the consultation such as openings, history taking and making diagnoses. Recent studies have looked at the typical ways in which doctors deal with patients' potential or actual resistances, such as on-line commentary when examining the patient and designing the diagnosis to overcome possible disagreements (Drew / Chatwin / Collins 2001).

While these continuities are clearly reflected in the patterns of interaction analysed, some are the product of the methodology used. Discourse and conversation analysis have focussed on 'frontstage' events such as patient-health professional interaction. They have tended to look for patterns and continuities across, in discourse terms, quite large data bases. The commonalities of 'typical' consultations therefore get played up and the discontinuities played down. And, until recently, Conversation Analysis, in particular, has set aside the wider ethnographic contexts which produce, as well as being produced by, the bounded front-stage events (see Collins 2005 for an alternative position). As well as taking account of the 'communicative ecologies' (Gumperz 1999) and wider contexts which give 'ecological validity' to interactional research (Cicourel 1987), the wider organisational processes and discourses of the 'new work order' mentioned above need to be traced in the analysis of talk. By taking a lens with a wider focus, which looks at change as well as continuity, some of the tensions in practice and how that practice is developed can be illuminated.

Discontinuities, arising from the global cities of to-day, are also masked in the training and development of family doctors. 'Patient-centeredness', 'decision-making' and 'communication skills' (Silverman *et al.* 1998) tend to be dealt with in a generic way in textbooks and continuing professional development. 'Patient-centeredness' is generally interpreted as eliciting and being responsive to the concerns, beliefs and expectations of the patient, including shared-decision making. These behaviours are underpinned by assumptions that the consultation should be more egalitarian, less bio-medical. Yet patient-centeredness, defined in this way, is not a universal and, as Example 5 (below) shows, can produce its own discontinuities and misunderstandings. Similarly, communication skills textbooks assume that more talk and more metatalk contribute to improved communication and the prevention and repair of misunderstandings. Recommended skills in the communication skills literature invariably entail the family doctor talking more, at more abstract levels and meta-communicating more (e.g. "There are two possibilities which explain your symptoms. I'm trying to decide between two ways forward …"; "What I've suggested makes sense to me but if it isn't right for you, we'll need to think again" (Silverman *et al.* 1998: 121)). However, if talk constitutes a communication problem, rather then contributing to its solution, as is frequently the case in contexts of 'superdiversity', then what counts as good communication becomes problematic (Moss / Roberts 2005).

4. Doctor–patient consultations in multilingual settings

The rest of this chapter uses a research study carried out in London between 2001-3 to explore some of the issues raised above. The study was based on 232 video recordings of family doctor–patient consultations in four settings in South London. The aim of the study was to find out how patients, who had limited English or with a very different communicative style from the doctor's, and doctors managed the consultation in English together. By charting the misunderstandings that occur on both sides (Roberts *et al.* 2005), it is possible to see how some of the continuities and stabilities of modern times are challenged by the demands of accountability and efficiency on the one hand and the globalised patient population on the other. The following table suggests some of these tensions which are illustrated in the examples below:

New work order discourses	*Globalised patient population*
Audit and measurement culture	Ambiguities and misunderstandings
Protocols and other texts for planning	Different styles of the presentation of self
Multiple targets	Multiple topics
Consumer-centred, self-disclosure	Different assumptions about Dr/patient relationship

5. Audit culture versus the potential for ambiguities and misunderstandings

The increasing surveillance and auditing of individual practices which are part of the more self-managed new work order, leave less room for the professional management of ambiguities. Yet as more patients from linguistically diverse backgrounds appear on patient lists, ambiguities and misunderstandings become a routine occurrence. These misunderstandings can be at several levels simultaneously, some of them to do with overall rhetorical styles of self-presentation and others at a more micro level. For example, many of the misunderstandings are the result of subtly different conventions in prosodic features. The tunes, rhythm and stress in speech help to chunk information into units, distinguish what is important, make the contrast between given and new information and establish speaker perspective. In the example below, the patient from Nigeria uses contrastive stress to show his perspective on the neighbour's trustworthiness or not. However, this is one of the conventions of Nigerian English which differs from the standard variety of English. An ambiguity is created which is never resolved.

GP	what kind of dog was that (.) it was somebody's (.) =dog=
Pt	=yes= somebody's
GP	it was a stray dog
Pt	no no it was somebody's dog
GP	right
Pt	yes I:: made an enquiry they said that- *they *they told me the dog go to the vet regular*
GP	*right *okay
Pt	*but that's *what they said*
GP	right (.) *right right so did you know the owner or =did=
Pt	=I= know the owner= =
GP	= =oh fair enough (.) so
Pt	*erm:: ((laughs)) [but]*
GP	did you see any doctor then
Pt	no

Example 1. Dog bite. (See appendix for transcription conventions)

The patient was bitten by a dog when on holiday in Nigeria and the doctor explores whether a rabies vaccination is necessary (lines 1 & 3). Told the dog reportedly sees a veterinary surgeon regularly (lines 6-7), and the patient knows its owner (line 11), the GP appears satisfied the evidence is authoritative – he says 'oh fair enough so' (line 12). Later in the consultation he suggests to the patient that a vaccination is not indicated. However, the patient has implied that he is not convinced that the dog is free from rabies ('*they* told me the dog go to the vet regular but that's *what* they said'; lines 6, 7 & 9). In British English, contrastive stress to convey this suspicion would emphasise the *verbs* 'told' and 'said': "they *told* me the dog goes to the vet regular, but that's what they *said*" (implication: and not what they actually *do*). Instead, the patient's intonation system focuses on the *agent* (the acquaintance, 'they'), and the *content* of the agent's utterance – the 'what'. The patient hints at his sceptical perspective by using the word 'but' twice and at line 13, by the use of a hesitation marker and laughter. Yet the difference between the participants' intonation systems means the hint is not consolidated categorically and the matter remains unresolved. As the patient leaves the room, the doctor puts on line the apparently unambiguous outcome of the consultation.

Such apparently minor misunderstandings, cumulatively, both within a consultation and across consultations can contribute to a widening gap between the managerialist practices of public health and patients' expectations of professional care. The time required to solve misunderstandings and listen more is eaten away by the increasing demand on doctors to present and document themselves both orally and in texts to auditors. Organisational discourses erode professional ones (Sarangi / Roberts 1999).

6. Protocols and other texts for planning versus different ways of presenting the self

The 'audit culture' encourages the use of protocols and other forms, plans and checklists to structure the doctors' practices and integrate and 'fix' the patients' treatment. For example, multidisciplinary care plans require a range of health care professionals to negotiate the text to be agreed by all, where different health care discourses have to be mitigated and mediated by the participants in the meeting (Cook-Gumperz / Messerman 1999; Iedema 2003). Protocols are designed to help plan and structure the consultation and like most new texts for self-management and surveillance are generic – assuming a patterned and predictable journey for the consultation. The idea that the medical consultation is an orderly event has been reinforced by studies in conversation analysis. Patterns across large data sets are identified which suggest that the consultation follows a particular sequential order and that phases of the consultation are organised in predictable ways (Byrne / Long 1976; Heath 1981; ten Have 1995). However, the usual pattern for the consultation starting with complaints/symptoms presentation and ending with agreeing a plan of action can be fractured by very different patient expectations of how to present both symptoms and self. In the next two examples, a comparison is made between how local or standard speakers of English present themselves in the opening stage of the consultation and the different forms of self-presentation used by patients from linguistic minorities.

Local and standard varieties of speakers do present their symptoms in predictable ways (Roberts *et al.* 2004). There are three aspects to this initial self-reporting: the description of symptoms, the context in which the symptoms occurred and the patient's stance. By stance here we include both 'affective stance' and 'epistemic stance' (Ochs 1996). These patients foreground their symptoms and keep in the background the context for those symptoms and stance. The relationship between these elements is conveyed through 'contextualisation cues' (Gumperz 1982) and the adequacy of the self-reporting is assessed by the doctor's first response.

1	D	right so how can I help =you=
2	M	=o:h= =erm=
3	D	=I'm sorry= you've had to come
4	M	oh it's ok / (. .) I think he's got conjuncti*vitis but =I'm not=sure (.) hes had
5	D	=oh dear=
6	M	it since la:st (..) he had a *gummy eye this side but {[ac]when he was born that was quite *gummy so I tolerated it}(.) then it *travelled to this one and got {[dc]progressively worse (. .) over the weekend we were in Germany for a wedding so }= =
7	D	= =oh right [nice time]
8	M	yeah it was good
9	D	ok
10	M	erm it went *red underneath *there and *red just a*bove
11	D	right
12	M	{[dc]and it's been very *gunky}
13	D	mm= =
14	M	= = {[ac] [lo]as you can see I've sort of left it (.) erm }= =
15	D	= =so this is for how many days now

Example 2. Conjunctivitis. (A young white woman who speaks a standard variety of English has brought her toddler to the surgery to have his infected eye checked out)

The mother focuses on the symptom and puts in the background the child's history of such infection. She does this by putting emphatic stress on key syllables 'conjunctiVITis', 'GUMmy' 'RED' and so on and by speeding up her utterance at turn 6 when giving some of the background detail and then slowing down when she returns to the symptoms at turns 6 (later in the turn) and turn 12. The repetition 'red' and the rhythmic stress in this turn and the next when she refers to the 'gunky' eye reinforces the display of symptoms as the foreground. The focus is on the presentation of symptoms, and the rest is in the background.

She also uses her epistemic stance to align herself to the doctor and present her moral self – as a caring but not over anxious mother. She says she 'thinks', but is not sure and later how she 'tolerated' the gummy eye as he has had it before. The combination of her words 'so I tolerated it' with accelerated pace, serve to illustrate her worth as a rational mother and one who is not too dependent on medical advice while recognising that it is the symptom telling which is the main focal event. Then again, later, she explains that she is not treating the child's infected eye at the moment and frames this with 'as you can see' with accelerated speech, thus bringing the GP on board and subtly defending her decision making position – with a hedge 'I've sort of left it' – against any potential criticism that she has been too autonomous. Through her predictable structure, mitigated assertions and prosody, she provides a routine pattern to the family doctor which she can readily process.

By contrast, the patient in the next example uses a less predictable structure, no mitigation and different contextualisation conventions.

1 D come in come in please come in [ ] good morning
2 P good morning
3 D have a seat
4 P thank you
5 D how are you today
6 P oh: {[dc] [creaky voice] not very good}
7 D not very good (.) what's happening
8 P I *pain here (.) *too much (.) I can't cope you know
9 D right
10 P *yesterday (.) *whole day
11 D right

12	P	and I eat (.) *three times (.) paracetamol
13	D	right
14	P	two three hours it will be *all *right and then (.) *come *pain again (.) I *can't cope (.) pain like
15	D	you can't cope with this pain
16	P	yeah very very bad (.) I don't know what's the wrong with me
17	D	sure how * long you have this

Example 3. Too much pain. (An elderly Gujerati woman has come to see her doctor who comes originally from the Panjab, India)

The patient slows down her speech with 'not very good' and speaks in a creaky, tremulous voice as if acting out the pain in her talk. The rest of her initial self report is delivered in short, quite sharply contoured, units with little distinction made prosodically between the different aspects of the report. So, the symptom giving does not stand out from her self-treatment remarks. The doctor does not immediately bring her back to the focus on symptoms but instead repeats what she has said "you can't cope with this pain" which elicits more affective talk. And when he does ask about the symptoms, the question is, prosodically, more like a comment than a question and does not seem to function as refocussing the patient on the facts of the condition. Why is this example different? One reason may be that the doctor is also of South Asian origin, a Panjabi speaker, and is willing to stay with the affective stance as the focus of this self report, rather than moving immediately to eliciting more detail of the symptoms.

Because doctor and patient share similar cultural resources for making meaning out of her self-presentation, the unpredictable way in which she deals with the opening stage of the consultation is managed in an orderly way. However, globalisation and the 'superdiversity' of global cities means that such sharedness is increasingly unlikely. So, there is a tension between the audit and surveillance demands of professional practice and the increasingly unpredictable nature of doctor–patient consultations. The culture of individual accountability produces more documentation which, in turn, requires more protocols and other recording procedures which structure and reduce communicative possibilities. And at the same time, the intercultural nature of consultations requires more creativity, flexibility and tolerance of ambiguity that disrupts the fixedness of the documentation. Ironically, the response to globalisation at an organisational level critiques the response to it at a local, face to face level.

7. Multiple targets versus multiple topics

Part of the surveillance of family doctors and the criteria for assessing their efficiency relates to targets. The 'target culture' is part of the increase in auditing and accountability of the new work order. Many of these targets relate to the diagnosing and prevention of diseases and screening processes which are part of the family doctors' routine repertoire. Typically, in Britain, family doctors are assessed on how they have reached targets in checking patients for such diseases as diabetes and cancer and monitoring cholesterol levels, weight, smoking and so on. They are expected to raise these issues with patients who may be at risk, even if the patient presents with quite unrelated symptoms or concerns. Once raised, the fact that the topic has been discussed is entered on the computer and helps to reach the target on which additional payments to the doctors are calculated.

These multiple targets are different from the multiple topics which patients, used to a different style of consulting, often bring to family doctors. It is a frequent complaint from them that patients from overseas raise several topics at each consultation. While many patients take a holistic view of themselves and their complaints, doctors still prefer a bio-medical model in which a particular disease is dealt with in one encounter. As well as their professional orientation to one-at-a-time concerns, the institutional demands of the health service put strict limits on how long a consultation should last. Patients who raise multiple topics will go beyond their allotted time and so undermine the time-keeping constraints of the practice.

In the next example, an elderly Italian woman comes with numerous problems: thinning hair, an allergy to dust mites, stiff fingers and a gynaecological problem. The strict time limits and protocols of the highly managed family health service are disrupted by her introduction and re-introduction of the different topics over the course of the consultation.

1	D	yes so (.) I think the next step is to: get you to see the: skin specialist
2		who deal with problems of the hair (.) =and=
3	P	=yeah=
4	D	em ask their opinion (. .) would you be happy to go and see the
5		spe=cial=ist
6	P	=yes= (.) please darling =yeah=
7	D	=yeah= cos =I think=
8	P	=I- I= sneezes (.) lot I sneeze lot
9	D	you sneeze a lot (.) ri:ght
10	P	((laughs)) cos =er=
11	D	=that's= something different is it

....

(later in the consultation)

12	D	it's the- to do with the joints
13	P	=ah the joints=
14	D	=and as= we get a bit older they get a bit =worn=
15	P	=gett=ing old too no
16	D	old*er ((laughs)) but it's erm (.) it's really important to: erm
17	(.)	
18	P	and =the- the- (.) listen this this this er=
19	D	=keep your fingers moving (.) do some exercises=
20	P	this dust mite is e:r (.) is *danger for the house you know
21	D	it's not dangerous no: it's nothing (.) that will do harm to your h- home

Example 4. Dust mites.

The doctor suggests that the patient should see a skin specialist but just as she is trying to be 'patient-centred' and explain why, the patient overlaps with another complaint that she sneezes a lot (line 8). The doctor breaks off her explanation to establish that this is new topic. Later on in the consultation, when again the doctor is trying to involve the patient more in her own treatment, she again overlaps the doctor to reprise an earlier discussion about dust mites. She assumes, from the enlarged picture of these microscopic insects that she has seen on a bottle, that these are dangerous beasts that can damage her house.

8. Consumer-centred, self-disclosure versus different assumptions about doctor–patient relationships

Part of the discursive environment of the new work order is the increased amount of self-disclosure required of employees. This can be seen as part of a wider 'confessional' (Foucault 1978) mode in which ordinary people disclose private and intimate details of their lives in the media. A redefinition of the boundary between public and private is developing. This new trend reinforces the late twentieth century value of 'patient-centeredness' which assumes that patients want their beliefs, concerns and expectations elicited and accounted for in the consultation. However, the shared decision making ideals of recent textbooks and articles (Gwyn 2002) assume a universal notion of what patients want and expect which is not born out in our data on diversity. In the next example, the family doctor uses widely accepted patient-centred questions with a young Somali woman who has brought her baby to the clinic because she had diarrhoea. The doctor has taken a brief history and then has asked about breast-feeding.

1	D	little bit (.) right so you're virtually stopped (.)
2		so what sort of questions have you got in your mind for me today (.)
3		what do you want me to do
4		(. .)
5	M	mm no: =she say=
6	D	=today=
7	M	eh: the lady she say if you want to contacting doctor eh: you want eh: talk him
8	D	yeah=
9	M	=I say yes I am happy with e- with =you=
10	D	=right= right ok=
11	M	=because (.) definitely when I am coming with you
12		when I go back I will go back happy
13	D	((laughs)) I hope so
14	M	because I will look to see you and your doctor K (.) I like it
15	D	good=
16	M	= [cos] when when I come in will come in the you know ((tut))
17		when I go back my home I'm happy
18	D	right
19	M	((laughs))
20	D	so you want me to- (.) check her over

At line 2, the doctor attempts to involve the baby's mother in the diagnosis and treatment of her baby. However, the mother seems to interpret the elicitation as a request to find out how she came to see this particular doctor. She then emphasises how satisfied she is with the doctor. This may be because she thinks the doctor is asking her whether she is questioning the doctor's competence or she thinks that it is generally culturally appropriate to praise the doctor. The doctor's minimal response at line 18 and then speaking *for* the patient at line 20 suggests that the doctor's early elicitation did not receive the expected answer. In this example we can see how more talk, and specifically more metatalk here at line 2, is part of the communicative problem rather than the solution. This metatalk is a more abstract formulation than the here and now of discussing symptoms and thus more difficult for a limited speaker of English. But it is the unexpected framing in line 2 which seems to be at the heart of the problem. It is likely that this Somali woman has only had experience of strictly hierarchical relationships between doctors and their patients. So, a question giving the patient some power (however circumscribed) to share in the decision making process may not be interpretable to her. Again, it is the generic nature of textbook precepts about patient power and involvement that fails to be sufficiently attuned to the diversity of patient populations.

9. Conclusion

The 'new work order' with its flattened hierarchies, increased surveillance and accountability means that day-to-day practices are becoming more rigid and formalised so that they are more readily subject to scrutiny. This is happening at a time when other effects of globalisation are producing 'superdiverse' societies in large cities such as London. Ironically, the increased rigidity, performance by targets and generic documentation produce conditions for medical practice which are incommensurable with the highly unstable population in terms of language and ethnicity. Just when flexible, creative and local solutions are required to respond to such a diverse patient population, more systems, auditing and business solutions are being put in place. Systems which cut down waiting time to see a doctor also, and unfortunately, undermine the principle and practice of 'continuity of care'. This allowed each patient to see 'their' doctor regularly so that conditions for shared understanding could be gradually developed over time (Freeman / Hjortdahl 1997). Now family doctors and their patients are increasingly unfamiliar to each other and the highly linguistically diverse settings which are typical in inner city clinics compound the difficulty and lead to more misunderstandings.

Many doctors are responding to this situation by becoming ethnographers of communication or 'bricoleurs'. As ethnographers, they are learning to tune into patients' communicative styles and so develop empathetic relationships despite differences in style (Mercer / Watt / Reilly 2001). As 'bricoleurs', they and their patients are finding creative, linguistic and non-linguistic ways of negotiating meaning together (Roberts / Moss 2003). 'Tuneful' doctors find ways of preventing and repairing misunderstandings and resourceful patients bring to the encounter props, such as empty cans to show what they have eaten, to animate the consultation. Yet much of this is despite of the new work order practices and discourses and the discontinuities they produce. This chapter has painted quite a typical picture of the tension between the old continuities – some of which need restoring and some changing – and the discontinuities arising from globalisation. There is an irony in the fact that the institutional responses to the new globalised times are, in the main, disruptive of just those continuities which need to be maintained because of the effects of superdiversity on the family doctor consultation.

Appendix: Transcription conventions

=word=	overlapping talk
word= =	latching (one speaker following another with no pause)
(.)	micro pause, less than one second

(2.0)	estimated length of pause of one second or more, to nearest 0.5 of a second
wor:d	segmental lengthening
wor-	truncation
[ ]	inaudible speech
[word]	unclear speech
((laughs))	non-lexical occurrence
{[word]}	talk overlayed by non-lexical occurrence
*word	stressed syllable
ac	speeding up
dc	slowing down
/	rising pitch
\	falling pitch
lo	shift to low register
hi	shift to high register

References

Ahmad, Wagar 1993. Making Black People Sick: 'Race' Ideology and Health Research. In Ahmad, Wagar (ed.) *'Race' and Health in Contemporary Britain*. Buckingham: Open University Press.

Ainsworth-Vaughn, Nancy 2003. *Claiming Power in Doctor–Patient Talk*. Oxford: Oxford University Press.

Baker, Philip / Eversley, John (eds) 2000. *Multi-lingual Capital. The Languages of London's School Children and the Relevance to Economic, Social and Educational Policies.* London: Corporation of London.

Barton, Ellen 2004. Discourse Methods and Critical Practice in Professional Communication: the Front-stage and Back-stage Discourse of Prognosis in Medicine. *Journal of Business and Technical Communication* 18, 67-111.

Byrne, Patrick / Long, Barrie 1976. *Doctors Talking to Patients: a Study of the Verbal Behaviours of Doctors in the Consultation.* London: HMSO.

Cicourel, Aaron 1987. The Interpenetration of Communicative Contexts: Examples from Medical Encounters. *Social Psychology Quarterly* 50/2, 217-26.

Collins, Sarah 2005. Communicating for a Clinical Purpose: Strategy in Interaction in Healthcare Consultations. *Communication and Medicine* 2/2, 111-22.

Cook-Gumperz, Jenny / Messerman, Lawrence 1999. Local Identities and Institutional Practices: Constructing the Record of Professional Collaboration. In Sarangi / Roberts (eds), 145-81.

Dent, Mike 2001. *Managing Professional Identities: Knowledge, Performativity and the New Professional.* London: Routledge.

Drew, Paul / Chatwin, John / Collins, Sarah 2001. Conversation Analysis: A Method for Research into Interactions between Patients and Health-Care Professionals. *Health Expectations* 4/1, 58-70.

Du Gay, Paul 1996. *Consumption and Identity at Work.* London: Sage.

Fisher, Sue / Todd, Alexandra (eds) 1983. *The Social Organisation of Doctor–patient Communication.* Washington DC: Centre for Applied Linguistics.

Foucault, Michel 1978. *History of Sexuality. Volume One: An Introduction.* Translator Robert Hurley. New York: Vintage Books.

Freeman, George / Hjortdahl, Per 1997. What Future for Continuity of Care in General Practice? *British Medical Journal* 314, 1870-3.

Freeman, Sarah / Heller, Monica (eds) 1987. *Medical Discourse* Special Issue of *Text* 7/1.

Gee, James / Hull, Glynda / Lankshear, Colin 1996. *The New Work Order: Behind the Language of the New Capitalism.* St Leonards: Allen and Unwin.

Gumperz, John 1982. *Discourse Strategies.* Cambridge: Cambridge University Press.

Gumperz, John 1999. On Interactional Sociolinguistic Method. In Sarangi / Roberts (eds), 453-71.

Gwyn, Richard 2002. *Communicating Health and Illness* London: Sage.

Halford, Susan / Leonard, Pauline 1999. New Identities? Professionalism, Managerialism and the Construction of Self. In Exworthy, Mark / Halford, Susan (eds) *Professionals and the New Managerialism in the Public Sector.* Milton Keynes: Open University, 102-20.

Heath, Christian 1981. The Opening Sequence in Doctor–Patient. In Atkinson, Paul / Heath, Christian (eds) *Medical Work: Realities and Routines*. Aldershot: Gower, 71-90.

Hoff, Timothy / Jamerson, Lottie / Hannen, Edward / Flink, Ellen 2004. A Review of the Literature Examining Linkages between Organisational Factors, Medical Errors and Patient Safety. *Medical Care, Research and Review* 61/1, 3-37.

Iedema, Rick 2003. *Discourses of Post-Bureaucratic Organisation*. Amsterdam: Benjamins.

Iedema, Rick / Degeling, Pieter / Braithwaite, Jeffrey / White, Les 2004. 'It's an Interesting Conversation I'm Hearing': The Doctor as Manager. *Organization Studies* 25, 15-34.

Iedema, Rick / Scheeres, Hermine 2003. From Doing to Talking Work: Renegotiating Knowing, Doing and Identity. *Applied Linguistics* 24, 316-37.

Mercer, Stewart / Watt, Graham / Reilly, David 2001. Empathy is Important for Enablement. *British Medical Journal* 322, 865.

Mishler, Elliot 1984. *The Discourse of Medicine: Dialectics of Medical Interviews*. Norwood, NJ: Ablex.

Moss, Becky / Roberts, Celia 2005. Explanations, Explanations, Explanations: How do Patients with Limited English Construct Narrative Accounts? *Family Practice* 22/4, 412-8.

Ochs, Eleanor 1996. Linguistic Resources for Socialising Humanity. In Gumperz, John / Levinson, Stephen (eds) *Rethinking Linguistic Relativity*. Cambridge: Cambridge University Press, 407-37.

Roberts, Celia / Moss, Becky / Wass, Valerie / Sarangi, Srikant / Jones, Roger 2003. *Patients with Limited English and Doctors in General Practice: Education Issues*. Final Report submitted to the Sir Siegmund Warburg Voluntary Settlement. King's College London.

Roberts, Celia / Moss, Becky / Wass, Valerie / Sarangi, Srikant / Roger Jones 2005. Misunderstandings: a Qualitative Study of Primary Care Consultations in Multilingual Settings, and Educational Implications. *Medical Education* 39, 465-75.

Roberts, Celia / Sarangi, Srikant / Moss, Becky 2004. Presentation of Self and Symptoms in Primary Care Consultations Involving

Patients from Non-English Speaking Backgrounds. *Communication and Medicine* 1/2, 159-69.

Sarangi, Srikant / Roberts, Celia (eds) 1999. *Talk, Work and Institutional Order: Discourse in Medical, Mediation and Management Settings.* Berlin: Mouton de Gruyter.

Silverman, Jonathan / Kurtz, Suzanne / Draper, Juliet 1998. *Skills for Communicating with Patients*. Oxford: Radcliffe Medical Press.

Smaje, Chris 1995. *Health, Race and Ethnicity: Making Sense of the Evidence.* London: King's Fund Institute.

Ten Have, Paul 1995. Medical Ethnomethodology: An Overview. *Human Studies* 18, 245-61.

West, Candace 1984. *Routine Complications: Troubles in Talk between Doctors and Patients.* Bloomington: Indiana University Press.

Wodak, Ruth 1997. Discourse-sociolinguistics and the Study of Doctor–Patient Interaction. In Gunnarsson, Britt-Louise / Linell, Per / Nordberg, Bengt (eds) *The Construction of Professional Discourse.* London: Longman, 173-200.

SRIKANT SARANGI / LUCY BROOKES-HOWELL

Recontextualising the Familial Lifeworld in Genetic Counselling Case Notes

1. Introduction: Case notes as institutionally framed professional accounts

Keeping records about clients is a routine professional activity in many institutional sites: education, health, social welfare, inland revenue, police etc (Weed 1971; Wheeler 1969; Raffel 1979). It is through such record-keeping professionals across institutions construct and manage cases. As Agar (1985) suggests, institutional discourse is constituted in three key stages: diagnosis of the client, directives targeted at the client's problems, and case notes which encompass both diagnoses and the directives.

Generally speaking, case notes can be seen as institutionally framed professional accounts. They constitute an institutional requirement, while retaining the status of a useful professional resource. One can argue that they are a site where the professional and institutional modes overlay on one another (Sarangi / Roberts 1999). Through case notes professionals with institutional authority are "in a position to give official imprint to versions of reality" (Goffman 1983: 17). As Mehan (1993) has pointed out in the context of special needs assessment in educational settings, the meeting talk is selectively filtered before it becomes case record – and it is this document which then represents the institutional reality for future action as far as the client is concerned. What is recorded in case notes – and how it is recorded – as well as what is left out are based on professional judgement and routine practice. Cicourel (1974) has shown this both in legal and medical settings. For him, recording of 'what happened' and next course of action are both to be accomplished within "the organisational rules and practices for 'making sense' of 'what happened' and 'preparing the scene for further inference and action" (1974: 85). This echoes Raffel's (1979: 48) observation that "it is not that the records record things but that the very idea of recording determines in advance how things will have to appear".

Case notes are therefore not just about categorisation of clients; they also offer a window on professional competencies and organisational procedures. As documents they turn subjective assessments into 'objective facts' and thus carry a stamp of authority by embodying professional autonomy and consensus. Their objective, reliable status is what Zimmerman (1969) refers to as the 'plain fact' character of records.

2. Recording cases in the healthcare setting

Given the nature and purpose of case notes, each profession develops its own way of constructing and using case notes. Case notes across professions vary a great deal, but perhaps less so intra-professionally across institutions. One could attribute genre-like quality to case notes. Variations can be identified, for example, in the use of language in the broadest sense – technical jargons, specific abbreviations, use of reported speech etc. Social work case notes tend to be very descriptive, but mixed with general, evaluative statements (Hall *et al.* 2006). In the legal setting, delinquent types are produced in case records by assuming 'inside' knowledge – what Cicourel (1974: 95) refers to as the "more managed language of official report". A patient record across hospital settings will share a great deal of properties, although these would be different across sub-specialities. For instance, Pettinari's (1988) exhaustive study reveals the reporting practices specific to surgery. And as we will argue in this chapter, case notes in the genetic counselling setting are rather different in content and character in relation to other medical sub-specialities.

Unlike mainstream bureaucratic record keeping which may primarily have a surveillance agenda, medical case notes may be seen as more pragmatically orientated but perhaps not without an element of surveillance. They are part of professional accountability realised as a means of communication, closely tied up with specific tasks that healthcare professionals have to coordinate between themselves in managing events. According to Pettinari (1988: 16), "the patient's medical record is the intervening document between one practitioner and another and this document is, no doubt, often accorded more credibility than the actual patient". Hobbs (2002, 2003) discusses how background knowledge is signalled through the use of evidential markers in order to express the writer's attitudes towards the information selected for entry. A subjective stance has to be balanced against 'objective facts' of the case so as not to distort future readings (Cicourel 1983). One can extend this to argue that over time the records become cases. In the context of psychiatric clinics, as Barrett (1996: 265) points out, "the record represents the patient as object, but, through ceaseless repetition, the record itself becomes an object which the patient strives to represent". This viewpoint is attested by Berg (1996) in his claim that the medical record as an artefact is constitutive of medical practice beyond its local production. The medical record is not the *record* of medical practice, it *is* the medical practice (Weed 1971).

In the healthcare setting, case notes are primarily a documentation of the contractual relationship between the patient and the practitioner. For Garfinkel (1967), the medical record represents a compromise between the therapeutic and the actuarial purposes, although the former generally takes priority over the latter. He thus emphasises the situatedness of medical records. According to him, these records are "results of self-reporting procedures" and are inevitably selective with regard to the activities of the professionals as they "actively seek to act in compliance with rules of the clinic's operating procedures that for them and from their point of view are more or less taken for granted as right ways of doing things" (Garfinkel 1967: 191). This underlines Garfinkel's classic slogan – "good organisational reasons for 'bad' clinical records".

3. Analytic challenges in interpreting case notes

There are two senses in which interpretation of case notes remains a challenge. In the first sense, although case records are primarily addressed to fellow professionals, their interpretation may be variable depending upon a shared understanding of the context and specialities. Following Garfinkel's (1967) documentary method of interpretation, the case in 'case notes' stands not for an individual case, but as a 'documented representation' of professional and institutional practice. However, the particular case under considera-tion is equally important.

This points to a tension in different types of ratified audiences of medical case records. Garfinkel (1967) suggests that interpretation of such records is indeterminate from the perspective of the writer in view of an 'elected scheme of interpretation'. "The present circumstances of the reader in deciding their appropriate present use" override "the circumstances that accompanied the original writing" (1967: 202). This is the occasionality dimension of interpretation.

In its second sense, we refer to the challenges faced by social researchers, discourse analysts included, in interpreting case notes. Garfinkel (1967) alerts us to the fact that case notes defy easy interpretation, especially from an outsider perspective. Following Garfinkel, Scott (1990: 124) notes:

> The clinical folder is elliptical and vague, resting on a vast body of taken-for-granted assumptions, and its therapeutic meaning can only be grasped by participants who understand the situation in which it was produced. The record is constructed so as to allow medical staff to reconstruct the therapy and so legitimate their actions.

Healthcare and other professionals do not overtly apply institutional rules when dealing with individual cases, and thus many of the recording practices may be guided by their stock of tacit knowledge, or what Cicourel (1975) calls 'folk practice'. In this sense, case notes involve both competent writers and competent readers. Coherence between parts is not given but arrived at through informed interpretation.

In light of the analytic difficulties posed in interpreting case records, our interest in this chapter is to offer an account of how written case notes derive from situated talk/interaction. Our interpretation of the case notes was no doubt facilitated by having access to the corresponding transcripts of the counselling sessions. Our analytic focus is on genetic counsellors' own selection of the counselling trajectory which then forms the basis for case notes entry. In other words, we set out to examine the linkage between the talk component of the counselling and its textual manifestation in case records, and what such a tracking might reveal about professional practice and the overall goal of genetic counselling. Before we do so, we would like to provide a brief overview of studies dealing with the talk-text interface in case notes by appealing to the notion of recontextualisation.

4. Talk and text interface: recontextualisation practices in documentation

Case notes, by default, can be seen as part of a recontextualisation process. By recontextualisation, we refer to the broader process of how prior talk, text and context are reproduced and transformed in a dynamic, dialogic fashion, with consequences for meaning making (Linell 1998; Sarangi 1998). According to Linell (1998: 144-5):

> Recontextualisation may be defined as the dynamic transfer-and-transformation of something from one discourse/text-in-context (the context being in reality a matrix or field of contexts) to another. Recontextualisation involves the extrication of some part or aspect from a text or discourse, or from a genre of texts or discourses, and the fitting of this part or aspect into another context, i.e., another text or discourse (or discourse genre) and its use and environment.

For our present purposes, recontextualisation is taken narrowly to apply to the transformation of counselling talk into case notes as text. Case notes are primarily written documents, but these are occasioned by talk-in-interaction. As a discursive event, case notes are situated between prior talk and future talk/text. They serve as institutional memory, both in the short term and in the long term. This form of institutional memory is then drawn upon strategically for future action, which can take the form of either talk or text. Barrett (1996) rightly shows how doctors routinely consult previously recorded case notes in an ongoing consultation (this also applies to how case notes are utilised in case conferences and multiprofessional team meetings). Moreover, case notes have a future orientation – they provide the basis for follow-up letters addressed to clients (Howell 2002) as well as for any formal assessment documents (Hak 1992; Ravotas / Berkenkotter 1998). It is through such recontextualising practices that professionals underpin institutional categories and realities, while legitimating their interventions and decision-making. The written record, in most institutional settings, becomes the credible account when the talk is no longer accessible.

Many researchers draw attention to the actual production of case records, i.e., how they fit into institutional routines and practices (e.g., Barrett 1996; Cicourel 1983; Cook-Gumperz / Messerman 1999; Coulthard 1996; Hak 1989; Jönsson / Linell 1991; Mehan 1991; Slembrouck 1992). In what follows, we offer a selective overview of some of these studies by paying particular attention to different layers of recontextualisation.

One obvious aspect of recontextualisation is the use of jargons which transforms what has actually been said. Cicourel (1983) draws our attention to how doctors' use of a specialised register in case notes is indicative of the imposition of the medical perspective over the patients' narratives. According to Cicourel (1983: 227-8), "the physician recodes the patient's often ambiguous, rambling, and somewhat emotional language into fairly abstract categories". The medical terminology is supposed to produce `objective' factual statements for the benefit of the ratified readers of case notes. Emotionally charged statements made by individual patients in a dialogic setting if reported in their original form can perhaps lead to misunderstandings or over- and under-statements.

Cook-Gumperz and Messerman (1999) examine the transition between decision-making talk and written records in the actual context of a multiprofessional meeting. They demonstrate the extent to which professional concerns about patients are reformulated and reported by appealing constantly to institutionally available categories. In the psychotherapeutic setting, Ravotas and Berkenkotter (1998: 211) show how such transformation always amounts to the production of an 'institutionally viable account': the report is "designed to provide readers with a clinical picture of the client's problems, justifies the therapist's particular diagnosis of mental disorder which, in turn, supports the therapist's treatment choice".

According to Hak (1989), the psychiatric case is systematically constructed through the case notes in the form of three types of statements (Hak 1989: 86-7):

1. contextual information: statements that are not transpositions of elements from the 'reality' described nor refer to psychiatric 'knowledge';
2. references to psychiatric 'knowledge': statements paraphrasing psychiatric textbooks; and
3. references to interview(s) with the patient: statements that are the product of procedures in which elements of the interview(s) are transformed into elements of the psychiatric report.

What this suggests is that case notes are primarily agenda-led, so the overall coherence of these notes may derive from what professionals choose to record and how.

Another significant aspect concerns how case notes are contextualised and recontextualised *in situ* and for what purpose. In the psychiatric clinical setting, Barrett (1996) discusses how recording of events happens during the interaction – what he calls 'record-speech event' to refer to the act of writing while talking, which may have a mediating effect on interaction.

In the police interview setting, as Coulthard (1996) points out, the very practice of recording, where a co-present transcribing officer is expected to write down verbatim what transpires between the interviewing officer and the suspect, is bound to render the records partial, but such partial reports acquire the status of credibility in the institutional process. As if such partial, selective recording is not distortion of reality already, Coulthard (1996) goes further to argue how case records can deliberately be tampered with, and thus become more inaccurate.

Jönsson and Linell (1991) compare police reports and police interviews along the written/spoken continuum and find how the medium contributes to the construction of two different versions of the same story. According to them (1991: 419):

> [T]he monological text has a more clearly elaborated narrative structure and a legally relevant perspective. In addition, the transformation from spoken dialogue to written text involves changes from vagueness to precision, from relative incoherence to coherence and a clear chronology, from emotionality to an objectively identified sequence of events and actions etc.

Some of these differences can be attributed to the contingent nature of talk in an interrogative setting. As Garfinkel (1967) points out, there are constraints of a general nature on self-reporting in the institutional context mainly because of the uncertainties about how an entry will be interpreted in the future.

As we can see from the above summary, recontextualisation practices are necessarily selective, and often this selectivity favours the professional perspective. Although these records are variably called 'patient records' and 'client case notes', there may be very little of the client's lifeworld that gets recorded. In the context of total institutions such as asylums, Goffman (1968) points out that case records are an important expression of the institutional mandate, and goes on to warn that all of us can be made into records with denigrating statements, and thus into deviant cases. This explains obvious omissions made in case notes, for instance, the rare mention of what mental patients are able to do, or their past. According to Goffman (1968: 14):

> One of its purposes is to show the ways in which the patient is 'sick' and the reasons why it was right to commit him and is right currently to keep him committed; and this is done by extracting from his whole life course a list of those incidents that have or might have had 'symptomatic significance'.

This draws our attention to the fact that case notes are not really about people, but about specific institutional practices of processing people. It follows then that several aspects of a patient's life are left out of the record.

One of the main deficiencies of medical records, according to Cassell (1987: 194), is that they do not provide a description of the patients – "what kind of people they are, how they have behaved in sickness, and the nature of their relationships with others". He writes:

> between abbreviations and technical jargon, it is difficult to recognise who they are writing about. Nobody ever seems to be sad, unhappy, sulky, gloomy, moody, mean, or even, happy, high-strung, jumpy, enthusiastic, quick-tempered, and so on. In attempting to exclude value judgements from descriptive statements, we have gone so far as to make our descriptions valueless! (Cassell 1987: 195)

Indeed this point extends to the clinical encounter itself, as Mishler (1984) has shown with regard to the dominance of the voice of medicine over the voice of the lifeworld. Cassell above is obviously alluding to the general clinical encounter. If we were to consider the psychiatric setting, we would no doubt have descriptions of clients' emotional states, although these would have a diagnostic overtone. Our interest in looking at case notes in the genetic counselling setting is to explore whether these case notes select and report clients' lifeword adequately given that much of counselling centres around psychosocial concerns that underpin decisions about predictive genetic testing and disclosure of genetic test results (Sarangi *et al.* 2004, 2005).

5. Inscribing the lifeworld in genetic counselling

Genetic counselling is generally characterised as a hybrid activity which combines a range of topics along the medical-lifeworld continuum, and a range of communicative formats ranging from explanation to advice giving (Sarangi 2000). In a given session, the genetic counsellor attempts a clear understanding of clients' reasons for their decision to undergo a predictive genetic test as well as their preliminary thoughts concerning disclosure of test results. Inevitably, the lifeworlds of families come to the fore and the complex familial relationships need to be accounted for with regard to both testing and disclosing test results. Based on one case study of a client at risk of

Huntington's Disease[1] spanning four clinic visits, we adopt the methodology of activity analysis as a way of uncovering the discoursal devices through which familial lifeworld characters and events are recontextualised in case notes. Central to activity analysis (Sarangi 2005, Roberts / Sarangi 2005) is the notion of thematic and interactional mapping. We begin with a mapping of the thematic episodes in the counselling session (AF2) as a way of signalling the topic range and topic progression. This is followed by tracking the themes on to the case notes. In a further analysis, we select two extended extracts and pay particular attention to the details of decision about testing (e.g., circumstantial triggers, reflective talk, self vs. other motivations, knowledge of testing services and procedure).

5.1. Analysis 1: Thematic mapping of the lifeworld across clinic talk and case note text

Thematic mapping of the clinic interaction for the counselling session shows clearly the occurrence of lifeworld topics (see Appendix 1). This is not surprising given that one of core objectives of genetic counselling is to lay bare the lifeworld concerns throughout the testing protocol. In the case of AF2, the lifeworld events go beyond the genetic concerns: she has problems with her knee and spine, and is also currently undergoing ultrascan on her womb.

In tracking the clinic interaction on to the case notes, we can identify some form of thematic correspondence. The sequence of topics in the clinics and corresponding case notes do not necessarily match chronologically. A different organising principle can be discerned from the case notes: decisions about testing are recorded first, followed by decisions about dissemination, although the clinic transcript (which is not shown fully here) does not provide such a neat

---

1 Huntigton's Disease is an inherited late onset degenerative neuropsychiatric disorder which affects both body and mind. The pattern of inheritance is autosomal dominant, i.e., there is a 50% chance that the child of an affected parent will have inherited the disease-associated mutation. There is currently no effective treatment or cure available for HD and clients typically die from the condition some 10 to 15 years after onset.

thematic order. We can account for this by the fact that the counsellor, when writing up the case notes, tries to maintain the topic focus, particularly when talk can easily be more fragmented and a single topic may have been recycled on a number of occasions within a clinic session. There is thus a 'good reason' for such 'bad' record keeping – whereby themes are grouped together in preference to the maintenance of a strict sequential/temporal order.

In considering the thematic mapping of the clinic interaction and the case notes, we can identify three aspects of the clients' lifeworld which are analytically distinguishable. Our position here is parallel to Mishler's (1984) attempt to characterise the voice of medicine as constituting different voices, e.g., the voice of cumulative personal experience and the voice of science: "the distinctions between personal experience and text-book science, captured in notions like the 'clinical mentality', hint at the possibility of competing voices in medical discourse" (Atkinson 1995: 130).

In a similar fashion, different lifeworld voices are likely to be involved in a genetic counselling setting. The first aspect is what we would call 'the medical lifeworld' which refers to clients' current or past medical problems, independent of their genetic condition, that need to be reported and attended to. An example of this can be seen at the beginning of the thematic map: "biopsy/ultrascan of womb, screws in leg, asthma, mood swings, hot flushes".

The second aspect, which is central to our argument here, can be labelled 'the familial lifeworld' which encompasses decisions about testing and dissemination and the potential consequences such decisions may have for family members. This can include immediate family members, e.g. daughters/sons, and extended family members, e.g. siblings and parents. An example of this can be seen in the thematic map: "AF2 is having the test to remove uncertainty for her children". In the case study, the familial lifeworld prevails: 13 out of 26 clinic episodes and 6 out of 11 case note episodes.

The third and final aspect is what we call 'other lifeworld events' which are family-related, but not familial in the technical sense. These lifeworld events may incorporate two elements: (i) the individual client's emotional, psychological feelings and mechanisms for coping with them while preparing for testing and dissemination of results; and (ii) the physical/social realities of the client, involving situations which prepare the ground for decisions to be made about testing and dissemination ("the couple appear more settled since moving house").

As can be seen from Appendix 1, there is a constant shift back and forth between different aspects of the lifeworld: the medical, the familial and the other. By distinguishing these different aspects and by mapping them across the counselling session and the case notes we get a clearer picture about the topic flow at any given time and what may be potentially salient for future uptake. It is worth acknowledging that in many of these counselling sessions, the physical examination of the client is often carried out by the counsellor in another room, while the client's partner and family members may choose to continue discussion of all or any aspects of their lifeworld with the co-present genetic nurse (in AF2, the discussion spanned turns 578-782). However, such discussions, despite their relevance, do not get recorded in the case notes as the counsellor is the one who usually has sole responsibility for writing the case notes. This seems to be another layer of selection in terms of what becomes accessible via case notes.

In what follows, we focus on two extended extracts, where we examine in detail how different aspects of the client's lifeworld, with particular reference to decisions about testing, are articulated in the interaction and are then recorded (or not) in the corresponding case notes.

5.2. Analysis 2: Recontextualisation of different lifeworlds

This case involves a female client (AF2) in her forties who attends the clinic together with her husband (MP). This is an Appointment 1 session, which follows a preliminary session in which the client has confirmed that they want to go ahead and discuss the testing procedure further. The genetic counsellor (GC) is a middle-aged woman and a genetic nurse is also present. The first extract occurs approximately two thirds of the way through the appointment, half an hour in (transcript lines 538-558), but with regard to the corresponding case note, this is the second entry (see Appendix 1). In

Extract 1 we reproduce the talk first, followed by the corresponding written component from the case note (see Appendix 2 for transcription conventions).

		Clinic
01	GC:	= I must say that you you seem much (.) sort of more settled in actually since we saw you in May
02	MP:	well as I say we've (.) we got a new house [living in a new house] =
03	AF2:	[living in a new house]
04	MP:	= we haven't got our noisy neighbours any more [and it's a better =
05	AF2:	[(we ^^^^)]
06	MP:	= house] and we can actually sit now in the living room and sleep in our own bedroom because we haven't got the noisy neighbours (.) which has taken a lot and we've just moved in the house and we're all settled and it's a better house it's just (.) better part (.) same estate but just better neighbours it's just (.) generally that's made life a lot better (.) 'cause g- g- given us chance to actually sit back and have a bit of peace and quiet and think [(.)] and just be able to sit there and listen to =
07	GC:	[yeah]
08	MP:	= nothing (.) and not next door and to be able to think (.) and talk things over without being wound up by the neighbours it's (.) oh it's been so much better (.) this last few months since we've moved
09	GC:	yes you seem (.) much [different] to me from when we saw you in =
10	MP:	[mm]
11	GC:	= [May] so I think even though it has been a delay *I sort of sort of =
12	MP:	[yes]
13	GC:	= [you seem]*
14	AF2:	[we're getting there]
15	MP:	yeah we are (.) [well]
Case note entry		In general much more settled than in May ((month of Prelimary Interview)). Especially since they moved house.

Extract 1.

This extract follows from MP's description of the reasons underlying AF2's decision to test (not shown in the transcript): "she won't have to worry any more she'll know" and "she'll just be able to live her life around knowing and this is what we've discussed". At this point in the interaction, GC offers an evaluation of AF2's and MP's overall situation as "more settled" (turn 01), when contrasted with the last visit ("since we actually saw you in May"). This can be seen as an orientation on the part of GC to the 'other lifeworld events' of the client. The case notes from the preliminary interview that preceded this first appointment had the following three entries which signal AF2's emotional state: "Have had a lot on their plate since home visit", "AF2 quite tearful" and AF2 "feels badly and gets upset". This is evidence that the previous case notes will have been read immediately prior to the current clinic appointment and will have acted as institutional memory.

As the interaction unfolds, we see MP offering an extended narrative, in turns 02-08, accompanied by collaborative cues from AF2 (see especially turn 03). "Living in a new house" is foregrounded as a significant contributing factor, especially in light of AF2's ongoing medical problems and anxieties associated with them. Although the details included in MP's account – better house, better part of the same estate, better neighbours – are not directly linked to their decision to go ahead with the test, the account does emphasise the physical conditions necessary to engage dialogically in the process of decision making and to reflect on potential consequences. Of interest here are the formulations: "[it's just] given us chance to actually sit back and have a bit of peace and quiet and think"; "to be able to think (.) and talk things over" (turns 06 and 08). The move to the new house thus affords the client and her partner to do the homework of thinking and talking which is what GC wants to bring off, as we can also see in the next extract when she reintroduces this format of self-reflection as part of the counselling process. The slight delay in appointments (turns 11 and 13) seems to have facilitated the process of self-reflection, and there is some consensus that "we're getting there" (turns 14 and 15). The justification of a delay in the testing protocol may have something to do with MP's eagerness and preference for not wanting to wait for the test results, but rather receive them the very next day (not shown in transcript here). From GC's viewpoint, AF2's wellbeing and preparedness are particularly important when the HD predictive test is imminent.

Although the case note does not indicate these procedural matters, it does make salient two key issues concerning the clients' 'other lifeworld events' – "more settled" and "moved house". This entry serves to consolidate this state of affairs, despite the fact that the topic was treated in a fragmented fashion in the clinic interaction, being recycled on three occasions. Interestingly, the case note entry relating to this lifeworld event occurs early in the sequence of coded episodes in the case notes (2nd out of 11 episodes), considering that the topic was raised relatively late in the clinic interaction (22nd out of 26 episodes). GC uses the opening summarising phrase "In general" as a way of indexing the lengthy clinic discussion. The core entry provides an evaluation of the current situation ("much more settled"), followed by an identification of the cause ("since they moved house"). This evaluation is carried out with reference to the previous visit, and thus indicates GC's awareness of clients' lifeworld events over a specific time span, which helps to anticipate that the client is now prepared to go ahead with the test, with relevant assistance through the genetic counselling process.

We may conclude from the above that not only is the lifeworld event of moving house judged significant enough to be attested in the case notes, but also that it provides a valuable function. By accommodating in this entry the psychological state of the client near the beginning of the notes, and preceded by a list of AF2's medical lifeworld involving non-genetic problems, it makes up a coherent overview of the patient's circumstances. Having established the current scenario, the notes then move on to a more lengthy record of the crux of the discussion – the familial lifeworld issues surrounding decision about testing.

The second extract below occurs earlier in the same consultation, about 10 minutes in (corresponding lines in transcription, 89-117), but constitutes a later entry in the case notes.

Clinic		
01	GC:	the other (.) issue talked that we talked a (.) a bit about last time (.) um (.) was (.) having children ((coughs)) (.) your feelings or both of your feelings about that has (.) has that still been something that you sort of been (.) talking about or something that you've been [(.) thinking about]
02	MP:	[funnily enough] we had er (.) a conversation about it in the kitchen (.) the other day when I turned around and said that (.) there's probably a lot of people out there who think that (.) not have that

		having children is (.) is an important thing but (.) I'm one of those people that (.) the way the world is believes that er (.) it's probably better off (.) I'm glad I didn't in in a lot of ways so (.) I think we've come to accept it now (.) haven't we it's (.) ten years down the line and she was more worried for *me* (.) her because she's got two two girls by the previous marriage and it was like *me* (.) but I've just come to accept it now and accept the two girls I mean I've been bringing them up for the best part of ten years it counts for a lot .hh (.) AND as for bringing a small child into the world we live in now I couldn't be so heartless (.) I really don't think I could (.) because it's not exactly the (.) the (.) most ideal world to (.) to bring children in to so (.) gives me a little bit of peace of mind (0.5) at the end of the day
03	GC:	how and how do you feel about it
04	AF2:	I a lot of it was worried the fact that he hasn't got children (.) but (.) I've always wanted three (.) three children I it's something about it (.) [always wanted three] and (.) but (.) looking on it no (.) =
05	MP:	[yeah always said that]
06	AF2:	= cause (.) I'm too old and (.) everything but (.) if I could have gone back yes I would have love loved another child (.) but it's STILL it's still like when I see babies there's still hurt there (.) but (.) you never know I might become a grandmother (.) in a couple of year
07	GC:	um so you sound like you're feeling (.) little bit sort of (.) sort of more settled about things (.) and I think I think you're right that (.) y- you know you always will feel that if you see a little baby and I think [(.)] even people who've decided actually they're going to =
08	AF2:	[y:::eah]
09	GC:	= finish their family when they see their last ones growing up you think [that you know everyone does] (.) feel that
10	AF2:	[well my friend now] my friend now just gone sterile (.) and I tried talking her out of it she was a single parent with three children (.) and I said to her don't do it (.) and erm (.) behold she had it done (.) a year down the line now she's with a new (.) partner and she's going through this (.) he've got children by his marriage (.) she've got children (.) but she wants one with him [(.)] s:o
11	GC:	[mm] (1.0)
12	AF2:	but I I wouldn't advise anyone or anything like that I had it done to me (.) under protest [(.)] but this is why I'm going ahead (.) with =
13	GC:	[yeah]
14	AF2:	= this because (.) I've got two girls (.) and I don't want it happening to them
15	GC:	*right* (.) 'cause last time we talked part of the reason that you were (.) wanting to go through for the test was [(.)] because you =
16	AF2:	[*yes*]

17	GC:	= were hoping that you yourself might want to have children but (.) now you're thinking it's (.) because of the girls
18	AF2:	the *girls* more than anything 'cause like I said I was sterilised (.) at eighteen (.) they wanted to sterilise me at sixteen (.) I didn't even sign the consent forms my (.) (^^^) and my ex husband signed the forms (.) and (.) I woke up from giving birth to (.) ((daughter)) (.) and went straight into theatre (.) having it taken away you know (.) and (.) from that day I felt like (.) my womanhood had been taken (.) away from me under protest [(.)] so but I don't want my girls =
19	GC:	[mm]
20	AF2:	= going through it (.) if they want six children (.) let them have six children with the knowledge that no they're not going to have Huntington's
Case note entry		Have now decided that they have come to terms with not having children. Whichever way the test goes. Want to know to remove uncertainty and for their children.

Extract 2.

This extract begins with a hedged initiation of familial lifeworld issues by GC. She once again refers back to the previous clinic session and the accompanying case notes. The following entry from the earlier case notes is of interest:

> Issues raised [...] having children resigned ((MP)) to not having a family. This issue *has not* been resolved for ((AF2)), feels badly and gets upset. Realises having children is probably not practical but suffering (about it).

This entry appears to have played a part in the current discussion. The knowledge of the unresolved nature of AF2's feelings may account for GC's explicit attempt to draw out AF2's own perspective in turn 03, as well as for her increased supportive feedback (turns 11, 13, 19) once AF2 begins to talk about her own feelings concerning future reproductive plans.

As in Extract 1, MP becomes involved by producing an extended narrative. He draws on a series of 'other lifeworld events' to account for the shift in his decision to not have children. He orients his story within his own lifeworld, providing minute details of his decision-making process. This account culminates in the following statements: "I'm one of those people that... the way the world is believes... it's probably better off [not having a child]" and "as for bringing a small child into the world we live in now I couldn't be so heartless" (turn 02).

GC, in turn 03, explicitly directs the next question to AF2. AF2 elaborates her own personal perspective with a very honest and open response: "I've always wanted three [children]" (turn 04) and "I would have loved another child" (turn 06). She describes the emotional pain she feels triggered by seeing babies: "it's still like when I see babies there's still hurt there" (turn 06). GC uses this occasion to normalise AF2's desire to have another baby as something that all mothers feel, including "even people who've decided... they're going to finish their family". This is reflection-in-action, which embodies other people's desires and experiences, from both clients' and professional perspectives.

AF2 recalls the story of her friend who was sterilised and later regretted it when she met a new partner (turn 10). This leads AF2 to recount her own experience of being sterilised against her will (turn 18). Such lifeworld events and experiences function rhetorically to give weight to the decision to have the test, and thereby have access to knowledge and to be in control. Here we see a shift to the familial lifeworld, as the decision to test is explicitly framed in relation to the potential consequences for AF2's daughters (turns 14 and 20).

This lengthy discussion finds its way into the case notes in the form of three sentences, which succinctly demonstrate the shift from previously stated reasons for testing (the couple's own reproductive plans) to the current need to "remove uncertainty and for their children". This shift of perspective is very well articulated by GC in turns 15 and 17. The couples' difficult decision to not have children is captured in the case notes as "come to terms with", which is a direct reformulation of MP's framing in turn 02: "we've come to accept it". There is the suggestion that this is not only an informed decision taken by the clients themselves ("Have now decided"), but also that it is a robust one, as is evident in the case note entry: "whichever way the test goes". Not that this is a stand-alone statement. It is not clear whether it refers to the preceding sentence (that the couple have decided not to have children whatever the result) or the following sentence (that they want the test result whether it is positive or negative in order to remove uncertainty for their daughters). The sequential positioning of the statement however inclines us to prefer the former interpretation as the latter cannot be discerned from the corresponding clinic discussion.

It is possible that the openness from both MP and AF2 has created a definitive closure of this topic, thus requiring no further details in the case notes (indeed the issue of reproduction is not brought up again in subsequent appointments). The detailed lifeworld events that have led to the decision to not have children are omitted in the case notes, as are the discussions about AF2's and her friend's sterilisation experiences. However, the familial lifeworld is clearly captured in the case notes as the decision about testing is explicitly linked with future consequences for the children. The entry "to remove uncertainty" turns out to be a formulaic summary statement, devoid of all the rich and complex lifeworld contours that make one individual story so different from another's.

6. Conclusion

In this chapter we have examined the record keeping practices in the context of genetic counselling where, unlike in other medical settings, case notes have to go beyond simple categorisation of a patient's illness and the outlining of necessary intervention. Our method of mapping the counselling sessions and the case notes, complemented by the thematic tracking of what gets recorded, when, and how, shows the multiple layering of recontextualisation practices involved. We have also drawn attention to different aspects of clients' lifeworld that come to the surface in the clinic and how several 'significant' bits of these lifeworld experiences have to be necessarily left out of the case notes, thus constructing a version of institutional reality which frames future readings and interpretations.

Important decisions have to be made about striking a balance between the familial lifeworld and other lifeworld events, including descriptions of people (their psychosocial disposition) and their relationship with others. Generally speaking, this may partly be due to the uncertainties surrounding the test result, the consequences of decisions made about testing and disclosure as far as different family members are concerned. The tensions are not just manifestly visible at the levels of the voice of medicine and the voice of the lifeworld, but also across different aspects of lifeworld – familial and other. One may equate the familial lifeworld or familial genetics with the voice of medicine, because the understanding of transmission of genetic conditions within the family constitutes the core of genetic counselling. The articulation and recording of such familial and other lifeworld events accord genetic counselling and the corresponding case notes a distinct character and set them aside from the mainstream medical consultations and the associated recording practices.

Acknowledgements

This paper is based on the project titled 'Communicative Frames in Counselling for Predictive Genetic Testing', funded by The Wellcome Trust (2000-2004).

References

Agar, Michael 1985. Institutional Discourse. *Text* 5/3, 147-68.

Atkinson, Paul 1995. *Medical Talk and Medical Work*. London: Sage.

Barrett, Robert 1996. *The Psychiatric Team and the Social Definition of Schizophrenia*. Cambridge: Cambridge University Press.

Berg, Marc 1996. Practices of Reading and Writing: The Constitutive Role of the Patient Record in Medical Work. *Sociology of Health and Illness* 18, 499-524.

Cassell, Eric J. 1987. *Talking with Patients*, vol 1: *The Theory of Doctor-Patient Communication*. Cambridge, Mass: The MIT Press.

Cicourel, Aaron 1974. Police Practices and Official Records. In Turner, Roy (ed.) *Ethnomethodology*. Harmondsworth: Penguin, 85-95.

Cicourel, Aaron 1975. Discourse and Text: Cognitive and Linguistic Processes in Studies of Social Structure. *Versus* 12/2, 33-84.

Cicourel, Aaron 1983. Hearing is not Believing: Language and the Structure of Belief in Medical Communication. In Fisher, Sue / Todd, Alexandra (eds) *The Social Organisation of Doctor-Patient Communication*. Washington DC: Centre for Applied Linguistics, 138-55.

Cook-Gumperz, Jenny / Messerman, Lawrence 1999. Local Identities and Institutional Practices: Constructing the Record of Professional Collaboration. In Sarangi / Roberts (eds), 145-81.

Coulthard, Malcolm 1996. The Official Version: Audience Manipulation in Police Records of Interviews with Suspects. In Caldas-Coulthard, Carmen Rosa / Coulthard, Malcolm (eds) *Texts and Practices: Readings in Critical Discourse Analysis*. London: Routledge, 166-78.

Garfinkel, Harold 1967. *Studies in Ethnomethodology*. Englewood Cliffs, NJ: Prentice Hall.

Goffman, Erving 1968 [1961]. *Asylums: Essays on the Social Situation of Mental Patients and Other Inmates*. Harmondsworth: Penguin.

Hak, Tony 1989. Constructing a Psychiatric Case. In Torode, Brian (ed.) *Text and Talk as Social Practice*. Dordrecht: Foris, 72-92.

Hak, Tony 1992. Psychiatric Records as Transformations of Other Texts. In Watson, Graham / Seiler, Robert M. (eds) *Text in Context: Contributions to Ethnomethodology*. Newbury Park, CA: Sage, 138-55.

Hall, Chris / Slembrouck, Stefaan / Sarangi, Srikant 2006. *Language Practices in Social Work: Categorisation and Accountability in Child Welfare*. London: Routledge.

Hobbs, Pamela 2002. Islands in a String: The Use of Background Knowledge in an Obstetrical Resident's Notes. *Journal of Sociolinguistics* 6, 267-74.

Hobbs, Pamela 2003. The Use of Evidentiality in Physicians' Progress Notes. *Discourse Studies* 5/4, 451-78.

Howell, Lucy 2002. An Investigation into Talk and Text about the Process of Diagnosis and Non-diagnosis in Genetic Counselling. Unpublished thesis. Cardiff University.

Jönsson, Linda / Linell, Per 1991. Story Generations: From Dialogical Interviews to Written Reports in Police Interrogations. *Text* 11/3, 419-40.

Linell, Per 1998. Discourse across Boundaries: On Recontextualisations and Blending of Voices in Professional Discourse. *Text* 18/2, 143-57.

Mehan, Hugh 1991. The School's Work of Sorting Students. In Boden, Deirdre / Zimmerman, Donald H. (eds) *Talk and Social Structure*. Cambridge: Polity Press, 71-90.

Mehan, Hugh 1993. Beneath the Skin and between the Ears: A Case Study in the Politics of Representation. In Chaiklin, Seth / Lave, Jean (eds) *Understanding Practice: Perspectives on Activity and Context*. Cambridge: Cambridge University Press, 241-68.

Mishler, Elliott G. 1984. *The Discourse of Medicine: Dialectics of Medical Interviews*. Norwood: Ablex.

Pettinari, Catherine J. 1988. *Task, Talk, and Text in the Operating Room: A Study in Medical Discourse*. Norwood, NJ: Ablex.

Raffel, Stanley 1979. *Matters of Fact: A Sociological Inquiry*. London: Routledge and Kegan Paul.

Ravotas, Doris / Berkenkotter, Carol 1998. Voice in the Text: The Uses of Reported Speech in a Psychotherapist's Notes and Initial Assessments. *Text* 18/2, 211-39.

Roberts, Celia / Sarangi, Srikant 2005. Theme-Oriented Discourse Analysis of Medical Encounters. *Medical Education* 39, 632-40.

Sarangi, Srikant 1998. Rethinking Recontextualisation in Professional Discourse Studies: An Epilogue. *Text* 18/2, 301-16.

Sarangi, Srikant 2000. Activity Types, Discourse Types and Interactional Hybridity: The Case of Genetic Counselling. In Sarangi, Srikant / Coulthard, Malcolm (eds) *Discourse and Social Life*. London: Pearson, 1-27.

Sarangi, Srikant 2005. Activity Analysis in Professional Discourse Settings: The Framing of Risk and Responsibility in Genetic Counselling. *Hermès* 41, 111-20.

Sarangi, Srikant / Bennert, K. / Howell, L. / Clarke, A. / Harper, P. / Gray, J. 2004. Initiation of Reflective Frames in Counselling for Huntington's Disease Predictive Testing. *Journal of Genetic Counselling* 13/2, 135-55.

Sarangi, Srikant / Bennert, K. / Howell, L. / Clarke, A. / Harper, P. / Gray, J. 2005. (Mis)alignments in Counselling for Huntington's Disease Predictive Testing: Clients' Responses to Reflective Frames. *Journal of Genetic Counselling* 14/1, 29-42.

Sarangi, Srikant / Roberts, Celia 1999. The Dynamics of Interactional and Institutional Orders in Work-related Settings. In Sarangi / Roberts (eds), 1-57.

Sarangi, Srikant / Roberts, Celia (eds) 1999. *Talk, Work and Institutional Order: Discourse in Medical, Mediation and Management Settings*. Berlin: Mouton de Gruyter.

Scott, John 1990. *A Matter of Record: Documentary Sources in Social Research*. Cambridge: Polity Press.

Slembrouck, Stefaan 1992. The Parliamentary Hansard 'Verbatim' Report: The Written Construction of Spoken Discourse. *Language and Literature* 1/2, 101-19.

Weed, Larry 1971. *Medical Records, Medical Education and Patient Care*. Cleveland: The Press of Case Western Reserve.

Wheeler, Stanton (ed.) 1969. *On Record: Files and Dossiers in American Life*. New York: Russell Sage Foundation.

Zimmerman, Don H. 1969. Record-keeping and the Intake Process in a Public Welfare Agency. In Wheeler (ed.), 319-45.

Appendices

Appendix 1: Thematic mapping of AF2-A1 clinic and case notes

Epi-sode	*THEMATIC MAPPING OF AF2-A1 CLINIC (line numbers indicated)*				*AF2-A1 NOTES*
	Medical Lifeworld	*Familial Lifeworld*	*Other Lifeworld Events*	*Procedural & other concerns*	
1				1-13 Opening	

				smalltalk about car problems	
2	14-84 GC initiates overview of AF2's non-genetic health problems under treatment/ investigation; discuss ultrascan on womb, screws in leg, crumbling of discs in back				1-9 Medical Lifeworld: Overview of AF2's non-genetic health problems; biopsy of womb, asthma, mood swings, hot flushes
3		85-88 GC initiates talk about couple's decisions to have a baby.			
4			89-117 MP feels that AF2's daughters are like his own, and the world is no longer an ideal place to bring a child into. AF2 always wanted another baby but feels she is too old. She still feels hurt when she sees babies but may be a grandmother soon.		12-13 Other Lifeworld Events: Couple have "come to terms" with not having another baby
5			118-124 AF2 tells story of a friend who regrets being sterilised.		
6		125-143 AF2 is having the test to give an answer for her daughters so they are not faced with being sterilised against their will like she			13-14 Familial Lifeworld: AF2 wants the test to remove uncertainty for her children (DAT).

		was (DAT). AF2 says test will let daughters' know they can have babies without worrying about HD			
7		144-165 GC asks if AF2's daughters are planning a pregnancy. AF2 provides an overview of her eldest daughter's gynaecological problems and effect on conception			15-16 Familial Lifeworld: Notes daughter is planning a pregnancy.
8		166-181 GC initiates talk about whether the daughters talk about HD (anxiety and awareness). AF2 explains that the daughters are involved in decision about test as they would rather know			15 Familial Lifeworld: AF2 will tell both daughters the test result (DAD)
9		182-219 GC initiates talk about the impact of the test result for AF2's daughters and their support for AF2 to have the test (DAT)			16 Familial Lifeworld: Daughters are keen to know test result (DAT)
10		220-251 GC initiates talk about impact of test result on AF2's brother and father. AF2 explains that she is not in contact			

		with her extended family and has not discussed her decisions with them (DAT).			
11		252-274 GC asks about decision about disclosure of test result to father and brother. AF2 explains that she is having the test purely for her immediate family. Explains that her extended family try not to think about HD			17-19 Familial Lifeworld: AF2 will not disclose test result to father and brother as they do not want to know and do not have contact with them.
12		275-308 GC explores extended family tree/info to find out whether brother might want to know for his own children			
13		309-338 AF2 explains that she wants the test to give certainty to her adult daughters so they do not have to live in uncertainty forever thinking about HD (DAT)			
14		339-371 AF2 explains that her daughter worried that AF2 might have HD recently and the not knowing is upsetting them greatly			
15			372-407 AF2 explains that		

			they cope with the thought of HD as it is just one of many medical problems AF2 might have. AF2 is "a fighter" and makes the best of what they have		
16		408-415 AF2 explains that she has talked about her decision to have the test with her friend who is also like a carer to AF2			
17		416-431 AF2 explains that she will tell her daughters when she gets home, on the day of the test results (planning DAD)			
18		432-469 N initiates talk of impact of result on extended family, father and brother, if they accidentally found out AF2's test result. AF2 explains that they have no contact with them so they will not find out			19 Familial Lifeworld: AF2 does not think her father and brother will find out her test result from another source (DAD)

19			470-504 AF2 and MP explain that they keep to themselves and do not mix socially with many people, therefore not many people will know the test result		
20				505-516 GC explains the appointment protocol, including blood taking and timescale for results	23-24 Procedural: Timescale for next clinic appointments set out
21			517-537 MP talks of AF2's level of anxiety and the feeling of calm that the result will bring		
22			538-558 GC initiates talk about how the couple seem more settled. AF2 and MP talk about how the move of house has allowed the couple peace to think and talk		10-11 Other Lifeworld Events: couple appear more settled since moving house
23			559-575 N explains she will set a date for the next appointment, so the couple will know when the results will be and plan some time off		
24				576-577 The physical examination is	20-22 Procedural: Results of

				conducted and blood-sample taken	examination and record that blood was taken
25				578-786 Nurse and Partner talk simultaneously while GC is conducting examination	
26				787-799 N checks contact details of AF2 and closes	

Appendix 2: Transcription conventions

GC: genetic counselor
N: genetic nurse
AF: adult female client
MP: male partner
(.): micropause;
(1, 2 etc.): timed pauses in seconds
Italic: indicates added emphasis;
CAPITAL LETTER: indicates increased volume;
Asterisked word: indicates decreased volume;
question mark [?]: rising intonation;
[:::::]: indicates lengthening sound;
[text in square brackets]: overlapping speech;
((text in double round brackets)): description or anonymised information;
(text in round brackets): transcriber's guess;
(^^^^^^): unrecognizable talk;
=: a continuous utterance and is used when a speaker's lengthy utterance is broken up arbitrarily for purposes of presentation.

Medical Discourse in Written Contexts

DIDIER CARNET / ANNE MAGNET

Editorials: An Intrinsic and/or Extrinsic Genre in Medical Journals

1. Introduction

Scientific discourse has been the source of much research endeavour over the past 40 years or so and a constant aim has been to describe it as a constrained and modelised mode of written communication. But this has mainly been evidenced for the research article, which was set up as a genre following Swales' archetypal studies (1990), and whose aim is to build scientific facts as evidenced by Bazerman (1988), Hopkins / Dudley-Evans (1988); Berkenkotter / Huckin (1995) to name but a few. However, scientific discourse cannot be limited to the research article, even if it is the dominant and most salient genre. It seems of interest to investigate genres which play a lesser part in the construction of scientific fact but interact with or against published articles. Two of the seven genres identified in medical journals (Webber 1994) involve the editor: letters to the editor and editorials, as opposed to research papers, review articles, book reviews, case studies and the news section. These modes of written scientific discourse represent either controversial reactions within the community toward published articles for the former (Carnet / Magnet 2006; Magnet / Carnet in press), or the opening onto new topics sometimes related to new themes of research for the latter (Salager Meyer 2002) or to societal problems at large.

Whereas letters to the editor tend to reduce a scientist's activity to his/her publishing pursuit, editorials aim to widen the scientific community's interests by commenting on general and even global issues. While letters to the editor represent some sort of aftermath in the process of publication, editorials represent an anticipating mode of expression. Perhaps an adequate way to understand the differences between these two genres is the metaphoric use of a traditional linguistic concept according to which letters to the editor could be described as an anaphoric mode of discourse, that is, referring to published articles in the past, while editorials could be qualified as cataphoric, since they herald what may or rather what should attract the community's attention in the near future.

2. General editorials

Unlike experimental research papers, scientific editorials cannot be perceived as a construct built by the scientific community since they have been a long-standing tradition in the general press, and especially in quality papers. The noun 'editorial' itself is worth commenting upon. Though the adjective 'editorial' was first introduced into the English language in the mid 18th century, meaning "pertaining to an editor or editing, written by or as by the editor, distinguished from news and advertising matter" (Brown 1993: 785), the use of the noun only appeared in the Anglo-American press in the mid 19th century, and was quickly borrowed by the international press. It is now understood as "a newspaper article written by or under the direct responsibility of the editor" (Brown 1993: 785). According to Rey / Rey-Debove (1984: 606), it also defines or reflects a general policy of the journal. For Sinclair (1991: 450), an editorial is "an article in a newspaper which gives the opinion of the editor or publisher on a topic or item of news".

The first linguistic and discursive studies of the genre 'editorials' were performed on editorials from the general press. They have led to extensive studies but often with special focus on themes (Hawes / Thomas 1995, 1996), structure and argumentative patterns (Bolivar 1994; Ansary / Babaii 2004), diachronic prospects (Hynds 1990), contents and ideologies (Van Dijk 1995), and contrastive rhetoric (Connor 1996; de Carvalho 1999). Following these generic studies, the present paper relies on the postulate that editorials can be considered as a genre. One should first, however, be reminded that "genre analysis is essentially based on two central assumptions. Firstly, the features of a similar group of texts depend on the social context of their creation and use. Secondly, these features can be described in a way that relates a text to other texts like it" (Hyland 2002: 114).

Le (2003: 478) argues that editorials play an important role in the definition of priorities in public agendas. She studied the argumentative structure of editorials and found that under the guise of bringing some objectivity to the editorials' argumentation, external sources of information are used to support and lend weight to subjective positions. Van Dijk (1995: 2) claims that "newspaper editorials not only play a role in the formation and change of public opinion, but also influence social debate, decision making, and other forms of social and political action".

3. Scientific and medical editorials

As far as scientific editorials are concerned, they appeared as early as the 19th century when they were first drafted to sketch the guiding line of a journal policy. It is thus possible to trace back the first editorial to *The Lancet*, published on October 5 1823, which presented the journal's editorial line. This initial editorial was called 'Preface', but it corresponds to the characteristic features of an editorial as defined above. Interestingly, today almost all scientific journals, even a vast majority of on-line journals, have kept this column.

We postulate, however, that some bias has prevailed in most studies on scientific or medical editorials, since it has been assumed that editorials in medical journals make up a solid and well-defined mode of communication within the community (Adams Smith 1984: 32-33; Salager-Meyer 2002: 47). Our overall investigation of editorials allows us to define two types of editorials. First, those found in journals which address general practitioners (GPs) and the general scientific community. These editorials (type 1 editorials) are written with a view to raising and tackling issues concerning the inner life of the medical community and its practitioners as well as its influence on society at large. They can be found in the leading scientific journals such as *Nature* and *Science,* but also in medical journals such as *The Lancet* and *The British Medical Journal (BMJ).* Second, editorials found in journals addressing specialists in which editors comment or highlight the research articles published in the same issue (type 2 editorials). This second type can be observed in journals such as *The New England Journal of Medicine (NEJM)* and *The Journal of the American Medical Association (JAMA*). One of the main differences between type 1 and type 2 editorials dealing with medical research is that type 1 editorials do not comment on one particular paper, but rather synthesize the results of several articles on the same subject, or report the trends in the research approach on a specific issue at a precise time. In contrast, type 2 editorials put the research results of one specific experiment into perspective. This chapter aims to analyse the first type, since it is a truly original genre, standing at the crossroads between scientific and general journalistic discourses. Our purpose is to evidence their potential similarities with those of quality newspapers and magazines from a linguistic and discursive point of view. In the general press, the authors of editorials tend to be the editors in chief, that is, senior journalists, who consider this task as a prestigious mission offering them the opportunity to vent moral/philosophical points of view on hot topics, and to be heard.

In the two journals we investigated, the editorial authorship policy is different from that of the general press. Moreover, each journal has its own rules. Though both journals publish type 1 editorials, *The Lancet* publishes unsigned editorials, which suggests that they are written either by the editor in chief, or by the editorial board as confirmed by Zoe Mullan, a senior editor contacted (through several electronic mails) in 2005:

> Editorials are always written by editors, but not necessarily the editor in chief. The topic is discussed by a group of us and a collective decision on the 'bottom line' arrived at. One editor will actually write the piece, with comments from others. [...] All of the editors are either medically qualified or have bioscience degrees, about fifty percent each. None of the editors are journalists as such.

The aim is to present the voice, not of one person, but of the journal at least, and perhaps even of the whole medical community.

On the other hand, *The British Medical Journal* offers editorials signed by one or several authors. They can be the editor in chief, members of the editorial board, senior lecturers as well as renowned researchers who have no direct link with the journal, but are famous in a specific field relevant to the topic addressed. In this case, the editorials are often co-signed, thus following the co-authoring process of research articles. In either journal, editorials are never written by journalists, not even science specialized journalists.

4. Purpose of the study

Editorials appear at the very beginning of medical journals. Type 1 editorials address the general community of GPs and those interested in medical issues. Yet, is the fact that type 1 editorials are written by scientists and address the scientific community sufficient to label them as scientific discourse? This is the first point to be addressed. Another goal of this chapter is to investigate whether the editors are just following the journalistic tradition or whether they are developing ideological strategies in order to justify their place, role (and cost) for society.

Since type 1 editorials have been little studied so far, we thought it interesting to account for their presence in medical journals. Our main interest is thus to highlight their rhetorical patterns, identify their macrostructure, and search for their linguistic specificities so as to define and characterize this particular genre.

5. Corpus, material and method

The corpus was based on editorials from the two leading non-specialist British medical journals according to the Journal Citation Report published by the International Science Index (ISI), *The Lancet* and *The British Medical Journal (BMJ)* whose impact factors are respectively 15 and 7.5 (type 1 editorials). We decided not to include editorials from the two leading American journals, *The New England Journal of Medicine (NEJM)* and *The Journal of the American Medical Association (JAMA),* impact factors: 31.5 and 16.5 respectively, since as said above, these are a different kind of editorial (type 2 editorials) which are labelled as such but should more appropriately be considered as short research articles rather than editorials.

When building the corpus, we planned to work on recent material. The year 2004 was selected with this idea in mind but also with the purpose of including the new editorial strategy clearly announced in the July 3rd issue of *the Lancet* that year. The format moved from the one page traditional general comment on one topic to a two-page genre presenting, on a weekly basis, one long editorial (one and a half pages) plus a short half-page editorial. This strategy corresponds to the general wish of the journal as stated in the July 3rd 2004 editorial: "The first third of the journal is devoted to analysis and interpretation of current issues in medicine. We have strengthened this material by doubling Editorials". Since our corpus is based on the year 2004, we have included both formats. In comparison, *The BMJ* did not alter its policy and continued to publish from three to five editorials in each issue. We thus chose to build a balanced corpus to allow us to compare the two journals' editorials as far as their strategies, choices and contents are concerned. A final corpus of 158 editorials (75 for *The Lancet* and 83 for *The BMJ)* was obtained.

6. Discursive analysis

6.1. The raison d'être of editorials

6.1.1. Opinions and ideologies of the medical community

British editors continue a long-lasting tradition of learned scientists who do not only deal with their patients' health but also consider themselves as humanists and philosophers dealing with man, his place and role in society. It corresponds more to a 19th century view of the medical practitioner than the pragmatic, efficient but somewhat restricted mission of the medical research community whose aim is to better understand human diseases and improve their treatments. Editorials help their readers make up their minds about global events related to the general well-being of people throughout the world. They play a role in the formation and evolution of the medical community's opinion, by setting the agenda and influencing social debate, decision making, and other forms of social and political action. Their influence may be based not so much on massive popular influence as on the influence on the elite. No consistent health policy in western countries and more specifically in the United Kingdom can ignore the recurrent critiques and attacks raised in the best ranked and most influential medical journals, which appear in the two journals we investigated. Before providing a comprehensive list of the topics tackled in the 2004 editorials, we can illustrate the trends in the choice of subjects by mentioning a few striking heads such as:

(1) The catastrophic failures of public health. (*The Lancet*, March 6)

(2) OTC statins: a bad decision for public health. (*The Lancet*, May 22)

(3) Why do doctors use treatments that do not work? For many reasons – including their inability to stand idle and do nothing. (*The BMJ*, February 28)

(4) Health tsars, more like Peter the Great than Ivan the Terrible – but only if they have money. (T*he BMJ*, January 17)

6.1.2. The medical community and society

These British journals try to keep alive a real link between the medical community and society as if their authors and readers felt they were indebted to society, which supports and funds research, as illustrated explicitly by one *BMJ* editorialist (February 14):

> An urgent need exists for the medical profession to enter into a dialogue with society – which is represented by consumers (patients and their families), health care managers, health care organizations, media, litigation lawyers, and the like – to agree on a compromise between these two opposite tendencies.

In contrast, most medical or even more hard-core scientific American journals tend to ignore society around them as if they did not have to account for their research choices. Today's editorials in British medical journals are like an open window onto the world enabling information transfer and communication in their professional community as already stated by Thomas Wakley, editor in chief of the first issue of *The Lancet,* though in a limited acceptation of the word at the time: "We purpose giving […] a correct description of all the important cases that may occur, whether in England or on any part of the civilized continent."

When editorialists now deal with health problems in Africa, or in Asia, it may be first to help improve the sanitary conditions on these continents, as developed in *The Lancet* May 15th editorial entitled *Political neglect in India's health*, but also because any health problem encountered *there* may influence public health *here*, due to globalization. For instance, the editorial on HIV/AIDS (*The Lancet*, July 3) stresses the fact that helping Africans fight the epidemic will also help the whole world to get rid of the disease. In the same way, some editorials illustrate how medical editorialists show an interest in health problems in developing countries, not only through ethical concern, but also to pinpoint the dangers for the rest of the world and especially western countries. Here are a few examples:

(5) Avian influenza: the threat looms. (*The Lancet*, January 24)

(6) Pandemic risks from bird flu, the risk to humans is small, but we need to be better prepared. (*The BMJ*, January 31)

(7) China: towards a 'xiaokang'[1] society, but still living dangerously. (*The Lancet*, February 7)

(8) Exchanging health lessons globally, BMJ issue will focus on lessons rich countries can learn from poor ones. (*The BMJ*, January 31).

As explicitly stated in this last editorial: "It is not just China that is seriously threatened by the country's weak disease-surveillance infrastructure. Nowhere is this wider risk more clearly true than for avian H5N1 influenza [...] On this pipedream rests the security of world health".

6.1.3. Editorialists' characteristics

Contrary to research articles whose authors are often non-native English speakers, it is worth mentioning that all *BMJ* editors are native English speakers. They are not necessarily British, but may be Australian, Canadian, American. As for *The Lancet*, the information provided by one of the senior editors confirms that all editors are British apart from two Americans and one German for the year 2004. Editorialists are required to follow a code of ethics to avoid conflicts of interest (Relman 1984: 1182-1183). Scientists who have been or who are consultants for private pharmaceutical companies are not allowed to write editorials and give opinions about drugs or treatments which could lead to conflicts of interest. As Angell and Kassirer (1996: 1055-1056) wrote:

> Editorialists who have worked with a company are also accustomed to seeing issues from that company's perspective, and this viewpoint can affect the focus of an editorial. [...] Readers should not have to go through the exercise of assessing editorials to decide which to trust.

6.2. Topics and subjects selected

Forbes noted about the general press that "Editorials are usually written on themes of the moment. When moment and matter pass, so does an editorial's relevance" (1974: 13). Those published in medical

---

1 As indicated in the text of the editorial, *xiaokang* means 'well off'.

journals also deal with current topics in the scientific community, but they tend to remain relevant for much longer as evidenced by the recurrence of some themes over the one-year period we studied. For example, our corpus contains three editorials on domestic violence, four on peer-reviewing, and five on adolescents' health problems.

The topics appearing in the editorials we analysed can be classified under the seven following headings: current medical issues in the UK, current medical issues in other countries, public health, scientific research implementation, ethical problems, regulations and health systems, medical training reforms. In fact, these different headings can also be considered as both factual and evaluative. These two categories were first defined by Van Dijk (1995: 15), who states that editorials can either deal with facts and/or opinions. Following this mode of categorization, our corpus presents topics that can be classified as *factual*, i.e. current medical issues in the UK, current medical issues in other countries, regulations and health systems, and *evaluative* i.e. public health, scientific research implementation, ethical problems and medical training reforms. Most of the time, however, the editorials from our corpus can be described as both factual and evaluative. Indeed, though starting with factual information, most editorials end up giving strong opinions and advice to improve current trends.

As appears in Table 1, general medical issues make up the first topic developed in both journals with around 55% of all editorials dealing with them, but with an interesting difference. In *The BMJ*, editorials generally focus on diseases and health problems encountered in the UK (40%), whereas *The Lancet* contains more editorials dealing with global health problems (37%) than with home medical issues (17.5%). As far as editorials are concerned, *The BMJ* can therefore be said to live up to its name. Here are a few titles from both journals that illustrate our point:

(9) Guidelines from the British hypertension society: the lower the pressure, the better. (*The BMJ*, March 13)

(10) Compulsory screening of immigrants for TB and HIV. (*The BMJ*, Feb 7)

(11) Europe's health priorities for the world. (*The Lancet*, November 27)

(12) Tropical medicine: a brittle tool of the new imperialism. (*The Lancet*, April 3)

Topics	*The Lancet*	*The BMJ*
Current medical issues in the UK	18.5%	40%
Current medical issues in other countries	37%	14.5%
Public health	16%	13%
Implementation of scientific research	11%	7.5%
Ethical problems	11%	7%
Regulations and health systems	5%	15.5%
Medical training reforms	1.5%	2.5%

Table 1. Topics treated in the editorials of *The Lancet* and *The BMJ* in 2004 expressed in percentages.

After medical issues in the UK or in other countries, the third leading theme developed in *The Lancet* is that of public health with 16% of editorials and a slightly lower percentage for *The BMJ* (13%), which illustrates the fact that public health and the prevention of diseases is a constant concern in the British medical community (cf. examples 13 and 14).

(13) The catastrophic failures of public-health. (*The Lancet*, March 6)

(14) Smoking and blindness: strong evidence for the link, but public awareness lags. (*The BMJ*, March 6)

In *The BMJ*, the third leading topic deals with regulations and the specificity of the health systems with 15.5% of editorials, whereas in *The Lancet*, this theme only represents 5% of all editorials, and is therefore among the least developed topics. This confirms that one of the aims of *The BMJ* editorials is to offer a forum to health professionals who want to take part in the shaping of health policies. It also justifies the fact that editorials in *The BMJ* are always written and signed by health professionals (cf. examples 15 and 16).

(15) A revised classification of headache disorders: regular updates are still necessary. (*The BMJ*, January 17)

(16) Reconfiguration of surgical, emergency, and trauma services in the UK: centralization of services is politically impossible. (*The BMJ*, January 24)

Finally, editorials commenting on problems encountered in the implementation of scientific research and general ethical issues are more frequent in *The Lancet* (11% for each theme) than in *The BMJ* (7.5% and 7% respectively). Examples 17 to 20 illustrate our point:

(17) Open access publishing takes off: the dream is now achievable. (*The BMJ*, January 3)

(18) Why are French scientists striking? (*The Lancet*, March 20)

(19) Facts versus ideology in the cloning debate. (*The Lancet*, February 21)

(20) Health tourism: where healthcare, ethics and the state collide. (*The BMJ*, January 10)

The concern about medical training reform is present, but it is not a recurrent topic, since it only appears in 2.5% of the editorials for *The BMJ*, and only 1.5% for *The Lancet.* However, whenever this subject is taken up, both journals are highly critical of the changing policies.

6.3. Argumentative patterns

The observation that editorials contain both facts and opinions leads to the study of the organization of ideas in this genre from a discursive point of view. This has been the subject of a lot of research in general editorials (Bolivar 1994: 276-279; Ansary / Babaii 2004: 11-12; Hynds 1990: 303-309), and it has resulted in the typifying of the writing devices used in editorials. As far as medical editorials are concerned, no common macrostructure can be detected, contrary to the genre 'Letters to the editor' where a clear-cut macrostructure could be identified (Magnet / Carnet in press).

In our corpus, each journal displays a different argumentative pattern. *The Lancet* tends to use a rather casual language with the recurrent use of rhetorical questions (especially in titles and conclusions), imperatives, orders and aphorisms, which produce a style close to that of sermons. It is as if the anonymous editorialist spoke in the name of his/her scientific community in the same way as a religious predicator speaks in the name of his/her church. *The*

Lancet's editorialists tend to use some of the common rhetorical tools, such as questions, repetitions and implied or stated calls for action (cf. examples 21 to 23).

(21) Who is responsible for adolescent health? ((June 19)

(22) Choose advice wisely for health. (September 11)

(23) Child protection: stop blaming doctors. (June 26)

Conversely, *The BMJ* tends to adopt a more formal style. Before developing the subject of the editorial, quotations from famous politicians or philosophers are sometimes used as implied calls for action. Questions and repetitions are much less frequently used. Quotations are for instance extracted from political speeches which may date back to the 18th and 19th centuries, as examples 24 and 25 clearly illustrate:

(24) You cannot fight against the future. Time is on our side. The great social forces which move onwards in their might and majesty, and which the tumult of our debates does not for the moment impede or disturb – those great social forces are against you; they are marshalled on our side; and the banner which we now carry in this fight, though perhaps at some moment it may droop over our sinking heads, yet it soon again will float in the eye of heaven, and it will be borne [...] perhaps not to an easy, but to a certain and to a not distant victory. (W.E. Gladstone 1866, January 3)

(25) Let us save what remains: not by vaults and locks which fence them from the public eye and use in consigning them to the waste of time, but by such a multiplication of copies, as shall place them beyond the reach of accident. (Thomas Jefferson 1791, January 10)

Adams Smith (1984: 31) notes about medical editorials that:

> a lack of subheadings makes their structure more difficult to follow, and they are the freest [within medical discourse] in form, the most heavily attitudinally marked, and syntactically and linguistically the most complex of the three categories: clinical case notes, research papers and editorials.

Though no common macrostructure as such can be evidenced from our corpus, similar rhetorical devices and persuasion strategies can be highlighted. All editorials are deeply rooted in current matters. They tend to use a pretext to deal with a specific matter and open a new debate that may lead to controversial exchanges. These pretexts can be understood as events occurring both inside and outside the medical community in the UK or anywhere else in the world. Examples of these are a scientific conference which has just taken place or is about to be held, the outbreak of an epidemic somewhere in the world, political or professional elections and their potential impact on health policies, wars and their sanitary impact.

Most editorials contain the discursive categories identified by Hulteng in his study on the construction of arguments in editorials from the general press (1973: 61-77), that is, the lead, the ending, the argumentative categories, and the writing device categories:

> *Lead categories* include statement of news or information, statement of opinion, combination of news and opinion, question, quotation, and other.
> *Ending categories* include summary of information, statement of reaction, call for action (implied), call for action (stated), question, quotation, and other.
> *Argumentative categories* include appeal to authority, evidence, analogies, examples, cause and effect relationship, and other.
> *Writing device categories* include narration, description, explanation, argumentation, direct quotes, indirect quotes, and other.

Numerous examples can be extracted from our corpus. Examples 26 to 28 are three illustrations of 'appeal to authority', 'statement of reaction', and 'statement of opinion', respectively:

(26) We call upon governments of the sub-Saharan African countries to ensure that their telecom networks are sold to the private sector. (*The Lancet,* July 17)

(27) We welcome this long overdue undertaking. However, several important questions remain. (*The Lancet,* August 28)

(28) Research is an essential component of a high quality health care system, not an optional extra. (*The BMJ*, January 31)

6.4. Editorials as scientific discourse

Their presence in scientific journals, the choice of topics, the authorship and readership allow us to consider editorials as scientific discourse, though in a very specific way. In the two British journals we investigated, editorials appear as highly ideological, and whether written anonymously or not, they stand for the medical community's viewpoint or at least part of it. We have not been able to obtain any definite explanation from the editorial board on the reasons why *The BMJ*'s editorials are always signed. But to our mind, these editorials tend to offer a forum to health professionals, in the same way as letters to the editor do, whereas *The Lancet*'s editorials are always written by a small committee made up of the journal's editorial board. Yet, in both cases, editorialists play a strong ideological role as they provide professional and ethical guidelines, and also act as watchdogs, monitoring the medical community's line of thought and behaviour. These features show that the editorials from our corpus share a strong polemical similarity with editorials from the general press.

In spite of common argumentative patterns, this genre is not characterized by a strong modelised structure. It is thus of interest to identify linguistic and stylistic constants and variables in the two journals we studied.

7. Linguistic characteristics

7.1. Heads

Following the rules observed in the general press, medical editorials in our corpus always begin with a head. These heads are generally composed of a few words (from 2 to 11) with a specificity for *The BMJ*, in which the heads are always followed by a subhead. In this journal, heads almost work as keywords introducing the topic, and subheads sum up the message the editorialist wants to convey.

(29) *Health tourism*
Where healthcare, ethics, and the state collide. (*The BMJ*, January 10)

(30) *Open access publishing takes off*
The dream is now achievable. (*The BMJ*, January 5)

(31) *Surgery in asymptomatic aortic stenosis*
Exercise testing is the key investigation. (*The BMJ*, January 10)

In *The Lancet*, there is no subhead as such. However, 25% of the heads contain a built-in subhead, with the use of a semicolon which precedes a sort of interpretation of the head. Here are a few examples:

(32) *Avian flu*: the threat looms. (*The Lancet,* January 24)

(33) *America 2004*: voting for a decent global society. (*The Lancet,* September 18)

On the whole, heads in *The Lancet* tend to be more eye-catching than those of *The BMJ,* with the recurrent use of catch-phrases, such as:

(34) China towards 'xiaokang', but still living dangerously. (*The Lancet,* Feb. 7)

The deliberate use of a Chinese word meaning 'well-off society', acts as a teaser for the reader of this head. In the same way, heads, such as:

(35) The catastrophic failures of public health. (*The Lancet,* March 6)

(36) Depressing research. *(The Lancet,* April 24)

induce the reader to go through the article to learn more about public health or research.

As seen in Figure 1, most heads are built in the form of an elliptical sentence, thus mimicking the editorials from the general press (Fløttum 1998: 221-230). When the head is not elliptical, the verbal form is systematically the simple present. In about 16% of the cases, a gerund is used, and its function is almost that of an injunction, a call for action. Here are a few examples:

(37) Facing up to surgical deaths. (*The BMJ*, February 14)

(38) Exchanging health lessons globally. (*The BMJ*, January 31)

(39) Kickstarting the revolution in health systems research. (*The Lancet*, May 29)

(40) Keeping ideology and bureaucracy out of science. (*The Lancet*, February 14)

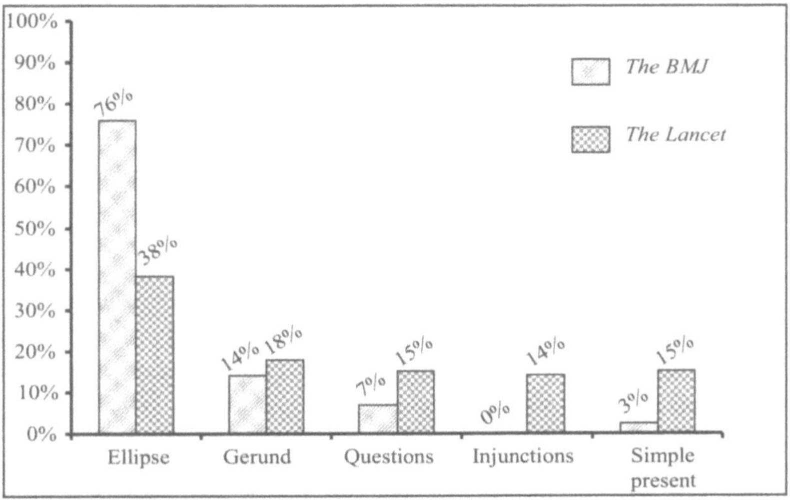

Figure 1. Verb forms in editorial heads of *The Lancet* and *The BMJ* in 2004 expressed in percentages.

As for real injunctions, it is worth noting that *The Lancet* is much more polemical than *The BMJ* since 14% of the heads use the imperative and 15% the simple present, which is an assertive verbal mode.

7.2. Tenses and modality

Verb forms are closely linked to the argumentative pattern of editorials. The largely dominant tense for both journals is the simple present used for statements of news or information, statements of opinion, combinations of news and opinion, questions, and quotations. It also applies to narration, description, explanation, and argumentation. The past tense only appears on a few occasions to report on a past event used to justify the topic addressed in the editorial.

As already observed by Forbes about editorials in the general press (1974: 5), editorialists constantly use active verb forms rather than passive ones. This trend is also confirmed by our corpus. However, passive verb forms can also be found, but with a higher prevalence in *The BMJ* than in *The Lancet*. In the latter, the authors' presence is more heavily asserted through direct endorsement expressed by the recurrent use of *we, in our view, in our opinion…* (cf. examples 41 and 42).

(41) *We* are not naive enough to […]. (*The Lancet*, September 4)

(42) *We strongly urge* those involved in these evaluations to […]. (*The Lancet*, August 28)

In both journals, the most common linguistic feature is the recurrent use of injunctions at the end of editorials. They can be expressed by verbs and modals and emphasized by adverbs. Modals most often express orders, though hedging is also present in *The BMJ* (cf. examples 43 to 47).

(43) Clearly, there is an *urgent need* to address the gap in essential knowledge about the size and nature of the problem and to suggest more specific solutions. (*The BMJ*, January 10)

(44) *It is now high time* that health-care workers took the lead in helping the victims of domestic violence. *(The Lancet*, October 30)

(45) Our public-health leaders *must* replace prevarication with imagination. *(The Lancet*, March 6)

(46) Good governance, like good medicine, *should* be evidence-based and proportionate. (*The BMJ*, January 10)

(47) The concepts of hypertension and hypercholesterolaemia *may* now be irrelevant or even harmful in this population. (*The BMJ*, February 7)

7.3. Syntactic and lexical features

In both journals, editorialists often use negations and restrictions as a way to formulate criticism (cf. examples 48 to 50).

(48) The status quo is *not* an option. (*The Lancet*, May 29)

(49) We would guess *not*. *(The Lancet*, July 20)

(50) Public health authorities *should not* advocate screening of unproved value. (*The BMJ*, February 7)

The evaluative aspect of editorials evidenced above can also be illustrated through the efficient use of adjectives which are mostly restrictive and derogatory. Forbes (1974: 5) also notes that

> Much of the difference between 'straight' reporting, as theoretically exemplified in articles, and 'interpretive' reporting as presumably exemplified in such publications as editorials, lies in the latter's sparing but vigorous use of adjectives.

The following adjectives and sentences found in our corpus (cf. examples 51 to 53 below) clearly support this finding: *unbelievable, unimaginable, impossible, questionable, inhumane, unsustainable, irrelevant, harmful, inefficient, acrimonious, destructive, murky...*

(51) Anything less is *inhumane* and *unsustainable*. (*The Lancet*, October 2)

(52) The concepts of hypotension and hypercholesterolaemia may now be *irrelevant* or even *harmful* in this population. (*The BMJ*, February 7)

(53) Thalassaemia major: the *murky* story of deferiprone. (*The BMJ*, February 14)

8. Conclusion

Editorials in medical journals do belong to scientific discourse. They are written by members of a well defined community, that is, health professionals writing for fellow doctors; they deal with health-related topics; they are published in medical journals only, and moreover they are very often quoted and commented upon in popularized scientific articles within the general press as representing the medical community's viewpoint. Nevertheless, unlike type 2 editorials and letters to the editor, type 1 editorials have but a loose link with scientific research.

Type 1 editorials should be considered as one of the genres making up scientific discourse. They share a common goal, that is, to inform the community and call for action, and also present common argumentative and linguistic features. They play an important role in the definition of priorities in the medical community's agenda. However, whereas research papers aim to export the results of scientists' activity from the laboratory to the specialists' community and then to society, type 1 editorials import problems and particularly health concerns into the medical community to make them a subject for debate, and eventually provide guidelines or suggest therapies and solutions.

Though type 1 editorials do belong to scientific discourse, their mode of writing borrows a lot from general press editorials. It can be concluded that type 1 editorials follow the journalistic tradition both by implementing ideological strategies or influencing societal choices and by using a stylistic mode close to that of editorials from the quality papers. They offer a great amount of freedom to editorialists within the limits of each journal's editorial style. Comparing the editorials of two leading British medical journals reveals that one of them, *The Lancet*, displays a much more polemical style than the more politically correct *BMJ*. Editorials thus represent a weakly modelised genre within scientific discourse. This is most certainly one of the reasons why they have been little studied so far by scientific discourse analysts.

Though our study strongly suggests that type 1 medical editorials can be labelled as both an intrinsic and an extrinsic genre in medical journals, we are well aware that further investigation needs to be done on a larger scale to confirm our results. This should especially be done from a corpus including American journals containing type 1 editorials, and with editorials written in other languages and in other disciplines.

References

Adams Smith, Diana E. 1984. Medical Discourse: Aspects of Author's Comments. *The ESP Journal* 3/1, 25-37.

Angell, Marcia / Kassirer, Jerome P. 1996. Editorials and Conflicts of Interest. *The New England Journal of Medicine* 335, 1055-6.

Ansary, Hasan / Babaii, Esmat 2004. The Generic Integrity of Newspaper Editorials: A Systemic Functional Perspective. *The Asian EFL Journal* 6/3.

Bazerman, Charles 1988. *Shaping Written Knowledge*. Madison: University of Wisconsin Press.

Berkenkotter, Carol / Huckin, Thomas 1995. *Genre Knowledge in Disciplinary Communication: Cognition, Culture, Power*. Hillsdale, NJ: Lawrence Erlbaum.

Bolivar, Adriana 1994. The Structure of Newspaper Editorials. In Coulthard, Malcolm (ed.) *Advances in Written Text Analysis*. London: Routledge, 276-94.

Brown, Lesley (ed.) 1993. *The New Shorter Oxford English Dictionary*. Oxford: Clarendon Press.

Carnet, Didier / Magnet, Anne 2006. Letters to the Editor. In Brown, Keith (ed.) *The Encyclopedia of Language and Linguistics*, 2nd ed. Oxford: Elsevier, 725-32.

Carvalho de, Gisele 1999. Contrastive Rhetoric and its Interface with EAP Reading. *The ESPecialist* 20/2, 143-55.

Connor, Ulla 1996. *Contrastive Rhetoric: Cross-Cultural Aspects of Second-Language Writing*. Cambridge: Cambridge University Press.

Fløttum, Kjersti 1998. The Editorial: A Heterogeneous Genre. In Lundquist, Pitch / Quistgaard, Jacques (eds) *LSP. Identity and Interface Research, Knowledge and Society*. Vol. I. Copenhagen: Business School, 221-30.

Forbes, Malcolm S 1974. *Fact and Comment*, New York: Knopf.

Hawes, Thomas / Thomas, Sarah 1995. Theme Choice and Lateral Verbs in Newspaper Editorials. *Hong Kong Papers in Linguistics and Language Teaching* 18, 103-13.

Hawes, Thomas / Thomas, Sarah 1996. Rhetorical Uses of Theme in Newspaper Editorials. *World Englishes* 15/2, 159-70.

Hopkins, Anthony / Dudley-Evans, Tony 1988. A Genre-based Investigation of the Discussion Sections in Articles and Dissertations. *English for Specific Purposes* 7/2, 113-21.

Hulteng, John 1973. *The Opinion Function.* New York: Harper and Row.

Hyland, Ken 2002. Genre: Language, Context and Literacy, *Annual Review of Applied Linguistics* 20, 113-35.

Hynds, Ernest 1990. Changes in Editorials: A Study of Three Newspapers, 1955-1985. *Journalism Quarterly* 67/2, 302-12.

Le, Elisabeth 2003. Information Sources as a Persuasive Strategy in Editorials. *Written Communication* 20/4, 478-510.

Magnet, Anne / Carnet Didier in press. Letters to the Editor: Still Vigorous after all These Years? A Presentation of the Genre and a Survey of its Use in a French-speaking Scientific Community. *English for Specific Purposes.*

Relman, Arnold 1984. Dealing with Conflicts of Interest. *New England Journal of Medicine* 310, 1182-3.

Rey, Alain / Rey-Debove Josette (eds) 1984. *Le Petit Robert. Dictionnaire de la Langue Française*. Paris: Robert.

Salager-Meyer, Françoise 2002. Market-place, Self Confidence and Criticism in Medical Editorials. *Revista Canaria de Estudios Ingleses* 44, 45-78.

Sinclair, John 1991. *Collins COBUILD English Language Dictionary.* London: Harper Collins.

Swales, John 1990. *Genre Analysis: English in Academic and Research Settings*. Cambridge: Cambridge University Press.

Van Dijk, Teun 1995. Opinions and Ideologies in Editorials. Paper for the 4th International Symposium of Critical Discourse Analysis. *Language, Social Life and Critical Thought*, Athens. Online on author's homepage, 1-30.

Webber, Pauline 1994. The Function of Questions in Different Medical Journal Genres. *English for Specific Purposes* 13/3, 257-68.

KJERSTI FLØTTUM

Medical Research Articles in the Comparative Perspectives of Discipline and Language[1]

1. Introduction

The main focus of this chapter is personal and polyphonic expressions as manifested in academic discourse. I will show in which ways and to what extent medical research articles may differ linguistically and rhetorically from research articles taken from the disciplines of economics and linguistics. As regards the nature of medical articles, isolated from the discipline perspective, I will also look at similarities and differences between articles written in three different languages: English, French and Norwegian.

The reported observations stem from the KIAP project (short for *Cultural Identities in Academic Prose: language versus discipline-specific*) where the key research issue is whether cultural identities may be identified in academic prose, and, if so, whether these identities are language or discipline-specific in nature. Studies of various linguistic and rhetorical features have been undertaken, with a point of departure in the hypothesis that discipline is more important than language as regards cultural identities.

In the next section, I will present the main research questions of the KIAP project as well as some characteristics of materials and methods. Section 3 will be devoted to quantitative results related to the main features studied, with a special focus on the medical

---

1 Many thanks to Trine Dahl and Torodd Kinn for inspiring and fruitful discussions and for their valuable contributions to the KIAP collaboration. Many thanks also to Sandra Halverson for helpful comments on the English manuscript.

discipline. In Section 4, the quantitative results will be discussed and related to various more qualitative investigations.

2. The KIAP project

2.1. Main research questions

As mentioned in the introduction, the analyses presented in this chapter derive from the KIAP project.[2] Some of the main findings of the project are reported, but with a special focus on medical discourse. The KIAP group has been inspired by many researchers focusing on various rhetorical aspects and contesting the traditional conception of academic discourse as neutral and objective (for instance Bazerman 1988; Swales 1990, 2004; Mauranen 1993; Berkenkotter / Huckin 1995; Hyland 1998, 2000; Salager-Meyer 1999; Salager-Meyer / Alcaraz Ariza / Zambrano 2003; Breivega 2003). Our key research interest is the identification of possible cultural identities as manifested by academic voices in scientific discourse, more specifically in the genre of the research article.

The central questions asked by the KIAP group are related to academic voices, more precisely to authorial presence and stance, to the manifestation of and interaction with other researchers' voices and to the author's presentation and promotion of his/her own research (summed up as *self* and *other* dimensions). We have studied various features such as first person and indefinite pronouns (e.g. Fløttum 2003a; Gjesdal 2003), verbs combined with these pronouns (Fløttum 2003b, 2004a, forthcoming a; Fløttum / Kinn / Dahl forthcoming),

2 KIAP, which is funded by the Norwegian research council (2002-2006), is located at the Department of Romance Studies, University of Bergen. In addition to the information and language technology unit AKSIS, the project has three main members (Trine Dahl, Torodd Kinn and Kjersti Fløttum (head)). We also have a number of national and international partners, as well as several important associated master and PhD candidates. For details and for the KIAP publication list, see our website http://kiap.aksis.uib.no. See also Fløttum / Rastier (2003).

markers of epistemic modality (Vold forthcoming), argumentative connectives (in particular French *donc* ('thus') (Didriksen 2004) and various adversative/concessive connectives (Fløttum 2005a), selected lexemes such as *result* (Fløttum 2004b), metatextual expressions (Dahl 2003, 2004), the construction *let us/let me* + infinitive (Kinn 2005; Fløttum / Kinn / Dahl forthcoming), polyphonic constructions (such as polemic negation and concession (Fløttum 2005a, 2005b) and bibliographical references (Fløttum 2003c, forthcoming b). For further references see Fløttum / Dahl / Kinn (forthcoming) and the KIAP publications list (see footnote 2). Some of the findings of these studies will be presented in Section 3.

In very general terms, our theoretical framework consists of the following orientations (from macro- to micro-level): Our point of departure is the rhetorical perspective on scientific discourse (Prelli 1989); at a more specific level, we take the genre perspective into consideration (Swales 1990; Hyland 2000; Breivega 2003). However, our main analyses are undertaken at the utterance level, to some extent inspired by the French enunciative approaches (Ducrot 1984); at this micro-level, one of our theoretical perspectives is the theory of linguistic polyphony, as developed in ScaPoLine (Nølke / Fløttum / Norén 2004).

With a polyphonic conception of meaning, it is essential to demonstrate how the presence of several voices are signalled in discourse. In the ScaPoLine linguistic version of the theory, the object of study is what is expressed by the utterance as utterance, and the polyphonic structure is to be found at 'langue' (or sentence) level. At the same time, the polyphonic structure gives us instructions as regards possible interpretations of the utterance, at the 'parole' and text level.

The relevance of the polyphonic perspective in the present context is that the author may set up a polyphonic play signalling the presence of both his / her own voice and the voices of others. Different voices are given the floor, if not explicitly (for example, by citation), then by some distinctive mark signalling polyphony. This is a play which the author of course sets up in his / her own way and which represents a subtle way of interaction, where the source of the different voices or points of view is not necessarily explicit. If we take an example like the utterance *The research article is not an interesting object of study,* two points of view are presented: one saying that 'the research article is an interesting object of study' and another qualifying this as 'not valid' – or as 'false'. While the author is responsible for this last (negative) point of view, the isolated utterance does not indicate who is the source of the first (positive) point of view; it might or might not be identified by the context. For the interpretation of the utterance it is of course important to try to determine the different points of view which are manifested and to identify the discourse individuals that are responsible for or constitute the source of these points of view (the author, another researcher, the scientific community, etc.).

2.2. Material and methods

The linguistic and doubly comparative KIAP investigations are based on an electronic corpus of 450 research articles written in English, French and Norwegian within the fields of economics, linguistics and medicine. There are 150 articles per language, and within each language subcorpus, there are 50 articles per discipline. Thus, there are nine subcorpora of refereed articles, from 35 different journals published between 1992 and 2003.[3] The subcorpora have been given labels based on combinations of abbreviations for language (English: eng, French: fr, Norwegian: no) and discipline (economics: econ, linguistics: ling, medicine: med); thus, for instance, engmed means English medicine. In addition, the individual articles are numbered from 01 to 50.

The total number of words is 3.15 million (complete articles). For each discipline and language subcorpus, the number of words of the body part of the text (i.e. the plain text, without abstracts, citations, examples, figures, references, etc.) is as shown in Table 1.

3 As regards the selection of leading specialized journals, we have consulted experts within the three disciplines in question. For more details on the selected journals and articles, see http://torvald.aksis.uib.no/kiap/KIAPCorpus.htm.

Economics subcorpus	907,028	English subcorpus	899,780
Linguistics subcorpus	939,007	French subcorpus	665,665
Medicine subcorpus	404,833	Norwegian subcorpus	685,423
Total for body part of texts:	2,250,868 words		

Table 1. Details of the subcorpora analysed.

For practical reasons, most examples in this chapter will be taken from the engmed subcorpus.

As regards methodological questions, the KIAP project has utilised various exploratory, quantitative and qualitative approaches; both automatic and manual investigations have been undertaken. For automatic searches in the corpus, the language technology unit AKSIS (see http://www.aksis.uib.no/) has developed a custom-made search program and interface that can be accessed over the internet. The corpus search interface allows searches for single words or collocations of two or three words. Without going into further details, I will just mention that searches can be restricted either to one particular article or to sets of articles defined by language, discipline and type of authorship. It is also possible to search in specified parts of the articles (such as the body, the abstract or the discussion) or the whole articles. (For further details, see Fløttum *et al.* forthcoming).

In Section 3.1 I will present the quantitative results of the main features studied, obtained through automatic searches made by the program mentioned above and accompanied by manual corrections. The relatively few features which are represented in Tables 2-6 have been selected through various exploratory and qualitative analyses. The search results have also been accompanied by analyses through statistical methods. Unless otherwise indicated, all differences between corpora that are mentioned are statistically significant ($p < 0.05$, two-tailed Mann-Whitney-Wilcoxon test; for further details, see Fløttum *et al.* forthcoming).

3. Quantitative results

3.1. Main features

In the presentation below, I will focus on the discipline of medicine in contrast to the two other disciplines investigated. Some aspects related to language will also be mentioned. However, for reasons of space, details concerning individual differences (hidden in the general figures) will not be commented on (for various case studies, see KIAP publication list, footnote 2).

In the tables, the relative frequency (%) – referring to the mean of every subcorpus – is calculated as the percentage of the number of occurrences in relation to the total number of words in each subcorpus (body part; see 2.2 above).

3.1.1. First person pronouns – singular and plural

The most direct and explicit indicator of author manifestation is the first person pronoun, singular or plural. Since medical research articles are normally multi-author articles, the first person singular becomes irrelevant here. Let us therefore look at a typical example of the use of first person plural *we*:

(1) We examined the potential role of fetuin on skin tumorigenesis by exploring the ability of fetuin to interact with MMP-3 and SCC cells. (engmed42)

Table 2 (where the subcorpora are ranked for relative frequency) shows that medical authors generally use fewer first person plural subject pronouns than both economists and linguists. I emphasise that the figures in this table are restricted to multi-author articles. Thus, the figures related to linguistics (especially French and Norwegian) are based on very few articles. Most of the articles in the linguistics subcorpora are single-author articles.[4] However, the relative frequency indicates that the discipline of medicine constitutes a cluster at the

4 In the KIAP Corpus, the relations between single-author and multi-author articles in the three disciplines are as follows: Economics: 87/63; Linguistics: 131/19; Medicine: 15/135.

bottom of the ranking displayed in the table (except for frling which comes in between). As regards language, we note that Norwegian and English medical authors use more first person plural pronouns than their French peers.

Subcorpora	*Occurrences*	*Relative frequency (%) Mean*
Noecon	1 230	1.110
Engecon	1 491	0.879
Engling	1 093	0.728
Noling	40	0.512
Frecon	441	0.392
Nomed	272	0.344
Engmed	470	0.303
Frling	21	0.273
Frmed	230	0.203
Total	5 288	0.463

Table 2. Frequency of first person plural personal pronouns (subject) in multi-author articles (*we, nous, vi/me*).

3.1.2. Indefinite pronouns

The use of indefinite pronouns (here: *one, on, man/en/ein* respectively in English, French and Norwegian) is not easily comparable between the three languages, since the use of English *one* is very limited compared to its French and Norwegian counterparts. However, Table 3 displays interesting figures for French and Norwegian.

Subcorpora	*Occurrences*	*Relative frequency (%) Mean*
Frling	1 564	0.680
Frecon	1 213	0.431
Noling	1 019	0.366
Nomed	296	0.277
Noecon	834	0.262
Frmed	238	0.169
Engling	210	0.049
Engecon	108	0.036
Engmed	4	0.001
Total	5 486	0.252

Table 3. Frequency of indefinite subject pronouns (*one, on, man/en/ein*).

The results support the traditional view considering French use of *on* as relatively frequent. However, Norwegian use of the indefinite pronoun is also quite considerable. In particular, we note that nomed uses it more than both noecon and frmed.

Of course, due to their often vague reference, indefinite pronouns constitute a less direct form of author manifestation than first person pronouns (Fløttum 2003a, 2004a). However, the pronoun is relevant since it always represents reference to a more or less indefinite person or group of persons, as in these examples:

(2) *On* peut considérer ces données comme [...]. (frmed03)
('One may consider these data as ...')

(3) *Man* må unngå manipulasjon av hjertet før [...]. (nomed15)
('One must avoid manipulation of the heart before ...')

3.1.3. Metatextextual expressions

Referring in different ways to (parts of) the text itself, metatextual expressions are also relevant as markers of author manifestation. By expressions like *in this article* the author guides the readers through the article itself (see Dahl 2004) and explains what will be done and where (for example *In section 4 we analyse ...*). For methodological reasons, the automatic search and the quantitative analyses were limited to the following expressions (and corresponding expressions in French and Norwegian): *article, paper, (sub)section, above, now, below.*[5] The results indicate very clearly that this feature is more or less absent in medical articles, in all the three languages. There are, however, 47 occurrences in engmed against 8 in frmed and 9 in nomed (in engling there are 1 230!). The following example is from engmed:

(4) This paper compares the characteristics of women who do and do not attend for breast cancer screening [...]. (engmed26)

5 Other metatextual or metadiscoursal expressions are studied in other contexts; see Fløttum *et al.* forthcoming.

3.1.4. Negation

The negation expressions studied are *not* in English, *ne ... pas* in French and *ikke/ikkje* in Norwegian. Let us first look at an example:

(5) The kidney is not, however, a major site of glycogen storage. (engmed45)

In this example a point of view ('The kidney is a major site of glycogen storage') is denied by another point of view, marked by the negation *not* (a contrast between two points of view emphasised by the connective *however*). The author is responsible for the latter point of view; the source of the former is not given. To the extent that negation is used polemically, to refute underlying points of view, it indicates author manifestation as well as the implicit presence of other 'voices'; in other words, there is polyphony in the text (Fløttum 2005b).

The results (cf. Table 4) show, roughly, that linguists use more negation than economists and economists more than medical researchers (however, the differences between economics and medicine are not statistically significant).

Subcorpora	*Occurrences*	*Relative frequency (%) Mean*
Noling	2 604	0.967
Frling	1 541	0.654
Noecon	2 059	0.646
Engling	2 822	0.623
Nomed	628	0.583
Engmed	717	0.442
Engecon	1 194	0.388
Frecon	1 084	0.371
Frmed	511	0.354
Total	13 160	0.559

Table 4. Frequency of negation (*not, ne pas, ikke/ikkje*).

We note that the language factor is also important here. Norwegian and English medical authors use negation more often than French medical authors.

3.1.5. Concessive constructions

The comparison of connectives in different languages necessitates particular semantic-pragmatic considerations. Even if connectives correspond more or less to each other, they often have particular semantic-pragmatic values in different languages. For this reason, we limited the automatic search to the adversative connective *but* and its corresponding connectives in French (*mais*) and Norwegian (*men*). These may also convey different meanings; however, they all have in common a concessive meaning. This is the meaning which is particularly interesting to the KIAP research questions. When concessive, these connectives function as markers of polyphony: the author first makes a concession related to a matter expressed in the sequence preceding *but* (the source of this matter may be different from the author, as indicated by the reference numbers in the example below). Then, the author contrasts it with a succeeding sequence, presented as the most important (the point of view of the author here and now):

(6) The evidence presented in this study of a hypometabolic state in exercising women with LPD is similar to the hypometabolic state observed in amenorrheic athletes (9, 10, 12), *but* it is not as comprehensive. (engmed46)

In this way, concessive constructions contribute to author manifestation and even author positioning. Table 5 presents the quantitative data related to the frequency of the connectives in question.

Subcorpora	*Occurrences*	*Relative frequency (%) Mean*
Noling	1 293	0.463
Frling	870	0.382
Nomed	337	0.325
Engling	1 428	0.319
Noecon	815	0.254
Engecon	592	0.197
Frmed	249	0.181
Engmed	276	0.171
Frecon	513	0.163
Total	6 373	0.273

Table 5. Frequency of adversative conjunctions (*but, mais, men*).

We see that linguistics is the discipline that displays the highest frequency of concessive constructions also. Except for nomed, medicine is at the bottom of the list (frecon, however, is the subcorpus which uses the least of such constructions). Nomed demonstrates a remarkably high frequency compared to engmed and frmed, which are quite close to each other. As regards language, we note that Norwegian has a higher frequency than English in all disciplines.

3.1.6. Bibliographical references

Here I only present the main figures related to the frequency of bibliographical references, without taking into consideration the different types of references and their place in the articles (see Fløttum 2003c, forthcoming b). Without going into details about the importance of bibliographical references in all kinds of academic discourse, I will just mention that medicine is a discipline with a relatively uniform standard.[6] References in a medical article are listed at the end of the article; they are indicated by numbers in the body of the text. In economics and linguistics, references are typically introduced (in different ways) in the text itself. When counting the references referred to (whether introduced by number or by author name + year of publication), we find that medical authors use more references than economists and linguists (this holds for all three languages).

Subcorpora	*Occurrences*	*Relative frequency (%) Mean*
Nomed	1 819	1.837
Engmed	2 663	1.630
Frmed	2 019	1.411
Engling	4 184	0.930
Noling	2 088	0.868
Noecon	1 583	0.493
Frling	1 040	0.485
Frecon	1 366	0.445
Engecon	1 279	0.437
Total	18 041	0.948

Table 6. Frequency of bibliographical references.

6 For interesting studies on medical discourse in general and bibliographical references in particular, see Salager-Meyer 1994, 1999, 2000.

We also see that Norwegian medical authors use more references than their English colleagues (however, this difference is not significant) and English more than French.

3.1.7. Presentation of 'results'

The main quantitative findings presented above have been complemented by different quantitative and qualitative analyses. Here I would like to mention the analyses of the use of words like *result* (verb and noun) and *conclude/conclusion* (and corresponding expressions in the two other languages) (see Fløttum 2004b). The purpose was to study how authors present their own final results, in particular how explicitly they are presented. Our observations show that *conclude/conclusion* are infrequent while *result* (especially as noun) is relatively frequent. As regards disciplinary differences, *result* with the meaning 'final result' is more or less absent in linguistics articles, but quite frequent in medical and especially in economics articles. As regards the language dimension, English authors use the noun *result* most frequently.[7] However, when *result* is used to refer to 'final results', the cotext is typically a 'neutral' one, with few or no colouring personal or evaluative elements:

(7) The results of this study demonstrate a number of such potential mediators. (engmed47)

3.1.8. Markers of epistemic modality

Finally I would like to mention a study undertaken within the KIAP-project (but not yet accomplished), concerning markers of epistemic modality (see Vold forthcoming). Vold's preliminary findings indicate considerable differences between languages (more use in English and Norwegian than in French) but relatively minor differences between disciplines. Some of the expressions studied in English are the following: *may, might, seem, suggest, appear, indicate, perhaps.*

---

7 For English, a search for the commonly used noun *finding(s)* was also undertaken to ensure a more correct picture of the situation. Its frequency was however much lower than for *result*; among the three disciplines studied, medicine was the one which used *finding(s)* most frequently (economics was second and linguistics third).

3.2. Discussion related to cultural identity

In general, our findings show that for cultural identities, discipline has greater influence than language. This means that, for example, there are more similarities between Norwegian and French medical articles than between Norwegian medical and linguistics articles. Statistically both discipline and language have an effect on the frequency of all the six main phenomena studied. However, for most of them, discipline seems to be more important than language. We have also found notable individual differences between articles, even within one discipline and one language.

As regards medical discourse, our findings indicate, in very general terms, that it is different from economics and linguistics discourse. The clearest difference seems to be related to author presence. Medical authors are not very visible in their texts, as compared to their economist and linguist peers. They 'hide' behind passive constructions and impersonal formulations of different kinds. Observations 'present themselves' to a larger extent than in economics and linguistics articles.

In an overall perspective, we may also conclude that medical articles resemble each other to a certain extent, whatever language they are written in. However, we have seen that Norwegian medical authors are more clearly and directly present than English and especially French colleagues as regards selected features (use of first person pronoun, indefinite pronoun, negation and concessive constructions). Nomed is also the subcorpus which displays the highest relative frequency of bibliographical references (however, as mentioned above, the difference between nomed and engmed is not significant).

4. Discussion

Let me start the discussion by relating academic discourse to rhetoric. Research articles are both argumentative and rhetorical, in the sense that, on the one hand, they represent a discourse created in order to induce cooperative attitudes and actions (see Prelli 1989). Academic discourse is created strategically with the purpose of being accepted as reasonable by a particular group. On the other hand, research articles provide the opportunity for the authors to position themselves in or in relation to a particular discourse community. This also implies the evident fact that the research article is addressed, i.e. it is directed towards someone. Given the present situation of tough competition in which research articles are produced, it seems reasonable to expect strategic positioning through explicit argumentation in the texts. However, we do not find much direct argumentation of the type *we argue* or *in this article we have shown* in medical articles. This does not mean that medical researchers do not argue. Argumentation is not to be found only in personal constructions introduced by personal pronouns. Strategies used to convince may also be realised by the presentation of facts or observations in 'neutral' utterances which at first glance appear as both objective and deprived of personal traces, as in *345 patients were included in the study.*

Between the two poles of formulations 1) *we argue that the water is polluted* and 2) *the water holds 15 degrees*, there are formulations such as 3) *the water is not cold* or 4) *the water is warm, but it is polluted.* The polyphonic formulations in 3) and 4) constitute subtle forms of argumentation, where other points of view are brought in and refuted (in 3) or conceded but not considered as important in the situation in question (4). As regards the negation and the concessive constructions investigated in KIAP, we have found that these are quite frequent also in medicine articles (see Tables 4 and 5); they are in fact important rhetorical elements, clearly manifesting author presence.

We can conceive of the research article as a drama, set up exclusively by the authors. Sometimes they assign explicit roles to themselves (as in *we argue*), sometimes they appear to be absent (as in 2 above). In still other cases, they are more clearly present, but with no overt reference to themselves (as in 3 and 4 above). In the latter case, they subtly extend the drama by introducing other players – players that also are only implicitly present.

However, the quantitative findings reported above leave no doubt that medical discourse in all the three languages studied here is less rhetorically explicit than economics and especially linguistics discourses are. Both personal presence and interaction with the readers are weaker in medical articles. This general observation is supported by the various qualitative studies undertaken.

I will first look briefly at the verbs combined with first person pronouns. These verbs indicate that the authors assume various roles, in what I have called the article drama, when referring to themselves by the pronoun *we*. Linguists play at least three different roles, i.e. arguers (*we argue*), writers or readers' guide (*in section 3 we will present)* and researchers (*we analyse, we find*). Economists generally take on only the researcher or the writer roles, while medical authors stick to the researcher role. A further illustration of this: the three most frequent verbs combined with *we* in the multi-author articles studied in KIAP are in engecon *find, assume, use*; in engling *find, argue, see*; in engmed *find, use, examine.*

When we look at how authors of cited articles are 'given the floor' (references to authors' names also occur in medical articles even though they are less frequent there than in economics and linguistics articles), a similar picture emerges. Cited linguists are allowed to *argue* and to *claim* something while cited medical authors (and also to a large extent cited economists) are typically only allowed to *find* or to *show* results and observations.

Various factors may explain this difference between linguistics (and to a certain extent economics) and medicine. I will just mention a few points here (for a more detailed discussion, see Fløttum *et al.* forthcoming). Medical research is more cumulative and need not discuss basic conceptual systems in the same way as linguistics often does. Second, in medicine, the reported research is typically presented as completed when the writing of the article starts; in linguistics, the research is often presented as if it is part of the writing process itself.[8] Third, by adhering strictly to the IMRAD article structure, medical authors need not guide the reader or make explicit transitions from one section to another in the same way as linguists and economists do in their often much more heterogeneously structured articles.

---

8 The form of presentation will of course also depend on whether the paper reports an experimental or a more theoretical research.

In this chapter, we have seen that medical articles are *different,* in the sense that their use of some selected features manifests clear differences in frequency in relation to the same features in articles from economics and linguistics. Unsurprisingly, the most obvious difference is to be found in the use of explicitly personal constructions. However, there are also differences in lexical choices. For example, there is not a single occurrence of the verbs *argue* and *claim* combined with a personal pronoun referring to the authors in KIAP's English medical corpus (all in all only 3 occurrences of *argue* and 1 of *claim*), while in the English linguistics corpus there are nearly 350 occurrences of *argue* used in both first (singular and plural) and third person constructions and nearly 570 occurrences of *claim* used as either verb or noun.

I have also maintained that these findings do not mean that the medical articles are deprived of argumentation. However, the argumentation is more subtle and implicit than in linguistics. There are two argumentative and rhetorical devices which deserve attention in this context: syntactic negation (*not*) and concessive constructions (with *but* and *however*). Authors use negation to position themselves; authors use concession to concede an external point of view (in rhetorical terms, to invite cooperative attitudes and actions) and, at the same time, to signal their own point of view as the most important one.

To conclude, I should point to some limitations of our results. The selection of features does not allow us to claim that the results present a general characterisation of the corpus. Nevertheless, we think that for our focus, i.e. person manifestation, the selection is relevant. Furthermore, our results confirm our main hypothesis: to the extent that it is possible to talk about cultural identities in academic discourse, discipline seems more important than language. However, much of the variation can be explained neither by discipline nor language. Variables such as age, position, subdisciplines, subject and journal instructions constitute other possible explanatory factors.

References

Bazerman, Charles 1988. *Shaping Written Knowledge. The Genre and Activity of the Experimental Article in Science*. Madison, WI: University of Wisconsin Press.

Berkenkotter, Carol / Huckin, Thomas N. 1995. *Genre Knowledge in Disciplinary Communication: Cognition / Culture / Power*. Hillsdale, NJ: Lawrence Erlbaum.

Breivega, Kjersti R. 2003. *Vitskapelege argumentasjonsstrategiar. Ein komparativ analyse av superstrukturelle konfigurasjonar i medisinske, historiske og språkvitskaplege artiklar*. Sakprosa 8. Oslo: Norsk sakprosa.

Dahl, Trine 2003. Metadiscourse in Research Articles. In Fløttum / Rastier (eds), 120-138.

Dahl, Trine 2004. Textual Metadiscourse in Research Articles: A Marker of National Culture or of Academic Discipline? *Journal of Pragmatics* 36/10, 1807-1825.

Didriksen, Anders A. 2004. *DONC et autres connecteurs argumentatifs dans les articles de recherche français*. Master's thesis. Department of Romance studies, University of Bergen.

Ducrot, Oswald 1984. *Le dire et le dit*. Paris: Minuit.

Fløttum, Kjersti 2003a. Personal English, Indefinite French and Plural Norwegian Scientific Authors? Pronominal Author Manifestation in Research Articles: A Cross-linguistic Disciplinary Study. *Norsk Lingvistisk Tidsskrift* 21/1, 21-55.

Fløttum, Kjersti 2003b. JE et le verbe. *Tribune* 14, 7-14.

Fløttum, Kjersti 2003c. Bibliographical References and Polyphony in Research Articles. In Fløttum / Rastier (eds), 97-119.

Fløttum, Kjersti 2004a. La présence de l'auteur dans les articles scientifiques: étude des pronoms *je, nous* et *on*. In Auchlin, A. *et al.* (eds) *Structures et discours*. Québec: Ed. Nota Bene, 401-416.

Fløttum, Kjersti 2004b. The Expression of 'Results' in Scientific Discourse – A Cross-linguistic and Cross-disciplinary Analysis. Paper given at Societas Linguistica Europaea 37th International Meeting, Kristiansand 29.07-01.08.2004.

Fløttum, Kjersti 2005a. The Self and the Others – Polyphonic Visibility in Research Articles. *International Journal of Applied Linguistics* 15/1, 29-44.

Fløttum, Kjersti 2005b. MOI et AUTRUI dans le discours scientifique: l'exemple de la négation NE...PAS. In Bres, J. *et al.* (eds) *Dialogisme, polyphonie: approches linguistiques.* De Boeck-Duculot, 323-337.

Fløttum, Kjersti forthcoming a. The Typical Research Article – Does it Exist? In E. Suomela-Salmi (ed.) *Cross-cultural and Cross-linguistic Perspectives on Academic Discourse.* Turku. University of Turku.

Fløttum, Kjersti forthcoming b. Interrelation de voix internes et externes dans le discours. In L. Perrin (éd.) *Dialogisme et polyphonie en langue et en discours.* Metz: Recherches Linguistiques.

Fløttum, Kjersti / Dahl, Trine / Kinn, Torodd forthcoming. *Academic Voices across Languages and Disciplines.*

Fløttum, Kjersti / Kinn, Torodd / Dahl, Trine forthcoming. 'We now report on …' versus 'Let us now see how …'. Author Roles and Interaction with Readers in Research Articles. In Hyland, Ken / Bondi, Marina (eds) *Academic Discourse across Disciplines.* Bern: Peter Lang.

Fløttum, Kjersti / Rastier, François (eds) 2003. *Academic Discourse. Multidisciplinary Approaches.* Oslo: Novus Press.

Gjesdal, Anje M. 2003. *L'emploi du pronom 'on' dans les articles de recherche. Une étude diachronique et qualitative.* Master thesis. Department of Romance studies, University of Bergen.

Hyland, Ken 1998. *Hedging in Scientific Research Articles.* Amsterdam: Benjamins.

Hyland, Ken 2000. *Disciplinary Discourses: Social Interactions in Academic Writing.* Harlow, UK: Longman.

Kinn, Torodd 2005. Tilbod og innbydingar: imperativ med *la* i forskingsartiklar. *Norsk Lingvistisk Tidsskrift* 23, 145-175.

Mauranen, Anna 1993. *Cultural Differences in Academic Rhetoric.* Frankfurt am Main: Peter Lang.

Nølke, Henning / Fløttum, Kjersti / Norén, Coco 2004. *ScaPoLine. La théorie scandinave de la polyphonie linguistique.* Paris: Kimé.

Prelli, Lawrence J. 1989. *A Rhetoric of Science: Inventing Scientific Discourse*. University of South Carolina Press.

Salager-Meyer, Françoise 1994. Hedges and Textual Communicative Function in Medical English Written Discourse. *English for Specific Purposes* 13/2, 149-170.

Salager-Meyer, Françoise 1999. Referential Behaviour in Scientific Writing: A Diachronic Study (1810-1995). *English for Specific Purposes* 18/3, 279-305.

Salager-Meyer, Françoise 2000. Debate-Creating vs. Accounting References in French Medical Journals. *Technical Communication Quarterly* 9/3, 291-310.

Salager-Meyer, Françoise / Alcaraz Ariza, María Ángeles / Zambrano, Nahirana 2003. The Scimitar, the Dagger and the Glove: Intercultural Differences in the Rhetoric of Criticism in Spanish, French and English Medical Discourse (1930-1995). *English for Specific Purposes* 22, 223-247.

Swales, John M. 1990. *Genre Analysis. English in Academic and Research Settings*. Cambridge: Cambridge University Press.

Swales, John M. 2004. *Research Genres. Explorations and Applications*. Cambridge: Cambridge University Press.

Vold, Eva Thue forthcoming. Epistemic Modality Markers in Research Articles: A Cross-linguistic and Cross-disciplinary Study. *International Journal of Applied Linguistics*.

DAVID R. HALL

Medical Leaflets, Empowerment and Disempowerment[1]

1. Introduction

In the medical field, there has been a major change in the last decade or so in the amount of information made available to people other than the traditional learned intermediaries – the doctors, pharmacists and other medical workers. Many countries have adopted policies which mandate that adequate information be made available about treatments, medication and surgical procedures so that people can participate in an informed way in the management of their own health. The growth of electronically-mediated information means that even where such policies do not exist, it is much easier now for people to find relevant (and irrelevant) data. The sources of data, however, whether electronic or print-based, and their reliability and objectivity are not always as transparent as they need to be. This chapter examines printed medical leaflets as one example of this lack of transparency and shows how they a play a role in the continuing struggle between the medical establishment and advocates of patient empowerment.

I have been involved for some time in the provision of written medical information, following an approach over ten years ago by various pharmaceutical companies and the Australian Pharmaceutical Manufacturers Association to help them meet the then new requirements that information about prescription drugs should be given in an 'easily readable' form. I have since worked not only with

1 I would like to thank the editors of this volume and Dr Alison Rotha Moore of Macquarie University for their perceptive and constructive comments on an early draft of this chapter.

this kind of mandatory information about pharmaceutical products, but also with general information leaflets (for example, for the Australian Association of Asthma Foundations), instructions for use, standard operating procedures, and internal company documents such as mission and vision statements.

Through all of this, my primary concern has been with the readability of the documents, and the underlying motivation has been empowerment. The notion of 'empowerment' has been called "the cornerstone of contemporary health care" (Brennan / Safran 2003: 301) and is often used as a theoretical and practical underpinning of moves towards greater disclosure:

> Patient empowerment is a high priority for healthcare policy makers in many countries. By increasing the role of patients, health care providers should become more responsive to patients' needs and preferences and deliver better quality care. (Wensing 2000: 200)

There have been many studies on the positive effects of patient empowerment in the management of particular conditions (eg Ayres *et al.* 1994; Anderson *et al.* 1995; Lorig *et al.* 1999; Trummer *et al.* 2003; Danholt *et al.* 2004). The idea has a long history and has deep roots in the sociology of medicine, though it has more recently come under attack, as will be shown below. The present research, however, points to a conclusion that empowerment has not always been the consequence of the more widespread availability of information. The original intention of those who have lobbied for greater transparency appears to have been taken over for other purposes, and the cloak of empowerment is used to hide the maintenance of control in the hands of the powerful.

This chapter will explore this issue in the context of the very real problems that face anyone involved in the preparation of documentation that attempts to link professional and lay discourse.

2. Data collection

There are at least three kinds of 'consumer information' documents that are available when a member of the public consults a medical practitioner and is prescribed a course of treatment. When the consumer buys the prescribed medication, it will normally be accompanied by documentation giving details of how the medication is used, what it does, what side-effects it might have, what contraindications there are, the name of the pharmaceutical company that produces the medication, and so on. There is a mandatory standard format for such information in Australia and in many other countries. I have concluded elsewhere that this standard format with its frequent exhortations to "see your doctor or pharmacist" militates against the effectiveness and usefulness of these consumer product information documents (Hall 1995).

Second, there is documentation that the doctor may have available in his or her office and may choose to give the consumer. This includes, for example, general printed material about diet, exercise, health management or information about specific conditions. This documentation is under the control of the doctor and is provided to the patient on the professional authority of the doctor. There is evidence that information given in this form is effective in improving communication between doctors and patients; Little *et al.* (2004: 441), for example, report that

> Among patients who received a general leaflet, satisfaction was increased, particularly when consultation time was short; the number of investigations was higher; and there was a small increase in consultation time.

Third, there is documentation available in the doctor's waiting-room, normally on display in racks and which the consumer may choose to pick up, take away and read. This is freely available. People waiting in the doctor's waiting-room may pick these leaflets up because they are relevant to their own condition or that of a friend or family member, because they are attracted by the glossy presentation or catchy 'tag-line', or simply because they want to have something to read as they wait.

Although I have worked as a co-author/editor on both of the first types of documentation, it is the last type that has attracted my interest in recent times, mainly because it is in these leaflets that the idea of the provision of disinterested empowering information is at its most questionable. In work that I had done previously with the Australian Association of Asthma Foundations on the production of a dozen different asthma leaflets aimed at different audiences (such as parents, teachers, children, sports trainers, etc), I believed that such leaflets were a good example where the stakeholders genuinely did want to communicate with their audience, providing useful information and, to an extent at least, empowering people by giving them the information they needed to talk with their doctor and combat the various myths about the illness. In examining the waiting-room leaflets in the present study, it was originally my intention to investigate the sorts of information presented, how easy that information is to understand and what action the leaflets are likely to provoke in the reader. In other words, the intention was to examine readability and effectiveness. Analysis, however, revealed something rather different.

The leaflets, about forty in all, were collected from various waiting-rooms in doctors' surgeries on the north shore of Sydney over the period 2004 to 2005. All were freely available from display-style racks.

3. Analysis of the leaflets

In looking at the leaflets, the most obvious thing is that they are, with a few exceptions, all glossy and all the same size. This similarity, however, hides some major differences. Far from offering empowering advice, many leaflets are in fact advertisements for the products of one company. Sometimes this is relatively obvious, as in one document that is quite clearly an advert for Flora margarine (see Appendix 1), with the name prominently displayed on the front page, and the products pictured on the back. In such cases, there is a link to claimed medical benefits, and this, accompanied by the placement of advertisements in the racks, carries the strong implication that the medical professionals endorse these claims. In the case of the Flora advertisement, the words *cholesterol* and *heart health* are in the largest font on the front page, while the internal pages of the leaflet have features such as medical-style diagrams of internal organs, a graph showing cholesterol, and prominent use of words such as *scientific*, *proven* and *research*.

Sometimes, however, the fact that the leaflet is in reality an advertisement is not so obvious. A leaflet called 'Acne can be cured' (see Appendix 2) is devoted to urging people to take medication for acne. The substance of the document points very strongly to the conclusion that only medication can cure acne. Washing, eating less fatty foods, sun-baking or other lifestyle modifications will not make any difference – only medication is effective. If over-the-counter treatments do not work, then you should go to your doctor and get more powerful medication, which may take "a few months" before you start noticing a difference. If that doesn't work, then the solution is an even more powerful product, available through a specialist dermatologist. Only in the fine print – and it is very fine print – do we see that the leaflet is produced by Roche Products Limited. There is a prominent link to a website – www.acnecanbecured.com.au – where much of the same information can be found, although the site is much more clearly targeted at adolescents, with images of young people in bathing suits, and where a page called 'Cool links' connects the reader to other product-oriented sites, including that of a magazine with a focus on selling cosmetics to pubescent girls.

Most leaflets have a certain ambiguity about them. A particularly pertinent example is a leaflet on Osteoporosis and Calcium (see Appendix 3). This leaflet has many of the accoutrements of a disinterested public-good information leaflet. It has a series of question-and-answer sections: 'Why do we need calcium?', 'Could I be at risk of developing Osteoporosis?', 'Can Osteoporosis be prevented?' and so on. These features are all typical of well-written documents designed to communicate, raise awareness and cause the reader to take action. At the same time, the leaflet asserts its authoritativeness and seriousness through the use of small-font footnotes referring to the medical literature.

On closer examination, however, the leaflet is as much a persuasive promotion for the products of the company as the acne brochure. The whole purpose of this leaflet is to persuade you that you need more calcium than you are currently getting, and that this should be in the form of the company's products. There are two key sections that push the reader to a 'solution' of taking the product that is being advertised. The first has this sentence:

(1) A lot of people think having a few cups of tea or coffee with milk per day plus a yoghurt is enough, but it isn't.

Note that this is very careful not to say: "A lot of people think that they can get enough calcium through their normal dietary intake, but they can't", because this wouldn't be true, but this conclusion is strongly implied by the actual sentence used. "A few cups of tea [...] plus a yoghurt" is treated in the second clause as though it were literally only this combination of dietary intake that is being talked about. From a legal point of view it would not be difficult to show that there is nothing dishonest about this sentence. From a pragmatic point of view, however, it is clear that the first part of the sentence is meant as an example of the sort of intake people might have in mind when they're thinking about calcium. By implication it therefore misleadingly extends to anything that the misguided reader might consider to be sufficient calcium intake as a normal part of dietary intake.

The last section of the leaflet poses the question: "Is your diet providing adequate calcium?" The implied answer to this is "No", but the question is not directly answered at all. Instead, there is this sentence:

(2) Many people limit their intake of these calcium rich foods due to personal dislikes, avoidance of fats, cholesterol, or lactose, or simply dieting for weight control.

In this way, calcium intake through normal diet is linked with undesirables such as weight gain, cholesterol and dislikeable food. The inevitable solution to this unsatisfactory state of affairs is then found:

(3) Taking a calcium supplement such as Caltrate is a simple, economical way to ensure you get adequate calcium every day.

A fourth leaflet – 'Caring for your eczema' (see Appendix 2) – comes very much closer to the idea of disinterested information. It is produced by the Eczema Association of Australia and contains information about bathing, clothing and itching as well as over-the-counter creams, pharmaceutical products and bandaging. It also has a section – albeit rather brief and casual – mentioning alternative treatments, including Chinese, naturopathic, homeopathic and stress-relief treatments. Even this leaflet, however, is not completely disinterested. On the first inside page, there is an announcement that the brochure is supported by a company that produces Eczema Cream and although the brand name is not mentioned anywhere else in the leaflet, the announcement is accompanied by a colour image of the company's products taking up about one third of the page, and the leaflet mentions that "sufferers now have a choice of products with all natural ingredients" of the kind produced by the sponsor.

4. Genre misrepresentation – a pragmatic fraud?

It might be argued that information cannot be free of bias and that everyone understands that a leaflet carrying the name of a pharmaceutical company is going to present information in a way that will promote the use of its products, but I believe that there is a cause for concern when one genre is presented in the clothing of another, and I believe that this is wider than the case of these leaflets.

In Australia, there have been several cases of such misrepresentation of genre. A series of television news stories about the dangers of bacteria in the kitchen – complete with a helpful remote video recording of a cat walking around the food-preparation surface of a kitchen while the owner's back was turned – turned out to have been placed by a company that was planning to introduce antibacterial kitchen wipes into the Australian market. Similarly there have been several exposés of so-called 'cash-for-comments' arrangements apparently common in talkback radio, whereby a company pays an announcer to make favourable comments about its products disguised as editorial comments (or private opinion) without revealing the payment. Similar also are those documents (most of them turning out to be from *Readers Digest*) that suggest you have won some major lucky draw, where the packaging as well as the language used attempt to hide the enticement to subscribe or to purchase behind the more alluring disguise of the announcement of a winning lottery number.

There is little doubt that large numbers of people are taken in by this kind of genre-bending. It is tempting to call it fraudulent, except that it is not fraud in any literal sense, since the authors are very careful not to make fraudulent claims. Phrases such as "you *may* be at risk", "it *can* proceed without symptoms", "a high level *can* cause problems", "these factors *may* increase your risk", "*usually* there are no serious complications, *but…*" (my emphases throughout) are common, and generally the leaflets use more hedging than Hampton Court Gardens. This certainly offers legal protection by putting limits (when read carefully) on the claims being made.

But it might be justified to call this sort of generic misrepresentation a *pragmatic fraud*, since its aim is to induce one kind of reaction when ostensibly it presents itself as reassuring or disinterested (and empowering) information.

5. Social models of medicine

It has long been contended that in the medical model of patient treatment, where a medical problem "is defined in terms of deviation from statistical norms" (White 2004: 29), it is insufficient for explanatory, diagnostic or treatment purposes to treat these norms purely as they relate to biological and anatomical features. Sociological and cultural norms play a large part in both the actual experience and occurrence of disease and the perception of that disease. Engels' contention in *The Condition of the Working Class in England* that sickness and disease are the product of social organisation is just as valid today as it was in the nineteenth century. Poverty maintains the social and physical conditions in which disease can flourish, with poor sanitation, cramped conditions, airless and polluted environments, unsafe or inadequate water supply, and food of inadequate nutritional value. This is compounded by a lack of adequate resources, with few doctors and other health workers, low levels of access to affordable medication and in many places little access to education. There is also a disempowerment "to make healthy decisions on such things as smoking, drugs, alcohol, diet or exercise" (Schrader 2004: 17). The efforts of international aid agencies and charity organisations and sporadic global campaigns to eradicate poverty appear to have made little impact.

These inequalities are not confined to global differences between the 'third world' and wealthy countries. The gap between rich and poor is also to be seen in the developed and prosperous west. As Schrader (2004: 17) points out, "Government socio-economic policies impact in myriad ways upon wealth distribution, inequalities and the health of the population". Wilkinson and Pickett suggest that in wealthy countries, the major determinant of different levels of health status is the degree of income inequality within the nation:

> [C]ountries with smaller differences in income enjoy longer life-expectancy and better educational standards. … [S]uch societies also enjoy better health, stronger social capital, and lower rates of violence and teenage births.
> (Wilkinson / Pickett 2006: 1127)

Many other writers have noted the relationship between neo-liberal policies, income inequality and health (e.g. Coburn 2000; Kelleher 2002; Schrader 2004; Labonte 2004; Franco *et al.* 2004).

Weber's notion of *Verstehen* has had considerable influence. By this term, he "meant that sociological research had to account not only for the regularities and observable patterns of social life but also for the meanings and intentions of the social actors" (White 2004: 30). This view has been followed up in many more recent studies, particularly, but by no means only, in feminist, black and queer studies. Susan Sontag's 1978 book *Illness as Metaphor* is one such study. Anyone who has studied medicine and health sciences in recent years will have noticed the increased emphasis on wellness, prevention, communication, social-psychological and political issues as an addition to the understanding of body systems and the treatment of disease. A book such as Schön's *The Reflective Practitioner* (1983) is one of many advocating the abandonment of a narrow medical view. His major concerns are characterised as follows:

> Professional practice – whether it be that of the lawyer, engineer or gerontologist – has been so grounded in instrumental rationalism and the science of convention that the actions of practitioners often become nothing more than the identification of a problem which is to be solved by applying one or other of the prescribed rules in the [...] 'store of professional knowledge'. (Battersby 1998: 24)

A similar broadening beyond the merely medical can be seen in attitudes towards mental health, where

> A full understanding [...] requires a research perspective that includes not only genetic, biochemical and neurological factors but also the interpersonal and cultural environments in which people live and the mental processes by which they comprehend that world, interpret their experiences, and plan their actions. (National Institute of Mental Health in the United States 1995, cited in Bloch / Singh 1997: 37)

At a global political level, similarly inclusive sentiments are constantly reiterated, and are enshrined in documents such as *The Ottawa Charter for Health Promotion* which adopted the following definition of health promotion:

> Health promotion is the process of enabling people to increase control over, and to improve, their health. To reach a state of complete physical, mental and social well-being, an individual or group must be able to identify and to realize aspirations, to satisfy needs, and to change or cope with the environment. Health is, therefore, seen as a resource for everyday life, not the objective of living. Health is a positive concept emphasizing social and personal resources, as well as physical capacities. Therefore, health promotion is not just the responsibility of the health sector, but goes beyond healthy life-styles to well-being. (Canadian Public Health Association 1986)

Despite this general endorsement, progress on the ground has not been as substantial as had been hoped:

> [W]hile the messages of lifestyle and personal behaviour have been taken on board by much of the population, and there is correspondingly greater awareness of the need for personal responsibility for health, the ability of many people to act upon this knowledge and understanding is generally severely limited by the absence of a conducive cultural, social and economic environment (Ziglio *et al.* 2000: 146).

I would contend that a powerful reason for the difficulty is that such health promotion attitudes, where individuals and their relationships to others are viewed as an integral part of a holistic approach to health and well-being, are constantly undermined by the medical establishment: "the technology of the pharmaceutical industry [and] the subtle compliance of medical practitioners" contribute to a feeling that "for every ailment there is a drug to cure it" (Carroll 2000: 26). While medical studies, sociology, psychology, gerontology, feminist studies and health promotion more generally are moving away from a uniquely medicalised view of the body, much of the medical establishment, and especially the pharmaceutical manufacturing industry, has a vested interest in undermining any approach that is not based on diagnosis of the disease followed by prescription of the medication. This is why "the balance of research effort is still tilted towards disease rather than health creation" (Ziglio *et al.* 2000: 146).

6. Information and empowerment

It is clear that the leaflets examined in this study not only promote particular pharmaceutical products, they more generally underline and reinforce the medicalised view. The Caltrate leaflet is a perfect illustration of the points made by Coney (1991). She points out that pharmaceutical companies promote the idea of a 'silent epidemic' of osteoporosis. As she says, "Osteoporosis sells things" such as calcium supplements and hormone replacement therapy, and it sells even more if we can be "persuaded to feel anxious, fragile and prey to a host of unpleasant diseases [thereby] [...] worrying ourselves half to death" (Coney 1991 cited in Sceriha 1996: 63).

Far from empowering readers, many of these leaflets have as one of their major goals the creation of fear and anxiety. For example, the Osteoporosis and Calcium leaflet has a nine-item yes-no "one-minute risk test" with questions such as "Have you broken a bone after a minor bump or fall?" and "Do you regularly drink heavily?" An affirmative answer to any one of the nine means that "you may be at risk of getting osteoporosis" (note the unobtrusive modality).

Consumer groups lobbying for greater access to information about treatments and medication have often invoked the concept of empowerment. The provision of information leaflets is to some degree a response to this consumer demand. The present analysis of medical leaflets supports some of the more theoretical critiques of empowerment that have been made in recent years. Such recent criticisms have arisen from Foucauldian conceptions of the nature of power and ownership. Payne (1991) says: "empowerment concentrates on developing clients' capacities and does not seek direct change in oppressive social structure", while Rees (1991) suggests that "empowerment may give the illusion of equality while in fact leaving the authoritarian nature of the practitioner-client relationship intact" (both cited in Solas 1996: 151). It seems to me that this is exactly what the advertising material dressed up as an information leaflet does. It creates the illusion – through misrepresentation of genre – that readers can self-diagnose, weigh risks and make informed choices through their access to authoritative information, but its real purpose is to persuade readers that whatever their health problem, whether they have a specific condition or are members of an at-risk population, the solution in the form of a purchasable product is at hand.

By presenting a relatively small number of circumscribed choices, the illusion of freedom is dangled before the consumer, but genuine freedom to examine the larger sociological and political issues is not even raised as a possibility. Those who campaign for more comprehensive approaches to health care have often had to turn to political action to have their voices heard. Frank Capra in the United States, for example, has devoted himself for the last twenty years to being an advocate for change in social, political, media and public health policy, following the publication of his 1983 book *Turning Point: Science, Society and the Rising Culture.* If the medical establishment and the vested interests of the pharmaceutical companies prefer to adopt the assumption that poor health is simply a matter of individual selection among a circumscribed set of prescribed treatments, then they ignore the evidence that social and political contexts are significant determinants of health. The notions of identity and control (our position in society and how we establish and maintain that position) are major factors in how we experience well-being (Labonte 1997: 15) and these are key issues that are ignored, marginalised or otherwise undermined by the relentless reification and commodification displayed in the leaflets examined in this study.

References

Anderson, R.M. / Funnell, M.M. / Butler, P.M. / Arnold, M.S. / Fitzgerald, J.T. / Feste, C.C. 1995. Patient Empowerment. Results of a Randomized Controlled Trial. *Diabetes Care* 18/7, 943-9.

Ayres, A. / Hoon, P.W. 1994. Influence of Mood and Adjustment to Cancer on Compliance with Chemotherapy among Breast Cancer Patients. *Journal of Psychosomatic Research* 38/5, 393-402.

Battersby, David 1998. Successful Ageing: Issues and Challenges. In Bevan, Celia / Jeeawody, Basseer (eds) *Successful Ageing: Perspectives on Health and Social Construction.* Artarmon: Mosby, 4-34.

Bloch, Sidney / Singh, Bruce S. 1997. *Understanding Troubled Minds*. Melbourne: Melbourne University Press.

Brennan, Patti / Safran, Charles 2003. Report of Conference Track 3: Patient Empowerment. *International Journal of Medical Informatics* March, 301-4.

Canadian Public Health Association 1986. *Ottawa Charter for Health Promotion.* Ottawa: World Health Organization, Health and Welfare Canada.

Capra, Frank 1983. *Turning Point: Science, Society and the Rising Culture.* New York: Bantam Books.

Carroll, Charles R. 2000. *Drugs in Modern Society.* Boston: McGraw-Hill.

Coburn, David 2000. Income Inequality, Social Cohesion and the Health Status of Populations: The Role of Neo-liberalism. *Social Science and Medicine* 51, 135-46.

Coney, Sandra 1991. *The Menopause Industry: How the Medical Establishment Exploits Women.* Alameda, CA: Hunter House.

Danholt, Peter / Bødker, Keld / Hertzum, Morten / Simonsen, Jesper 2004. Healthcare IT and Patient Empowerment : The Case of Diabetes Treatment. In van den Besselaar, P. / Bond, A. / de Cindio, F. / Clement, A. / Schuler, D. (eds) *Artful Integration : Interweaving Media, Materials and Practices.* PDC 2004 Proceedings. Volume II, Palo Alto, CA: 80-3.

Franco, Àlvaro / Álvarez-Dardet, Carlos / Ruiz, Maria Teresa 2004. Effect of Democracy on Health: Ecological Study. *British Medical Journal* 329, 1421-3.

Hall, David R. 1995. Technical Information for Consumers: The Case of the Pharmaceutical Industry. In Bruthiaux, Paul / Boswood, Tim / Du-Babcock, Bertha (eds) *Explorations in English for Professional Communication.* Hong Kong: City University Hong Kong, 187-96.

Kelleher, Cecily. 2002. How Exactly Do Politics Play a Part in Determining Health? New Perspectives on an Age Old Issue. *Journal of Epidemiology and Community Health* 56, 726.

Labonte, Ronald 2004. Social Inclusion/Exclusion: Dancing the Dialectic. *Health Promotion International* 19/1, 115-203.

Little, Paul / Dorward, Martina / Warner, Greg / Moore, Michael / Stephens, Katharine / Senior, Jane / Kendrick, Tony 2004. Randomised Controlled Trial of Effect of Leaflets to Empower Patients in Consultations in Primary Care. *British Medical Journal* 328, 441.

Lorig, K. / Sobel, D. / Stewart, A. / Brown Jr, B. / Ritter, P. / González, V / Laurent, D. / Holman, H. 1999. Evidence Suggesting that a Chronic Disease Self-management Program can Improve Health Status while Reducing Utilization and Costs: A Randomized Trial. *Medical Care* 37/1, 5-14.

Payne, Malcolm 1991. *Modern Social Work Theory: A Critical Introduction*. London: Macmillan.
Rees, Stuart 1991. *Achieving Power: Practice and Policy in Social Welfare*. Sydney: Hale & Iremonger.
Sceriha, Madge 1996. *Women and Violence. Working for Change.* Sydney: Hale & Iremonger.
Schön, Donald A. 1983. *The Reflective Practitioner: How Professionals Think in Action*. New York: Basic Books.
Schrader, Tracy 2004. Poverty and Health in Australia. *New Doctor* 80, 17-9.
Solas, John 1996. The Limits of Empowerment in Human Service Work. *Australian Journal of Social Issues* 31/2, 147-56.
Sontag, Susan 1978. *Illness as Metaphor*. New York: Farrar, Straus & Giroux.
Trummer, U. / Nowak, P. / Pelikan, J.M. 2003. Effects of Patient Empowerment on Health Outcome and Patient Satisfaction among Surgery Patients. *Quality of Life Research* 12/7, 801.
Wensing, M. 2000. Evidence-based Patient Empowerment. *Quality in Health Care* 9, 200-1.
White, Kevin. 2004. The Social Origins of Illness and the Development of the Sociology of Health. In Grbich, Carol (ed.) *Health in Australia: Sociological Concepts and Issues*. Sydney: Prentice Hall, 28-45.
Wilkinson, Richard 1996. *Unhealthy Societies: The Afflictions of Inequality* London: Routledge.
Wilkinson, Richard / Pickett, Kate 2006. Health Inequalities and the UK Presidency of the EU. *The Lancet* 367/9517, 1126-8.
Ziglio, E. / Hagard, S / Griffiths, J. 2000. Health Promotion Development in Europe: Achievements and Challenges. *Health Promotion International*. 15/2, 143-154.

Appendix 1

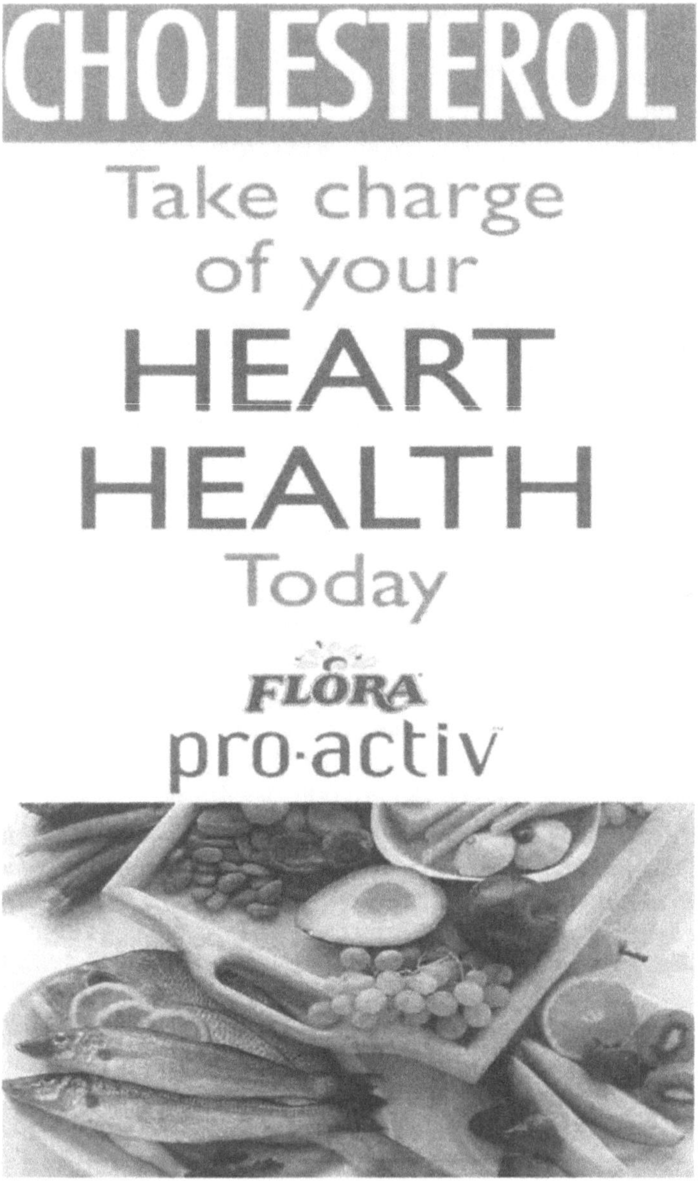
CHOLESTEROL
Take charge
of your
HEART
HEALTH
Today
FLORA
pro·activ

Appendix 2

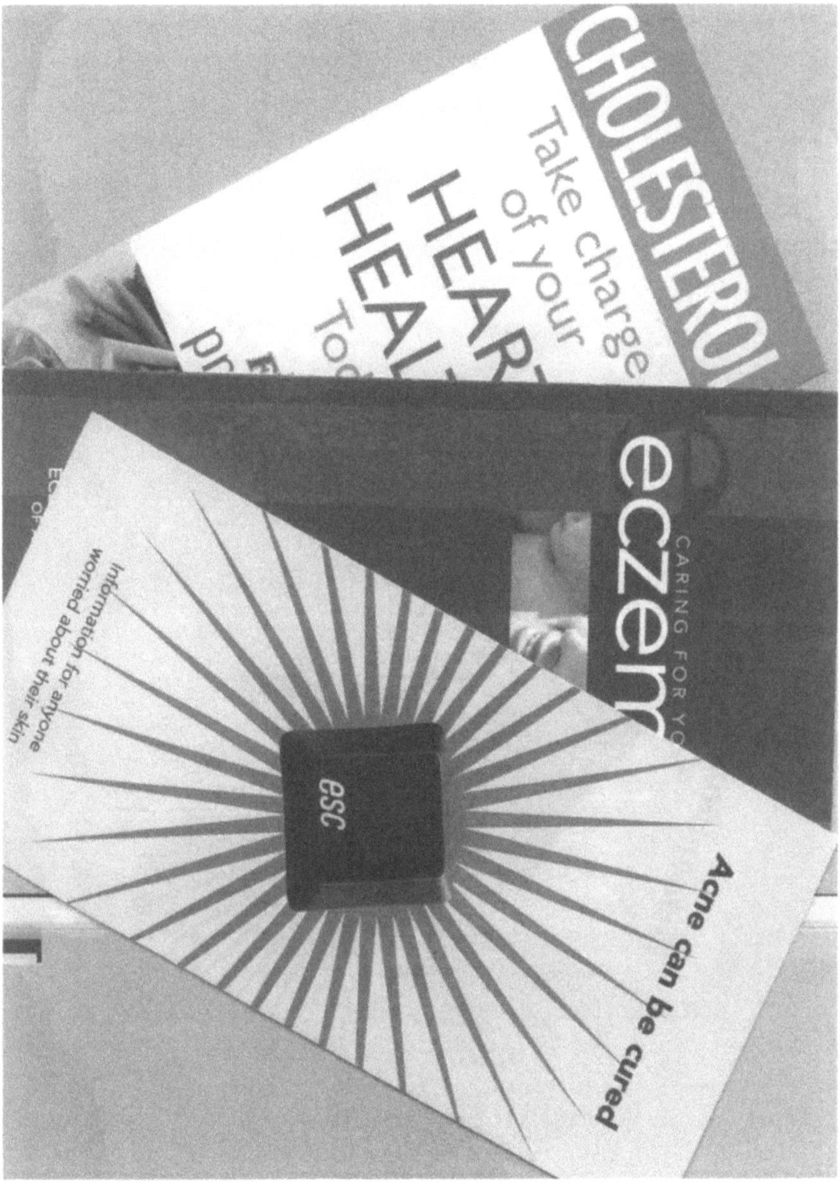
Take charge
of your
Acne can be cured
esc
Information for anyone
worried about their skin

Appendix 3

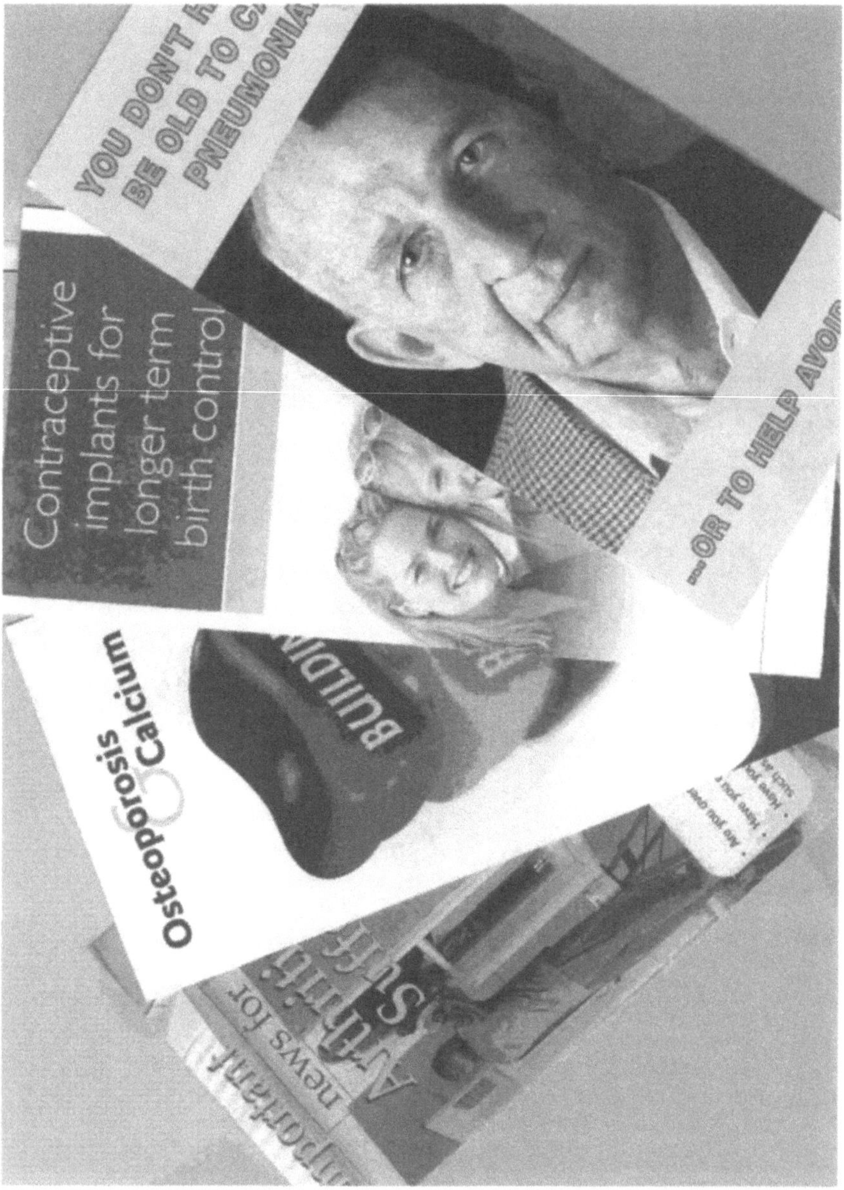
Contraceptive implants for longer term birth control
Osteoporosis & Calcium

ISABEL K. LEÓN / LOURDES DIVASSON

Nominal Domain in the Biomedical Research Paper: A Grammatico-rhetorical Study of Postmodification

1. Introduction and objectives

Those elements traditionally known as noun phrases (NP) or noun groups are defined as structural units used for referring to entities, i.e. the mental representations of extra-linguistic concepts, things or beings. While the prominent role of the nominal domain in scientific prose does not appear to have been questioned, the NP has been extensively dealt with in general and literary language, but has received relatively little attention in scientific, academic and professional discourse. This lack of attention is somehow surprising considering the pioneering role of scientific discourse studies in LSP research (see Varantola 1984, De Haan 1989).

A large number of the studies conducted so far on specialized languages, Medical English (ME) among them, have conventionally followed a lexical approach, focusing either on terminological aspects (Salager-Meyer 1985b, Cabré 1998, Percebois 1999, Esteve Ramos 2001) or on textual and discoursal ones (Crookes 1986, Bhatia 1993, Búllow-Møller 1995, Biber 2001), whereas the communicative potential of syntax (Gerbert 1970, Salager-Meyer 1985a, Jucker 1992) has been somehow neglected since Barber's paper (1962). Most syntactic research about special purpose languages have traditionally dealt with sentential or verbal features (Huddleston 1971, Swales 1976, Heslot 1982, Malcolm 1987, Tarone *et al.* 1998) to the detriment of nominal syntax.

The lack of research on this structural aspect has perhaps been motivated by the extremely complex and versatile nature of the NP.

Be that as it may, as has been observed by many (De Haan 1989, 1993, Giorgi / Longobardi 1991, Rijkhoff 1994; Jucker 1993, Varantola 1993, Expósito González 1996, Lerat 1997, Oostdijk / Aarts 1997), a better understanding of the role of nominal elements in scientific discourse is long overdue. According to Halliday and Martin (1993: 84), "learning science is the same thing as learning the language of science". Although there is as yet no research to substantiate such a claim, it is well established now that the NP provides a valuable tool for condensing communication in science, thanks to its structural and functional malleability which facilitates the use of multifunctional structural patterns (Jucker 1993). These can range from extremely brief units to exceedingly long word strings with intricate interconnections and the capacity to express complex ideas. Such structural patterns may be rhetorico-pragmatic in origin, a hypothesis that should be thoroughly investigated, quantified and interpreted.

In this regard, we believe that a comprehensive analysis of the NP may reveal whether its internal constituency, length and other formal features of its postnuclear modification (the least studied so far) are functionally connected with certain rhetorical characteristics at the discourse level. In her study of NPs in engineering English, Varantola (1984: 1) puts it as follows:

> Noun phrases are a powerful syntactic device. Their structure can vary from very simple forms to extremely complicated constructions with intricate *premodification* and *postmodification* patterns (i.e., modification previous and posterior to the nucleus). A noun phrase can incorporate a great deal of information in a compact, synthesized form.

Among the few comprehensive investigations of NP modifiers, prenuclear modification has been the predominant object of study. Postmodification or, as Varantola (1984: 175) calls it, "[the] tightly packed strings of postmodification" may thus deserve a systematic analysis. Therefore, with the aim of making a contribution to a more complete understanding of nominal syntax and its functions in scientific discourse, we carried out the present quantitative and qualitative study.

Our research is both syntactic and rhetorical. Firstly, we conducted a grammatical analysis of the structure (lexical and morphosyntactical features) of the NP in a corpus of medical research papers (RPs).[1] Secondly, we sought plausible connections between (some of) the structural NP features identified, the communicative function of the RP and of its standard rhetorical sections. The expected contribution of this study lies in this double perspective. The information obtained from both analyses may well prove useful for the writer's decisions (or the reader's expectations) about where, how often and why different traits of NP postmodification are to be used or are likely to appear. We decided to analyse the NP in the scientific RP because it is the preferred genre for dissemination of knowledge among medical researchers.

The objective of the present study is thus to analyse NP postmodification structure, both qualitatively and quantitatively, in a corpus of biomedical RPs written in English and published in leading medical journals from the beginning of 1994 to the end of 1995. Our study is part of a wider project involving other components of the NP, whose results are currently being contrasted and interpreted.

2. Corpus and method

To a corpus of 20 RPs (74,354 running words) a random stratified selection method and a freezing point analysis were applied in order to obtain a sample of 2,136 NP instances whose description we could afford. In this stratified random sampling method (Trochim 2002), the number of NPs taken from every section of the RP is proportional to the length of the different sections so that the resulting figures and statistical estimates are accordingly representative.

The freezing point analysis refers to Raumolin-Brunberg's claim (1991) that, when a corpus is a homogeneous compilation, the type and distribution of the NPs most relevant features get "frozen" (i.e. do not vary significantly) after examining some 200 or 300 instances per text (from 1,300 to 2,000 words). Such a selection

1 For space reasons, the corpus references are available at ikleon@ull.es and ldivass@ull.es.

procedure and sample size allowed us to identify general tendencies regarding NP behaviour in contemporary medical discourse written in English (Hakulinen *et al.* 1980, Valle 1993, Gunnarson 1994).

The length of the RP analyzed ranged from 1,004 words to 5,830, with an average of 3,717.7 words. The different sections of the RP macrostructure (Title and Abstract, Introduction, Materials & Method, Results and Discussion) also varied in length. The average length of each one was taken into consideration in the data recording and analysis. These data are relevant to both the sample selection and the freezing point analysis.

NPs may be potential constituents of the internal structure of another NP or any other type of phrase (phrase level), such as in *The median percentage changes [in the treated group [after 1 year]].* They can also be included in a clause modifying another NP or other kind of phrase (phrase-clause level), as in *Placebo treatments [given [during 2 consecutive months [in random order]]].* In addition, it can be embedded in a main clause or sentence (sentence level), as in *[Hormone treatment] is often recommended [to asymptomatic postmenopausal women].* Similarly included in the sample were the NPs forming part of prepositional phrases (PrepPs), following Dik's (1997a, 1997b) functionalist concept of *term*,[2] but only when the cited phrase belongs to the sentence level, as in *Bone loss occurs [with cessation [of ovarian function]].*

Thus, the NP analysed following this randomized experimental design belong to the sentence level as described above, that is to say with the maximal degree of expansion and complexity of the nominal domain. Instances of NPs within others were registered as part of their multiple modification, although not internally described. The following cases were considered for the analysis (emphasis given to excluded elements):

(1) Bone mineral density [at the spine and hip [*in postmenopausal women*]].

(2) The sum [of scores [*for the 10 days* [*of medroxy-progesterone*]]].

---

2 Any NP, regardless of its possible oblique syntactic functions (structurally introduced by prepositions).

Once the NP sample was obtained, after careful reading and analysis of the RPs, a manual codification process was employed, ranging from 10 codes needed for the simplest NPs up to 46 for the most complex ones, with some exceptionally dense cases demanding the use of as many as 83 different codes. Two thousand one hundred and thirty-six NP instances were thus codified according to a descriptive system designed and refined at a preliminary stage with the purpose of avoiding subjectivity in the analytic process, this being an important limitation of many earlier studies of the NP (as highlighted by Jucker 1992 and 1993, among others). Such a system allowed us to determine a number of correspondences between structural and functional features. The categories taken into account, with brief definitions, and their reference code numbers together with some examples are displayed in Table 1.

NP variables for describing POSTFIELD (LEXICAL) MODIFICATION		
Restrictors (*attributive material*): modifying expressions found posterior to the NP nucleus with the function of delimiting and specifying its referent		
Code	*Variable*	*Examples*
1	None	• *The study* • *The strongest and most consistent correlation*
2	Adjectival phrase (AdjP)	• *Data* ***suitable for the study*** • *Alcohol consumption* ***sufficient to produce a large population benefit for CHD***
3	Relation / Inclusion phrase (RelatP) (*of* phrase)	• *A study* ***of the whole population*** • *The clinical significance* ***of a possible synergistic effect***
4	Prepositional phrase (PrepP) (any but the *of* phrase)	• *Defense* ***against prolonged hypoglycemia*** • *Our previous work* ***on the natural history of genital herpes infection***
5	Relative clause (defining, non-defining)	• *The 26 countries* ***which met the GDP criterion*** • *An income cutoff level of US$ 9,500 per capita of gross domestic product (GDP)* ***which provided a clear bimodal separation of high-income and low-income countries***
6	Participial clause (present, past)	• *Beer drinkers* ***consuming less than 5g per day*** • *The risk of severe or fatal hypoglycemia* ***associated with the use of oral hypoglycemic agents and insulin***

7	Other restrictors (OtherRs) (appositive, infinitive, complement or other subordinate clauses; also adverbs or adverbial phrases, etc.)	• *Tests* ***to measure insulin and counterregulatory hormones*** • *Components of wine* ***other than ethanol (such as antioxidants)***
Length: measured in number of words		
8	1-2 words (minimum size)	• *Different types* ***of surgery*** • *The patients cohort* ***with HSV-2***
9	3 -5 words (medium size)	• *An increase* ***in readmission rates*** • *Other developed countries* ***with comparable dietary intake***
10	6 - 9 words (long size)	• *A fair comparison* ***of subtler dietary differences across the 21 countries*** • *The strikingly low rate* ***of mortality from coronary heart disease (CHD) in France***
11	10 or more words (maximum size)	• *The mechanism* ***for the increased susceptibility of the elderly patient with diabetes to hypoglycemia*** • *Increasing interest* ***in the study of nonpyroglyphid storage mites as a source of important environmental allergens***
Complexity: Internally connected constituents		
12	Composition and derivation (technical terms, abbreviations, acronyms, symbols, Greek and Latin fossilized words, comparatives and superlatives, etc.)	• *Men* ***older than 50 years*** • *Recurrence Rates in Genital Herpes after Symptomatic* ***First-Episode*** *Infection*
13	Coordination (parataxis of different kinds, juxtaposed constructions, asyndeton, correlations, etc.)	• *Insulin tests* ***before and after treatment*** • *Positive associations* ***for saturated and monounsaturated fat intake***
14	Subordination and multiple (recursive) modification (concatenated or embedded)	• *Participation* ***by many patients in studies of cell-mediated immunity after the primary episode*** • *The first study of which* ***we are aware that evaluates the symptomatic awareness of hypoglycemia in patients with diabetes***

15	Any combination of the previous (several concurrent sources of complexity)	• *457 consecutive patients* ***who did not have acute-phase serum antibodies to herpes simplex virus type 2 (HSV-2) but who did have herpes simplex virus (HSV) isolated from genital lesions*** • *Only patients* ***willing to participate in prospective studies with long-term follow-up or in therapeutic trials***

Table 1. Typology of properties and relations in NP postmodification.

By means of a systematic analysis, we then identified and described distinctive features of NP *postfield*, i.e., NP modification region posterior to its nuclear element. The so called postfield is usually occupied by modifiers, called *restrictors*, which are of the lexical type. Our analysis covered variation regarding postmodification constituency, degree of structural complexity, internal relations of the elements involved and length. The syntactic features identified were both quantitatively and qualitatively analysed.

Our working hypothesis was based on the assumption that nominal expression, as a key aspect of scientific discourse, may show profiles which might be dependent on – or at least conditioned by – a certain degree of interaction between the functional structure of the analysed units and the pragmatics of the RP rhetoric. We also assumed that postnuclear modification (postmodification) may show different degrees of structural complexity, internal constituency, recurrent combinations and length, which could be measured (quantified) and interpreted in relation to the IMRAD (Introductions, Methods, Results and Discussion) pattern characteristic of the experimental RP in medicine.

3. Results and discussion

3.1. Presence and absence of postnuclear NP modification

Our results show that postnuclear modification occurs in almost half (47.99%) of the NPs in the total sample of medical RP studied and that the number of simple NPs (i.e. with neither previous nor posterior modification to the nucleus) is very small: only 15.96% of the occurrences. In contrast, modified NPs are prevalent: 84.03% show some kind of (prenuclear or postnuclear) modifying structure. In addition, 35.72% of the NPs studied have modifiers both previous and posterior to the nucleus. We also observed that postmodification is usually both semantically and syntactically rich. This seems to be related to its role as a first-mention variant (it usually occurs earlier in the text than its prenuclear alternative), as has already been noted in previous works (Sørensen 1980, Dubois 1982). As can be seen in Table 2, Discussion and Materials & Method are the sections which exhibit the highest rates of NPs with no postmodification at all.[3]

Postnuclear modification. Restrictors.							
Code	*Vari-able*	*Title & Abstract*	*Intro-duction*	*Materials / Method*	*Results*	*Discus-sion*	*Total (raw data & percentages)*
49	None	8.55 58.28	8.91 55.30	27.81 65.32	17.10 37.03	37.62 51.73	1,111 (52.01)
•	Whole sampl e (raw data & percen tages)	163 (6.36)	179 (8.38)	473 (22.14)	513 (24.01)	808 (37.82)	2,136

Table 2. Absence of postmodifiers per rhetorical section and in the total NP sample.

3 This postmodification involved two concurrent levels of analysis: that referring to the total sample regarding the RP as a whole, and that referring to each rhetorical section. For space reasons, data on the former are displayed in the upper part of every table cell, and the latter, in the lower.

This tendency might be due to the complex and functionally rich nature of the former, which also contains one of the highest rates of postmodified NPs. Perhaps the more straightforward style of the MM section could account for the use of NPs without postmodification. The frequency and distribution of unpostmodified NPs are seen in Table 2.

The expression of nominal postmodification is heterogeneous both in its structure and distribution. This contributes to enhancing its complexity and variability. As Table 3 shows, various syntactic units are used as postmodifiers. The PrepP[4] is the most frequent of postnuclear modifiers, followed by the RelatP – i.e. the *of* phrase. OtherRs are less common and include NPs in apposition;[5] infinitive, complement and other subordinate clauses; adverbs or adverbial phrases (AdvP), etc. These all show a similar frequency of use. On the other hand, in decreasing order of frequency, we found participial clauses, both active and passive, relative clauses and, finally, adjectival phrases (AdjP). This last category was rare, as is to be expected in the genre under study.

In her study of NPs in literary language, Raumolin-Brunberg (1991) also emphasizes the predominance of PrepPs and of the relative clause, although the latter is not common in the scientific RP, as confirmed in our analysis and those of Varantola (1984) in engineering English, and Jucker (1992) in journalistic texts. In line with our data as well, Varantola (1984) found a frequent use of PrepPs and internal recurrent subordination, also described by Quirk *et al.* (1985: 1296). The prevalence of PrepPs is similarly corroborated by Expósito González in 15th century administrative documents (1996). However, regarding the total number of cases per category in the whole RP, we found a tendency to use them in the R (Results) and especially in D (Discussion) sections, whereas this construction is quite uncommon in the remaining sections of the paper.

---

4 In our taxonomy, any prepositional phrase except the *of* phrases.

5 The term *apposition* is understood as an element independent of the NP nucleus. For a simpler syntactic description, it was regarded as a postmodifier, due to its explaining or specifying function in relation to the nominal reference. Intra-nuclear distinctions between antecedent and constituents in apposition were thus unnecessary.

Table 3 presents the homogeneous distribution of RelatPs found throughout the RP, except for their lower frequency in MM. OtherRs are more frequent in R, and in MM and D. The relative, followed by the participial clause, scant in all the RP sections, is mostly used in D. This latter restrictor exhibits its highest frequency in literary texts, according to De Haan (1989) (although his research is based on clausal postmodification only). Participial clauses are only used in D, R and MM sections, and are barely present in the remainder of the RP. Finally, the AdjP shows the most variable pattern per rhetorical section: it is totally absent in the Title and Abstract (T&A), quite frequent in D, less common in the Introduction (I) and MM sections, and barely present in R.

Postnuclear modification. Restrictors (B).							
Code	*Variable*	*T&A*	*I*	*MM*	*R*	*D*	*Total (raw data & percentages)*
50	Adjective phrase	0	17.64*	17.64*	5.88*	58.82 *	17 (1.36)
		0	3.22*	1,5*	0.25*	2.16*	
51	Relation phrase	8.45	9.03	17.20	25.94	39.35	343 (27.46)
		30.52	33.33	29.50	22.30	29.22	
52	Prepositio n phrase	7.83	6.14	9.95	35.80	40.25	472 (37.79)
		38.94	31.18	23.5	42.35	41.12	
53	Relative clause	8.51*	4.25*	19.14*	25.53*	42.55	47 (3.76)
		4.21*	2.15*	4.5*	3*	4.32	
54	Participial clause	7.01*	7.01*	21.05	25.43	39.47	114 (9.12)
		8.42*	8.60*	12	7.26	9.74	
55	Other re-strictors	6.64	7.81	22.65	38.67	24.21	256 (20.49)
		17.89	21.50	29	24.81	13.41	
Total (raw data & percentages)		95 (7.60)	93 (7.44)	200 (16.01)	399 (31.94)	462 (37)	1,249

Table 3. NP postnuclear restrictors per rhetorical section and in the total sample.

To sum up, in relation to the total number of instances per type found, the highest rates of postmodifiers tend to accumulate in R, because of the large quantity of prepositional modification used (both of PrepP and RelatP), and D, for its structural complexity and highly specific content. On the contrary, the lowest rates are to be found in T&A and I. The following are examples of some postmodified NPs:

(3) The popliteal nodes *adjacent to the woven knee prosthesis* (15-R).[6]

(4) Children *who had secondary enuresis after the age of 10 years* (17-R).

(5) The low rate *of coronary heart disease (CHD) in France compared with other developed countries with comparable dietary intake* (8-T+A).

As previously stated, both the PrepP and the RelatP are the most frequently used restrictors per rhetorical section. The high incidence of these categories in the biomedical RP can be accounted for demands of linguistic economy. As in Varantola (1984), the remaining types of postmodifiers are far less common.

The category OtherRs includes all the instances of apposition. These have been defined in the widest sense of the term, i.e. any grammatical structure formed by two nominal elements, the latter having an explaining or specifying function in relation to the former (referent). We found that defining, explaining or clarifying are the most common functions of these NPs in the biomedical RP. The following are some examples:

(6) Fibrillin, *a microfibrillar glycoprotein component of the extracellular matrix* (14-T+A).

(7) Quality of life in four areas of particular concern to cancer patients – *physical function, psychosocial function, medical interaction, and sexual function* (20-MM).

3.2. Length and complexity of postnuclear NP modification

Postmodification length was measured by the number of words. It is another key factor for assessing NP structure. We considered four categories: minimum length (1 or 2 words); medium length (3 to 5

---

6 Information of the example source is given in brackets (both the text reference number and the RP section). This particular example has been taken from the Results section of RP number 15 in the corpus.

words); long (6 to 9 words), and maximum length (10 words or more). The results obtained (see Table 4) show that there is a marked tendency to use long modification chains (such was the case in 84% of postmodified NPs). There was, however, a small number of minimum length modifiers, mostly found in R and likely due to the rather straightforward style of this section. Postmodification of medium and maximum lengths was also recorded. This corroborates Varantola's (1984) findings concerning her special language (engineering) corpus.

Postnuclear modification. Length.							
Code	*Variable*	*T&A*	*I*	*MM*	*R*	*D*	*Total (raw data & percentages)*
56	Minimum	4.26*	9.75	18.29	42.68	25	164
		9.33*	18.39	17.75	22.01	10.76	(16)
57	Medium	5.53	8.74	17.20	29.44	39.06	343
		25.33	34.48	34.91	31.76	36.48	(33.46)
58	Long	8.04	8.81	11.87	26.81	44.44	261
		28	26.43	18.34	22.01	30.44	(25.46)
59	Maximum	10.89	7	19.06	29.96	33.07	257
		37.33	20.68	28.99	24.21	22.30	(25.07)
Total (raw data & percentages)		75 (7.31)	87 (8.48)	169 (16.48)	318 (31.02)	376 (36.68)	1,025

Table 4. Postmodification length per rhetorical section and in the whole sample.

The highest rates of lengthier postmodification was recorded in D. The second highest frequency was recorded in R, followed by MM. The remaining sections tend to use lengthy postmodifiers, especially the T&A, due perhaps to their synthetic function and high degree of specificity. In the following examples of postnuclear NP modifiers, we can observe not only their varying length, but also their semantic and structural complexity. Besides, their high postnuclear modification complexity does not always go in line with their length:

(8) The presence *of small but pervasive associations between the presence of secondary enuresis in childhood and rates of behavioural problems in early adolescence* (17-R).

(9) The questions *about a possible role for NC in producing the high incidence of neurological complications that follows vaccination in humans using rabies vaccines prepared in animal brain* (11-D).

(10) Previous studies *of acute symptomatic first-episode genital herpes infection* (5-D).

(11) Evaluation *of disease-targeted quality-of-life measures* (20-D).

As shown in Table 5, all postmodified NPs contain at least one instance of syntactical complexity (see examples below), structurally simple postmodifiers being rather unfrequent.

Postnuclear modification. Complexity.							
Code	*Variable*	*T&A*	*I*	*MM*	*R*	*D*	*Total (raw data & per-centages)*
60	Composition / Derivation	7.58 26.66	9.48 36.66	13.10 26.02	29.31 33.07	40.51 33.47	580 (31.81)
61	Coordination	9.83 14.54	6.96 11.33	20.08 16.78	29.50 14	33.60 11.68	244 (13.38)
62	Subordination / Multiple modification	9.35 30.90	7.70 28	17.43 32.53	27.15 28.79	38.34 29.77	545 (29.89)
63	Combination of several	10.13 27.87	7.92 24	15.85 24.65	27.31 24.12	38.76 25.07	454 (24.90)
Total (raw data & percentages)		165 (9.05)	150 (8.22)	292 (16.01)	514 (28.2)	702 (38.50)	1,823

Table 5. Postmodification complexity per rhetorical section and in the whole sample.

(12) Neonatal deletion and selective expansion *of mouse T cells by exposure to rabies virus nucleocapsid superantigen* (11-D).

(13) Large number *of non-caseating, epithelioid cell granulomata which replaced much of the parenchyma* (15-R).

(14) With the hypothesis *that this increased susceptiblility to hypoglycemia is caused by alterations in release of counterregulatory hormones and psychomotor performance during hypoglycemia* (6-T+A).

In the 1,025 postmodified NPs (see Table 4), which represent 47.98% of the total number of NPs recorded, 1,823 structurally complex components (1,369 individual occurrences and 454 combinations of different types) were found, as shown in Table 5. This accounts for the considerable syntactico-semantic density of postmodification, an average of almost 2 cases (1.77) of complex components in postmodification per NP. The expression of complexity in postmodification per rhetorical sections is characterized by the homogeneous distribution and high frequency of certain grammatical resources, particularly morpholexical composition and derivation, subordination and the combination of these. The three possibilities show a similar distribution in all the sections of the paper. Coordination is the least frequent source of postmodification complexity.

3.3. Rhetorical analysis

The results of the present study confirm the nominal nature of the RP (Dubois 1982, Salager-Meyer 1983, Adams Smith 1984, Varantola 1984, Lerat 1997). They also corroborate what is already known about the NP in general and contribute to a better understanding of the behaviour of its postnuclear modification in scientific English prose in the sense that the NP proves to be a suitable tool for the expression of the communicative function of the biomedical RP in general, and of its sections, in particular.

We were able to identify three NP syntactico-rhetorical patterns corresponding to the different RP sections: the economical style of the RP Title and Abstract; the argumentative and persuasive discourse of the Introduction and Discussion and the factual prose of the Materials & Method and the Results sections (Swales 1990, Nwogu 1997).

3.3.1. Title and Abstract: summarizing topical information

Perhaps the most conceptually condensed RP sections are the Title and Abstract. Their concision calls, as we have seen, for the use of semantically dense nominal units (with few linking elements). The prose of the Abstract is mostly informative and expository and aims at extracting the essential content of the reported research. It also has a somehow persuasive function, enticing, as it does, the potential reader to consider reading the whole paper.

The fact that there is not a single AdjP in the Abstract and that participial or relative clauses are rare could be accounted for by the Abstract informative function. Complexity of postnuclear modification appears to be a highly functional linguistic tool in the scientific RP and in the Abstract it is usually long, often formed by prepositional phrases. As a first-mention variant, it readily transmits specific (semantically new) information by means of (structurally transparent) more explicit connections.

3.3.2. Introduction and Discussion: arguing and persuading

Although they are primarily argumentative and persuasive, the Introduction and Discussion sections also present an informative component. Both are the most conceptually dense and more subjective (author-oriented) sections, as seen in their NPs. They display not only the most nominal and specialized expression but are also the sections with a more complex and variable form in the nominal structures used both from a formal and functional point of view. Cohesion here is often achieved through NP internal juxtaposing or subordinating elements. The typical prose of the Discussion is based on argumentation and speculation. These imply numerous communicative functions, such as explaining, summarizing, interpreting, contrasting, or claiming, among others. This explains the frequent use of long complex syntactic structures and the highest rate of different types of postmodification (from prepositional phrases to relative and participial clauses).

3.3.3. Materials & Method and Results: communicating facts and data

The Materials & Method and Results sections present data and features in a narrative form by using an object-centred discourse. NP postnuclear modifiers in these two sections clearly illustrate their informative and expository nature, with a highly specialized use of terminology, mostly in Results. They exhibit a limited degree of complexity but a considerable variation. Therefore, in spite of the high frequency of occurrence of postmodifiers in Results, these correspond to the mostly prepositional categories and are thus, functionally speaking, the closest to premodifiers because they are structurally and semantically the least explicit postmodifiers.

The sequenced presentation of information is very common in both sections. It is illustrated by the predominant use in their NPs of juxtaposing and paratactic structures, categorization and classification (qualifying and evaluative expressions), exposition and ordering instead of synthesis and analysis, etc. The features of these two rhetorical sections, due to the factual nature of their contents and the expository kind of their reporting discourse, justify the high frequency of the recorded NP structures. Table 6 summarizes the functional load of NP postmodification features in the different sections of the biomedical RP.

SCIENTIFIC RESEARCH PAPER: NP POSTMODIFICATION AND THE IMRAD PATTERN			
Expression of communicative functions	**Title & Abstract**	**Introduction Discussion**	**Materials & Method Results**
Rhetorical features of discourse	+ Information conciseness	+ Author-oriented text	+/- Information conciseness
	+ Lexical condensation & conceptual density	+ Conceptual density	- Conceptual density
	+ Object-centred discourse	+ Object / author centred discourse	+ Object-centred discourse
	+ Structural density and complexity	+ Structural complexity	- Structural complexity
	+ Synthetic, expository & informative style	+ Arguing & persuasive style	+ Expository & informative style
	+ Nominal expression	+ Highly nominal expression	+/- Nominal expression
	+ Specialized vocabulary	+ Specialized vocabulary (particularly in the Introduction)	- Specialized vocabulary (except in Recults)
	POSTFIELD NP MODIFICATION		
	- Frequency of postmodifiers	- Simple NPs with only one type of postmodifier	+ Prevalence of postmodification in Results
	- Adjectival restrictors	+ Frequency of possesive restrictors (in the Introuction) & adjectival, nominal, participial and adverbial	+ Frequency of postnuclear prepositional restrictors (lower in Materials and Method than in Results)
	+ Prepositional postmodifiers	+ Frequency and extension of postmodification (especially in the Discussion)	- Frequency of adjectival and participial postnuclear restrictors
	+ Lengthy & complex postmodification	+ Prepositional, relative and participial restrictors (both active & passive)	+/- Lengthy postmodification
Summary	**Three functional patterns of synctactic-rhetorical correspondences**		

Table 6. NP structural features and functions in the scientific RP.

4. Conclusions

Our results allow us to conclude that there is a close connection between some of the structural NP features identified in postmodification and the communicative function of the RP rhetorical sections. We reached the conclusion that, firstly, the synthetic pattern of the Title and the Abstract parallels with a low occurrence of postmodifiers, a lack of adjectival restrictors, and a remarkable prevalence of prepositional modification within usually lengthy and highly complex expressions. Secondly, the arguing and persuading style of the Introduction and the Discussion sections gives rise to a highly frequent NP postmodification, which is dense in form and function, and generally complex in structure, often made up of several types of restrictors in combination. Such postnuclear modification generally shows a higher presence of adjectival, nominal, participial and adverbial components (some possessive restrictors may also appear in the Introduction), and it is made up of lengthy chains of constituents with multilevel interconnections (especially in the Discussion). Lastly, the factual language of the Materials & Method and the Results sections is shown with variable frequency in both the use (more common in Results) and the length of postmodifiers. In these sections we noticed a great amount of concise prepositional restrictors (particularly in the Results section), while more subjective postnuclear elements (adjectives and participles) were found to be rather scarce.

Further cross-generic, cross-disciplinary, cross-cultural and cross-linguistic studies may well answer questions the present study only partially addresses. More grammatical units could also be described in order to obtain a more comprehensive picture of the interconnections between form and function in other non nominal domains. Finally, a diachronic perspective could also be considered to prove the relevance of these or other variables regarding the nominality of scientific discourse, the spoken form of which would also be worth analysing. Part of this research is presently being undertaken with the analysis of the other constituents of the NP, i.e. the prefield elements (lexical and grammatical modification) and the

NP nucleus. The results obtained could then be compared and would add to our understanding of the nominal domain in the biomedical RP.

References

Adams Smith, Diana E. 1984. Medical Discourse: Aspects of Author's Comment. *The ESP Journal* 3/1, 25-36.

Barber, Charles 1962. Some Measurable Characteristics of Modern Scientific Prose. In Behre, Frank (ed.) *Contributions to English Syntax and Philology. Gothenburg Studies in English* 14. Gothenburg: Almqvist and Wiksell, 21-43.

Bhatia, Vijay K. 1993. *Analysing Genre: Language Use in Professional Settings*. London / New York: Longman.

Biber, Douglas 2001. Intra-textual Variation within Medical Research Articles. In Conrad, Susan / Biber, Douglas (eds) *Variation in English: Multi-Dimensional Studies*. Harlow: Longman, 108-23.

Búllow-Møller, Anne Marie 1995. Discourse Organization in English, German and Russian Medical Texts. In Budin, Gerhard (ed.) *LSP. Proceedings of the 10th European Symposium of Language for Special Purposes*. Vienna: *TermNet*, 114-48.

Cabré, María Teresa 1998. *La Terminologie, Théorie, Méthode et Applications*. Presses de l'Université d'Ottawa, Armand Colin. Translated from Catalan and adapted by Monique C. Cormier and John Humbley.

Crookes, Graham 1986. Towards a Validated Analysis of Scientific Text Structure. *Applied Linguistics* 7/1, 57-70.

De Haan, Pieter 1989. Postmodifying Clauses in the English Noun Phrase. A Corpus-Based Study. In Aarts, Jan / Meijs, Willem (eds) *Language and Computers*. Amsterdam: Rodopi.

De Haan, Pieter 1993. Noun Phrase Structure as an Indication of Text Variety. In Jucker (ed.), 85-106.

Dik, Simon C. 1997a. *The Theory of Functional Grammar. Part I.* Hengeveld, Kees (ed.) Berlin: Mouton.

Dik, Simon C. 1997b. *The Theory of Functional Grammar. Part II.* Hengeveld, Kees (ed.) Berlin: Mouton.

Dubois, Betty Lou 1982. The Construction of Noun Phrases in Biomedical Journal Articles. In Høedt, Jørgen / Lundquist, Lita / Picht, Heribert / Qvistgaard, Jacques (eds) *Pragmatics and LSP. Proceedings of the 3rd European Symposium on LSP.* Copenhagen, 49-67.

Esteve Ramos, María-José 2001. New Perspectives in LSP: Diachronic Evidence of Medical Lexicon. In Palmer, Juan Carlos / Posteguillo, Santiago / Fortanet, Inmaculada (eds) *Discourse Analysis and Terminology in Languages for Specific Purposes.* Castelló de la Plana: Publicacions de la Universitat Jaume I, 25-31.

Expósito González, M. de la Cruz 1996. *La Estructura del Sintagma Nominal en el Inglés de la Cancillería: 1400-1450.* Barcelona: Kadle Books.

Gerbert, Martin 1970. *Besonderheiten der Syntax in der Technischen Fachsprache des Englischen.* Halle/S.

Giorgi, Alessandra / Longobardi, Giuseppe 1991. *The Syntax of Noun Phrases.* Cambridge: Cambridge University Press.

Gunnarson, Britt-Louise 1994. Textual Patterns and the Discourse Community: A Socio-Semantic Approach to the History of LSP. In Brekke, Magnar (ed.) *Applications and Implications of Current LSP Research.* Bergen: Fagbokforlaget, 888-99.

Hakulinen, Auli / Karlsson, Fred / Vilkuna, Maria 1980. *Suomen Tekstilauseiden Piirteitä: Cvantitatiivinen Tutkimus.* Helsinki: University of Helsinki.

Halliday, Michael A.K. / Martin, James R. 1993. *Writing Science: Literacy and Discursive Power.* London: The Falmer Press.

Heslot, J. 1982. Tense and Other Indexical Markers in the Typology of Scientific Texts in English. In Hoedt, J. (ed.) *Pragmatics and LSP.* Copenhagen: Copenhagen School of Economics, 83-103.

Huddleston, Rodney D. 1971. *The Sentence in Written English. A Syntactic Study Based on an Analysis of Scientific Texts.* Cambridge: Cambridge University Press.

Jucker, Andreas H. 1992. *Stylistic Variation in the Syntax of British Newspaper Language.* Berlin: Mouton.

Jucker, Andreas H. (ed.) 1993. *The Noun Phrase in English: Its Structure and Variability*. Heidelberg: Universitätsverlag C. Winter.

Lerat, Pierre 1997. *Las Lenguas Especializadas*. Barcelona: Ariel.

Malcolm, Lois 1987. What Rules over Tense Usage in Scientific Articles? *English for Specific Purposes* 6, 31-44.

Nwogu, Kevin Ngozi 1997. The Medical Research Paper: Structure and Function. *The ESP Journal* 16/2, 119-38.

Oostdijk, Nelleke / Aarts, Jan M. 1997. Multiple Postmodification in the English Noun Phrase. In Aarts, Jan M. / Mönnink, I. de / Wekker, H. (eds) *Studies in English Language and Teaching*. Amsterdam: Rodopi, 107-22.

Percebois, Jacqueline 1999. *L'Interconnector*: un Réseau de Transmission de Gaz Européen. Approche Lexicologique Comparative du Français et de l'Anglais des Réseaux et Contrats Gaziers. *ASp* 23-26, 223-252.

Quirk, Randolph *et al.* 1985. *A Comprehensive Grammar of the English Language*. London: Longman.

Raumolin-Brunberg, Helena 1991. *The Noun Phrase in Early Sixteenth-Century English. A Study Based on Sir Thomas More's Writings*. Helsinki: Société Néophilologique.

Rijkhoff, Jan 1994. Word Order in the Languages of Europe: The Simple Noun Phrase (A Preliminary Report). *Working Papers in Functional Grammar. EUROTYP Working Paper* II/5, 64-100.

Salager-Meyer, Françoise 1983. Compound Nominal Phrases in Scientific-Technical Literature: Proportion and Rationale. In Pugh, A. J. K. / Ulijn, J. M. (eds) *Reading for Professional Purposes: Studies and Practices in Native and Foreign Languages*. London: Heinemann, 136-46.

Salager-Meyer, Françoise 1985a. Syntax and Semantics of Compound Nominal Phrases in Medical English Literature: A Comparative Study with Spanish. *English for Specific Purposes* 95, 6-12.

Salager-Meyer, Françoise 1985b. Specialist Medical English Lexis: Classificatory Framework and Rhetorical Function – A Statistical Approach. *English for Medical Purposes Newsletter* 2/2, 5-18.

Sørensen, Kurt 1980. From Postmodification to Premodification. In Jacobson, S. (ed.) *Papers from the Scandinavian Symposium on Syntactic Variation: Stockholm Studies in English* LII, 77-84.

Swales, John M. 1976. Verb Frequencies in Scientific English. *ESPMENA Bulletin* 4, 28-31.

Swales, John M. 1990. *Genre Analysis: English in Academic and Research Settings*. Cambridge: Cambridge University Press.

Tarone, Elaine / Dwyer, S. / Gillette, S. / Icke, V. 1998. On the Use of Passive and Active Voice in Astrophysics Journal Articles with Extensions to other Languages and other Fields. *The ESP Journal* 17/1, 113-133.

Trochim, William M. K. 2002. *Research Methods Knowledge Base*. Web site: http://trochim.human.cornell.edu/kb/random.htm.

Valle, Ellen 1993. The Development of English Scientific Rhetoric in the Philosophical Transactions of the Royal Society of London. *FINNLANCE* 12, 94-124.

Varantola, Krista 1984. *On Noun Phrase Structure in Engineering English*. Turku: Turun Yliopiston Julkaisuja.

Varantola, Krista 1993. Modification of Nouns by Nouns. Bad by Definition? In Jucker (ed.), 69-84.

SUSAN MCKAY

The Discursive Construction of Health Risk in Magazines: Messages, Registers and Readers

Health information in the media is pervasive with television, radio, newspapers, magazines, and increasingly the internet, providing a constant and readily accessible supply of health care information and advice (Signorielli 1993; Seale 2002, 2004; Gwyn 2002). The media cover advances in medical treatments and new drugs; they alert their audiences to health risks; they promote the value of taking care of the self; and they act as advocates for change on socio-political issues like medical funding and health service delivery. The provision of health information is widely distributed across the media occurring in news stories, documentaries, medical and science programs, and health promotion campaigns. In addition, health and illness are major themes in entertainment media forms like television dramas, lifestyle shows, and from time to time, soap operas too. Advertisements also feature health promotion, cures and treatments. Magazines, especially women's magazines, carry significant health content. Health and medical websites on the internet provide a range of health-related material, and chat rooms and newsgroups facilitate patient-to-patient interaction and discussion.

These media hold a unique position of influence over our understandings and expectations of health and medicine. The degree of that influence is notoriously difficult to assess given the complexity of the media / audience relationship as audiences interact with media texts, use what is relevant to them in their own social lives, construct their own meanings and draw their own understandings in a process where the media may shape perceptions of reality but where personal experience is important too. Health and well-being choices (insofar as they are choices) may be thought of in terms of other personal lifestyle choices like what to eat or drink, how to behave, who to be with etc. They are important in identity terms, of who we are and what we aspire to be, forming part of the way we work on our identity and in our capacity to maintain or revise it (Giddens 1991). Gauntlett (2002) contends that while the range of lifestyle ideals propagated in the media may be limited, it is broader than those we might come across by chance in everyday life. The significance of the media in offering advice and choices on lifestyle issues may be self-evident but the extent of the impact of that diversity is arguable. According to Petersen (1994: 123), "the argument is not that we are passive recipients of media information, but rather that the ideas and images conveyed by the media help to shape the context within which opinions are formed and decisions are made that ultimately affect health and well-being".

A major way in which the media add to the understanding of health and medicine in the lay public is through the coverage of risk. The identification of a huge raft of potential 'harms' and the associated projects to eliminate or minimise associated risks that have come to characterise western societies (in what Giddens (1991: 115) has termed a 'climate of risk' or in what Beck (1992: 19) has described as 'risk society') have become an integral part of mass media content. The media's role in profiling risks in modern society provides information for what Williams and Calnan (1996) label 'lay re-skilling' by which individuals can take back control over matters of health and illness and return to less technological forms of health and healing through non-compliance with medical treatments and advice, the use of complementary therapies, attending self-help groups and participating in environmental health movements. The media aid in this process of 'lay re-skilling' through the provision of information and advice.

Within the domain of magazine publishing, a significant number of titles are health-related, either as separate publications which are devoted to health and fitness, or, as part of their remit (like many women's magazines), take a responsibility for giving health advice of various kinds in the midst of fashion, beauty, gossip, recipes and interior decoration projects.

Women's magazines often detail personal battles with illness as both celebrities and ordinary people tell of their experience (McKay / Bonner 1999; 2002). Regardless of the outcome of the illness, the magazines emphasise positive elements like family love and support, the desire to help others, and the need to raise awareness about particular diseases both to aid in early detection and to raise research funds. This is particularly the case for breast cancer in Australia with several major women's magazines promoting awareness through personal stories, and even one title, *Pink Ribbon*, devoted entirely to articles about risks, detection, treatment and prognosis for breast cancer sufferers and interested readers and personal stories related to the experience of the disease.

One of the problems for the media in conveying risk information is the difficulty with a form of address that can only speak to a relatively anonymous subject, so that susceptibility and risk factors can only be dealt with in generalised terms rather than in anything approaching individual advice (Greco 1993). It is the nature of that advice, or more particularly the language of that advice, and its discursive construction that form the central discussion in this chapter.

The magazine industry's relationship with audiences is complex and the connection with health issues (like most topics) is tied as much to market share and advertising revenue as any desire to merely advise or inform. Rather, magazines operate at an intersection between consumption, desire and identity (Winship 1987) providing opportunities for readers to explore and negotiate the latter in a package of entertainment and information. This chapter takes into consideration some of the ways selected magazines provide health advice to particular audiences, within the context of increasing anxiety about a whole range of risks, but especially to those health consumers whose personal anxieties, and aspirations for self-improvement and self-actualisation are actively cultivated in demographically-specific titles.

Magazines may be mass-market publications but each title tries to achieve a brand distinctiveness based on a certain identity, however illusory, related to a certain lifestyle and a certain attitude. As Machin and Thornborrow point out in their 2003 study of *Cosmopolitan* magazine, this branding even persists across international editions. The so-called core values of a magazine can be promoted to potential advertisers to 'match' their products to a captive market with closely defined demographic characteristics, and so perhaps more than other forms of media, magazine publishers feel more confident in tailoring quite narrowly the form of address they use. This chapter does not attempt to survey the entire magazine market but focuses on two groups who for quite different reasons are routinely considered to be 'at risk' in terms of their health: teenage girls, and men, using two Australian teen magazines with a strong focus on health concerns and one of the most prominent men's lifestyle magazines, *Men's Health*. The period studied was 2002-2004.

1. Health advice for young women

Teenage girl magazines offer health advice along with the latest celebrity gossip, fashion, and advice on how to attract young men. Academic scholarship, especially feminist research, on teen magazines has focused on issues relating to role models for young women and how the magazines interpellate their readers in ways that might reinforce traditional femininity, and others have focused on body image noting the disjunctions between editorial content and advertisements depicting underweight models and airbrushed perfection. The long tradition of accounts of women's and girls' magazines and their readers includes work by Ferguson (1983); Winship (1987); Ballaster *et al.* (1991); McCracken (1993); Hermes (1995); McRobbie (1996, 2000); Currie (1999).

This section concentrates on magazines aimed at young women but looks more specifically at health, and at how the magazines construct risk messages associated with the leading causes of morbidity and mortality in this age group. For many, the adolescent years are a time of focusing on important goals like becoming more popular, being more successful, finding satisfying personal relationships, becoming more self-sufficient and gaining more self-confidence, but it is also a time when young people make choices involving health-related risky behaviour (Harris / Duncan / Boisjoly 2002). Medical researchers tell us that many of the major threats to health and well-being in adolescence are not biomedical in origin but social, and are the consequence of risk-taking behaviours including self-harming, substance use and abuse, unprotected sex, poor diet and physical inactivity (Millstein / Litt 1990).

Adolescence has become a segmented market for magazine publishers and advertisers, not just in Australia but in other countries as well, as publishers and advertisers recognize the spending power of this age group. It is a gendered market with boys targeted with titles on personal computing and games, music, sports and various motor vehicles, and girls offered titles resembling younger versions of women's 'lifestyle' and fashion magazines. The most prominent and long-running titles in the 'teenage girl' market in Australia are *Dolly* (started in 1970) and *Girlfriend* (from 1988) and both publish significant amounts of health-related information. The magazines' pitch at a group around 12-14 years and upwards becomes a significant point in research on health messages because many of the young women in the targeted age group are likely to be younger than the legal drinking age, not yet old enough to be able to buy cigarettes legally or to hold driving licence, and may be younger than the age of consent. Most are still likely to be been taken to see medical practitioners in the company of a parent. So what then are the implications of trying to deal with 'risky' topics like drinking, smoking, driving under the influence, having unprotected sex, many of which represent the inconsistencies in adult expectations for health behaviours in young people in contrast with those that are socially acceptable in older groups (McKay 2005)?

Both *Dolly* and *Girlfriend* see themselves as sources of advice providing a "guide to life" (quoted in both magazines' websites). They both aim to relate to their readers at their own level – *Dolly* as a "valued friend and confidante", and *Girlfriend* as the stereotypical best friend as implied in the masthead. In language terms, they do this by employing a range of linguistic devices which constitute the restricted codes and narrow register of 'teenspeak'. This is not an adult world and it is not male or even gender-neutral territory. The 'girls' (for that is how the magazines describe them) are addressed with a specific identity constructed for them embedded in a discourse of 'girl power' which incorporates the sometimes difficult conjunction between 'empowerment' (however minimal), assertiveness (which is often hard to substantiate when most of the time the articles are requiring readers to solicit male approval), with shades of moral authority, and being 'best friends' (sharing secrets, needing and offering support, being embarrassed, being cool).

2. Addressing the reader

The language of these magazines employs what Tincknell and her colleagues (2003: 53) describe in their study of teen sex in British magazines as the idiom of imitative speech, a kind of "'teen demotic' of feminised mateship" which mimics the codes teens use and incorporates them into the discursive structures of the texts. These Australian magazines employ this imitative register to frame their messages using:

- Imitations of teen slang like *bestie* for *best friend* as in "how to deal when your bestie gets a boy"; *fave* as in "your fave celeb mag"; *spesh* for *special* as in "hot celeb couple spesh".
- Prolongation of vowels as in the over-used *soooooooo* as in "Dolly Doctor Confidential SOOO Totally Sealed"; "tooooooo gross".
- Overuse of *cos* for *because.*
- First Person plural ("We love Guy! He's our idol"); "We all love chocolate" or "glowing sparkling skin".

But, they also make use of visual signs to emphasise, para-linguistically, the nature of teenspeak like:

- Representations of typescript which attempt to mimic conversation and 'scream' drama, concern, innuendo: exclamation marks, scare quotes, stress, question marks, dollar signs, bullet points and increasingly larger font size to indicate increasing importance.
- Overuse of highly saturated, very bright colours like neon pink and orange, acid green, cobalt blue.

The content of the articles reinforces the narrow concerns but also the alleged insecurities of this group, using:

- Questions like "How far are other girls going?"; "The ugly disease, could you have it?"; "Will your year be magic or tragic?"; "What's wrong with my love handles?".
- Directives like "Fix your freaked out skin;" "Be the girl everyone wants to hang out with"; "Read this now".

- Celebrities, like Britney Spears, Hilary Duff, Mary-Kate and Ashley Olsen, and Paris Hilton, are used for comparison, compassion or criticism.

The language and form of address used is a construction of the magazine industry and tries to convey a conversation-like quality as in advice from peers or perhaps an older sister. When looking at health information in feature articles in these magazines, this adolescent register or 'teenspeak' approach is maintained but on occasions a rather odd disjunction develops between 'real life' experience for 12-14 year olds and the moral authority of the magazines.

Both magazines cover the health risks outlined above, but not consistently or evenly. Unsurprisingly, because of the nature of the magazines and their emphasis on relationships and heterosexual teen angst, sexual behaviour is at the centre of the magazines' concerns with many articles devoted to basic information, anatomical detail and explanations, decisions about when to start, and the hazards of unprotected sex. Teen pregnancy and abortion are covered. The message is gendered and, just as in Tincknell *et al.*'s UK study (2003), tends to suggest that regulating sexual behaviour is the girls' responsibility while initiating sex remains what boys do.

Dietary behaviours too, as expected, are regularly covered, with many stories related to anorexia and bulimia, but also warnings about obesity too. The magazines tend to relate physical inactivity to obesity rather than to other health risks. While the dangers of alcohol, binge-drinking, and drugs are dealt with, they are often not put in the context of straightforward health risk as such, but discussed as contributing factors to date rape. One story about the dangers of hitch-hiking turned out to be a story about two girls who had been drinking accepting a ride home with boys whom they actually knew and then being raped. Tobacco and smoking are covered but probably not in proportion to the significance for this age group. Suicide and self-harm stories are prevalent and are often tied to information about depression.

To talk about these categories of risk the magazines do make use of a type of teenspeak. Its artificiality of course would become even more transparent if the magazines were to construct an all-knowing, highly reflective speaking *adult* position especially in the personal narratives in the 'reality' stories. Personal narratives are a favoured way for mass-market magazines right across the spectrum (with the possible exception of men's magazines, see below) to convey health information as those who have experienced a health threat or an illness share their experiences with an audience already intensely interested in personal, emotional details. Individuals' stories, especially when mediated through a magazine article, become recontextualised as meaningful so that readers can benefit from the experiences of others (McKay / Bonner 2002).

Health features in the teen magazines are often structured around personal narratives and 'reality' situations e.g. "How I beat anorexia"; "A shark tore off my arm"; "I got breast cancer when I was 4"; "I had a secret abortion at 16"; "How mental illness changed my life", but these are often complex texts with accompanying text boxes of additional information.

While adult personal narratives (related to, say, cancer survival, overcoming medical odds, or dealing with mental illness), may convincingly incorporate wider and wiser perspectives and evaluations of the meanings of the experience, teen narratives are less able to do this credibly, and need to extend other discursive strategies.

While both adult and teen personal stories often position the narrator as a victim and then a survivor, the adult narratives usually end with an empowering evaluation of the experience through emancipatory and enabling devices through which sufferers rationalise the experience of illness and give it meaning (McKay / Bonner 2002). These range from re-evaluating relationships and support, doing something for others, restoring self-identity, to explaining illness in terms of fate. Not unexpectedly perhaps, given the age group, this step of altruism and intense introspection verging on philosophizing, is missing in most of the teen 'real life' stories. They are more likely to end with a more self-focused statement bringing the reader up to date with the person's life and perhaps a statement about what they have learned.

What characterizes many of these teen personal stories is their format. Similar experiences are often clustered together in multiple mini-narratives. Like other magazine feature articles, most will be accompanied by a photograph, usually not of the person(s) concerned but of a low modality, 'generic' image of a young woman or a group. Like other articles, there may be sidebars or boxes with additional text. What distinguishes these features from those aimed at an older audience is the number and nature of those extra texts. For example, *Girlfriend's* "The Big Issue" (March 2004) included regular information on obesity and diet in a mix of personal experience, advice from dieticians, a separate personal narrative in the sidebar, a block of information from weight management experts, and another of celebrity attitudes to weight and body shape. A URL for facts and advice is included. A later article in *Dolly*, "Obesity Crisis: How Not to be a Victim" (June 2004: 106-107) used advice from a health professional interspersed with short paragraphs of personal experience accompanied by editorial evaluations like "These days, Naomi's and Renee's low activity levels are seen as 'normal', but our weight problems are made worse because we're not eating any less to compensate for being 'couch potatoes'. Once again, weblinks are included, along with a box of quick tips. In another, "Jesslyn" tells of having an abortion without her mother's knowledge ("I had a Secret Abortion at 16", *Girlfriend*, March 2004: 106-07). The accompanying text box "It Could Happen to You" gives statistics on teen pregnancy, vague contraceptive advice, warnings about sexually transmitted infections, a directive to talk to an adult "you trust", and a website for more information. *Dolly's* feature on abortion, "Why are so Many Teenagers having Abortions" (Dec. 2003: 42-44) also used personal stories, weblinks and included text boxes on facts including cost, the legal situation and whether girls need to tell their parents, contraception, and another titled "The Case Against" offering alternatives to abortion from a Christian organisation.

The multi-faceted approach to teen health risk messages allows separate voices to come thorough where peers can tell it like it is, celebrities can be quoted, and where expert voices position young women together into seeking help, finding solutions, or dealing with friends who are taking risks.

3. Health advice for men

There are some similarities in the adoption of a specific register in health risk messages aimed at men. Magazine interest in mens' health is relatively recent, at least compared to interest in women's health. 'Men's health' is a much newer concept than 'women's health' (Baker 2001). It came into use as a term in the 1990s following the growth of the men's movement with its prevailing health discourse that men suffer health disadvantage comparable to, if not greater than, that suffered by women as promoted by the feminist movement and the associated women's health movement (Cameron / Bernardes 1998). One of the obstacles to improving men's health has been seen as their reluctance to seek medical help (Banks 2001; Griffiths 1996).

While many women's magazines have a long tradition of incorporating health information alongside features on fashion, food, family, home decoration, craft, careers, etiquette, social relationships, and entertainment, lifestyle magazines for men are much newer. Notable among the work undertaken on this genre of men's lifestyle magazines has been that of Stevenson, Jackson and Brooks (2000a, 2000b) which offers a critical perspective on the changing nature of contemporary masculinities in the UK. One of these men's lifestyle titles with a significant health component is *Men's Health* magazine. It was first published in the US in 1988 by Rodale Press, followed over the next 10 or so years by more than 20 international editions. As Gauntlett (2002) acknowledges, it has a broader remit than evidenced by the title, and closely parallels the content of women's lifestyle magazines. However, there are differences too. Jackson, Stevenson and Brooks (2001: 96) describe the magazine as offering advice with discernible rewards: "it is an attempt to gain a sense of masculine autonomy over a private world in a public culture which is increasingly fraught with risk and uncertainty" and where "men are encouraged to 'work the body' (in private) in order to be able to succeed in the (public) world of relationships and work".

Stylistically, there are similarities with other lifestyle magazines for both men and women, with articles ranging from fitness and health to relationship advice. Some of the items are presented as feature articles, some as advice columns, some as readers' letters and still others as small snippets of information from the latest research. However, workouts and fitness tips are the mainstay of this magazine and better health is promoted mainly through exercise and fitness.

In fact the fitness message is overwhelming in these texts with regimes of self-control presented as the universal answer to a range of health risks. The message is that fitness is both necessary (linked to sex appeal as much as good health) and achievable, even easy, with advice on how to "Build big arms in just a month" (cover, *Men's Health,* UK ed., April 2002) ; "Turn fat into muscle (at the beach)" (cover, *Men's Health,* Australia ed., February 2002); "Lose Weight Build Muscle" (cover, *Men's Health* Aust. ed., Jan. 2003); "Build muscle in 3 weeks" (cover, *Men's Health,* UK ed., Sept. 2002) or how to achieve a "Hard Body Now" (cover, *Men's Health,* Singapore ed., August 2003); and "The Easy Way to Hard Abs" (cover, *Men's Health,* US ed., February 2003).

Other health-related topics are covered including osteoporosis in an article titled "Skeleton Key" (*Men's Health,* US ed., June 2002: 88); dental health in "The Drill is Gone" (*Men's Health,* US ed., March 2002: 82); snoring and sleep apnoea in "The Snore War" (*Men's Health*, Aust. ed., Feb. 2003: 82-85); prostate cancer in "Cancer-proof your Prostate" (*Men's Health,* US ed., March 2004: 100-102); haemorrhages in "Bloody Hell" (*Men's Health*, UK ed., March 2002: 94-99); or the benefits of olive oil in "Extra-virgin Territory" (*Men's Health,* Aust. ed., June. 2003: 104-106).

Readers are exposed to a wide variety of health issues but they are swamped by articles telling how to double their muscle in half the time ("Weights Management", *Men's Health,* UK ed., June 2002: 67-70) or less ("Muscles in a Minute", *Men's Health*, US ed., April 2004: 92-92); lose their love handles ("Retrieving his Fitness", *Men's Health,* UK ed., June 2002: 46); build muscle without leaving the house ("The Genius of Dumbbells", *Men's Health,* Aust. ed., March 2002: 76-81).

4. Addressing the reader

Men's Health, like the teen girl magazines adopts a special register to address its readers. This time it is macho and ironic, although as Gauntlett explains, the irony is used defensively. The magazine acknowledges that many men may reject serious articles and so uses humour and irony to make the advice more palatable (Gauntlett, 2002). Unlike other men's lifestyle magazines like *Loaded* and *FHM*, there is a clear distinction made by *Men's Health* between the magazine as expert and the reader as someone who needs advice (Jackson *et al.* 2002), indeed who is ignorant, not just in health matters, but in most things especially in their relationships with women (Toerien / Durrheim 2001). This premise of ignorance underpins the way health advice is offered.

The language used is quite distinctive and relates to the magazine's use of 'macho' and 'new man' versions of masculine identities. As Petersen / Lupton (1996: 82) argue, "The meanings associated with 'health' and 'protective behaviours' are inextricably linked with the feminised discourses of 'looking after yourself', risk avoidance and caution, and are highly embodied. Such practices are also often coded as 'homosexual' rather than 'heterosexual', in their feminised interest in physical appearance". As a consequence, the magazine goes to great lengths to resolve any tension between "the imperative towards achieving the ideal of the hard, muscular body that bespeaks hegemonic masculinity and the desire to avoid an appearance of vanity" (Petersen / Lupton 1996: 84), and more feminised discourse. It approaches this possible tension in several ways:

- Through a pervasive use of *you* and *your* to personalise the information and make it sound accessible and easy to read. For example, "You know that the secret to good health is drinking in moderation, but you lost the plot a bit over the silly season. Here is how to save your system in 2003" (*Men's Health,* Aust. ed., Feb. 2003: 29), or "You might drop dead while reading this, even if you are a model *Men's Health* reader – you eat right, your blood pressure is great over excellent, and your LDL-cholesterol is post-it-on-the-refrigerator low – you might at any minute feel that gripping pain in your chest that tells you it's over" (*Men's Health*, US ed., Jan-Feb 2003: 78, 81).

- Through the use of language that is relatively plain and colloquial again imitating the slang of the assumed readership. For example, doctors can identify cases of diabetes in crowded shopping malls according to an article that told readers, "The giveaway is the belly, that bulging sack of fat lolling over a shopper's belt. Fat, especially belly fat, has been linked to an increasingly common and lethal form of diabetes, a disease that dumps toxic levels of sugar into the blood stream" (*Men's Health*, UK ed., July 2002: 116).
- Through the use of humour to frame even the most dire health message. In the article on Heart Attack, readers were told that "The surgeon won the argument to slice and dice me. The scan showed convincingly that my heart's big gun in front was a mere memory, and that the area it served was long dead. As bad as news was, I have to admit being somewhat relieved there would be no bypass. Having my chest cracked wide while my body is being run by machines is not my idea of a fun day" ("My Heart Attack: An Annotated Guide", *Men's Health*, US ed., Sept. 2002: 157).

These repetitive discursive constructions (using the second person form of address, using lay language, and framing risk messages with humour) allow the magazine to address men with a seamless group identity in a context of what might otherwise be a set of conflicting discourses. At the same time it uses a pragmatic form of instruction to distance itself from what might be perceived as a more feminine advice genre (Schirato / Yell 1999). In a six page feature article titled "Healthy Living Simplified" (*Men's Health,* US ed., March 2002: 112-117), readers were told "Ignoring things like fiber and floss doesn't make you a bad person, but it does put you at risk. Here 17 short cuts to perfect health for the less-than-perfect guy". The advice offered ranges from:

> If you don't eat fish twice a week (and thus risk heart disease) [...] take fish oil supplements.
> If you won't use sunscreen (and risk skin cancer) [...] drink iced green tea.

> If you avoid that annual flu shot (and risk respiratory illness) […] become a compulsive hand washer.

To:

> If you can't stand separating your laundry by whites and colors […] toss everything in together and select 'Permanent Press' and 'warm'.

Some are risks readers can do something about, others seem less easy to deal with. In the "Health Bulletin: Advice and Information You Can Use" column, snippets of health advice seemingly extracted from medical research were given. "Double Dose of Heart Help" said it is possible to reduce the risk of heart disease by taking both vitamin E and aspirin every day, even if cholesterol levels are high (*Men's Health*, Aust. ed., May 2002: 21. Also US ed., March 2002). Aspirin advice occurred several times in the period under consideration including in an article on DVT – "Bloody Jet-leg [sic]" (*Men's Health*, UK ed., March 2002: 98). A feature, " Multi-pill Choice" (*Mens' Health*, Aust. ed., Jan. 2003: 48-49), listed 13 benefits from a regular dose of aspirin including to guard against strokes, ward off prostate cancer, or reduce the risk of colon cancer.

In contrast, other examples provided information about risk that is harder to do something about. The risk of developing Alzheimer's disease was correlated to having a small head (less than 53cm in circumference) with advice given to "keep your brain active" ("Health Bulletin", *Men's Health,* Aust. ed., May 2002: 21. Also US ed., March 2002). In a similar vein, another "Health Bulletin" ("Some Men Sold Short on Heart Health", Aust. ed., February 2002: 22; also "Caught Short", *Men's' Health* , UK ed., June 2002: 29) told readers that "men with short legs have an increased risk of heart disease and diabetes" because leg length may be an indicator of poor nutritional and environmental circumstances during childhood, which makes the body prone to depositing excess fat tissue.

These are just a few examples of how the magazine communicates health risk to its readers. On one hand, some types of serious health risk seem to be able to be managed by merely taking an aspirin; but other conditions are beyond the individual's conscious control because unfortunately for them, they have small heads and/or short legs. However, this mix of readily available interventions and stories of odd correlations construct a discourse of risk that, while entertaining, is not necessarily helpful.

Occasionally, health information is conveyed through narrative. While narratives are used frequently in women's magazines to tell of the experience of severe illness, and very often in the teen girls' magazines too, there are comparatively few in *Men's Health.* One exception was a feature including stories from three men on how they dealt with panic attacks ("When Panic Attacks", *Men's Health*, Aust. ed., May 2002: 103-107. Another was "My Heart Attack: an Annotated Guide" (*Men's Health,* US ed., Sept. 2002: 157) where one man tells of the mistakes he made in not recognising the seriousness of his condition, not seeking help quickly and even having a whisky and smoking a cigar before going to hospital.

But there is another way that the magazine conveys health risks: through risk profiling in much the same way that the financial or insurance community profiles and then assesses risk, albeit using much more simplistic measures. For example, at one time and across most international editions, readers were able to assess all kinds of risks on the "Gameshow" page where three people were profiled and the readers asked to assess their risk of various diseases or conditions e.g. "Who will get colon cancer?" (*Men's Health,* Aust. ed., February 2002: 67); "Who will lower his cholesterol for good?" (*Men's Health,* Aust. ed., Feb. 2003: 41); "Who will get Alzheimer's first?" (*Men's Health,* Aust. ed., March 2002: 3); "Who will fight off a cold first?" (*Men's Health,* Aust. ed., June 2002: 69; UK ed., March 2002: 69; US ed., March 2002: 63). The latter was re-published across several editions to take account of the seasonal incidence of the common cold.

Readers are then routinely provided with information about the possible risks and defences for each person and asked to "take a few minutes to consider each contestant's prospects, then turn the page to meet this month's winner". In the Alzheimer's example, the three candidates were assessed by a doctor from the University of California's Centre on Ageing who decided Ron Reagan (son of the former American president) was the most at risk due to his family history, although all three had risk factors of serious concern. There is the opportunity for readers to score their own risk with the advice "if your score is –2 or less: write yourself a note so you don't forget to see your doctor – you have high risk of developing Alzheimer's disease. Need us to repeat that?"

In language terms, health issues are being re-contextualised into a discourse more commonly used in the insurance industry or in the financial pages. But more than that, in their re-contextualisation and with accompanying humour and irony, the health and protective behaviours mentioned are being distanced from more feminised discourses related to health mentioned earlier, and re-situated in a world more reminiscent of hegemonic masculinity.

5. Conclusion

These two quite different types of magazines present different opportunities to focus on the language of health risk and how it is conveyed.

On one level, the discursive repertoire of teenspeak and all that that entails in the teen girls' magazines supports the construction of a trusted friend to turn to for advice, experience and direction, all wrapped up in personal narratives, confidences and stories that could just happen to 'you' or 'someone you know'. If that is not enough, then celebrity experiences are invoked for role models, but they are usually not like 'you' at all. Celebrity health experiences are usually related to eating disorders and diets with very little on issues related to drug or alcohol addiction. It is perhaps cynical to think that celebrity promotional machines come into play here which permit focus on some issues but not others. At another level, this construction of sharing experiences with a trusted friend or reading about a celebrity is undermined by the advice that is possible to give from this perspective. It is here that the magazines find themselves in something of a moral dilemma of wanting to offer credible and qualified advice to young girls, and yet maintain an image of utility and value for advertisers, parents and the general public. Hence, the personal stories are moderated with extra advice such as further explanations of health risk, with recommendations to see a doctor, or very often to check a website or seek help via a telephone helpline.

The multi-layered approach to teen health risk both within individual feature articles, but also considered across an entire issue with the various sections and types of articles, allows separate voices to come through as a kind of multi-faceted approach, where peers can tell it like it is, celebrities can be quoted, and where expert voices can be heard. This approach is necessary firstly, to fit in with the teen register that the magazines use to address their readers, but more significantly, it is needed to minimize the disjunctions that occur between the 'real life' problems as experienced by very young women and the solutions that can be offered. The assumption underlying the magazines' discourse on health risk and which frames most of the health messages is that parents and doctors are not approached much for information and advice by this age group. The magazines then are attempting to fill this gap.

Men's Health works similarly to fill a gap on the assumption that many men are not much interested in health issues and rarely visit medical practitioners. It too uses an imitative register which is designed to reflect the vernacular of its readers. Its use of humour and irony works in anticipation of reader resistance to health advice while its pragmatism and appeal to rationalism evoke a business-like risk discourse. Like the attention the teen magazines pay to ensuring that their method of address does not 'talk down' to their readers but talks to them as peers, *Men's Health* uses its speaking position to instruct its readers in playful recognition of their ignorance of health matters. Both are of course in keeping with their respective audience identities and their assumed sensibilities in terms of health issues.

References

Baker, Peter 2001. The International Men's Health Movement has Grown to the Stage that it can Start to Influence International Bodies. *British Medical Journal* 323 /7320, 1014-1015.

Ballaster, Ros / Beetham, Margaret / Frazer, Elizabeth / Hebron, Sandra 1991. *Women's Worlds: Ideology, Femininity and the Woman's Magazine*. London: Macmillan.

Banks, Ian 2001. No Man's Land: Men, Illness, and the NHS. *British Medical Journal* 323/7320: 1058-1060.

Beck, Ulrich 1992. *Risk Society: Towards a New Modernity*. London: Sage.

Cameron, Elaine / Bernardes, Jon 1998. Gender and Disadvantage in Health: Men's Health for a Change. *Sociology of Health & Illness* 20/5, 673-693.

Currie, Dawn 1999. *Girl Talk: Adolescent Magazines and their Readers*. Toronto: University of Toronto Press.

Ferguson, Marjorie 1983. Forever Feminine: Women's Magazines and the Cult of Femininity. London: Heinemann.

Gauntlett, David 2002. *Media, Gender and Identity: An Introduction*. London: Routledge.

Giddens, Anthony 1991. *Modernity and Self-identity: Self and Society in the Late Modern Age*. Cambridge: Polity.

Greco, Monica 1993. Psychosomatic Subjects and the 'Duty to be Well': Personal Agency within Medical Rationality. *Economy and Society* 22/3, 357-372.

Griffiths, Sian 1996. Men's Health: Unhealthy Lifestyles and an Unwillingness to Seek Medical Help. *British Medical Journal* 312/7023: 69-70.

Gwyn, Richard 2002. *Communicating Health and Illness*. London: Sage.

Harris, Kathleen Mullan / Duncan, Greg J. / Boisjoly, Johanne 2002. Evaluating the Role of 'Nothing to Lose' Attitudes on Risky Behaviour in Adolescence. *Social Forces* 80/3, 1005-39.

Hermes, Joke 1995. *Reading Women's Magazines: An Analysis of Everyday Media Use*. Cambridge: Polity.

Jackson, Peter / Stevenson, Nick / Brooks, Kate 2001. *Making Sense of Men's Magazines*. Cambridge: Blackwell.

Machin, David / Thornborrow, Joanna 2003. Branding and Discourse: The Case of *Cosmopolitan*. *Discourse and Society* 14/4, 453-471.

McCracken, Ellen 1993. *Decoding Women's Magazines from 'Mademoiselle' to 'Ms'*. New York: St Martin's Press.

McKay, Susan 2005. Communication and 'Risky' Behaviour in Adolescence. In Williams, Angie / Thurlow, Crispin (eds) *Talking Adolescence: Perspectives on Communication in the Teenage Years*. New York: Peter Lang, 265-281.

McKay, Susan / Bonner, Frances 1999. Telling Stories: Breast Cancer Pathographies in Australian Women's Magazines. *Women's Studies International Forum* 22/5, 563-572.

McKay, Susan / Bonner, Frances 2002. Evaluating Illness: Health Narratives in Women's Magazines. *Journal of Language and Social Psychology* 21/1, 53-67.

McRobbie, Angela 1996. More!: New Sexualities in Girls' and Women's Magazines. In Curran, James / Morley, David / Walkerdine, Valerie (eds) *Cultural Studies and Communications*. London: Arnold, 172-94.

McRobbie, Angela [2]2000. *Feminism and Youth Culture*. Basingstoke: Macmillan.

Millstein, Susan G. / Litt, Iris F. 1990. Adolescent Health. In Feldman, S. Shirley/ Elliott, Glen R. (eds) *At the Threshold: The Developing Adolescent*. Cambridge MA: Harvard University Press, 431-456.

Petersen, Alan R. 1994. *In a Critical Condition: Health and Power Relations in Australia*. St Leonards, NSW: Allen & Unwin.

Petersen, Alan R. / Lupton, Deborah 1996. *The New Public Health: Health and Self in the Age of Risk*. St Leonards, NSW: Allen & Unwin.

Schirato, Tony / Yell, Susan 1999. The 'New' Men's Magazines and the Performance of Masculinity. *Media International Australia* 92, 81-90.

Seale, Clive 2002. *Media and Health*. London: Sage.

Seale, Clive 2004. Health and the Media: An Overview. In Seale, Clive (ed.) *Health and the Media*. Malden MA: Blackwell, 1-19.

Signorielli, Nancy 1993. *Mass Media Images and Impact on Health: A Sourcebook*. Westport, Connecticut: Greenwood Press.

Stevenson, Nick / Jackson, Peter / Brooks, Kate 2000a. Ambivalence in Men's Lifestyle Magazines. In Jackson, Peter / Lowe, Michelle / Miller, Daniel / Mort, Frank (eds) *Commercial Cultures: Economics, Practices, Spaces*. Oxford: Berg, 189-211.

Stevenson, Nick / Jackson, Peter / Brooks, Kate 2000b. The Politics of 'New' Men's Lifestyle Magazines. *European Journal of Cultural Studies* 3/3, 366-385.

Tincknell, Estelle / Chambers, Deborah / van Loon, Joost / Hudson, Nichola 2003. Begging for It: 'New Femininities', Social Agency and Moral Discourse in Contemporary Teenage and Men's Magazines. *Feminist Media Studies* 3/1, 47-63.

Toerien, Merran / Durrheim, Kevin 2001. Power through Knowledge: Ignorance and the 'Real Man'. *Feminism and Psychology* 11/1, 35-53.

Williams, Simon / Calnan, Michael 1996. Modern Medicine and the Lay Populace: Theoretical Perspectives and Methodological Issues. In Williams, Simon / Calnan, Michael (eds), *Modern Medicine: Lay Perspectives and Experiences*. London: UCL Press, 1-25.

Winship, Janice 1987. *Inside Women's Magazines*. London: Pandora.

PHILIPPA MUNGRA

Macrostructure and Rhetorical Moves in Secondary Research Articles: The Meta-Analysis and the Systematic Analysis

1. Introduction

With the proliferation of research publications in the middle of last century, a filing system had to be devised to cope with the enormous output of medical literature in English. This has led to the creation of several bibliography indexing services in the mid 1960s such as the Science Citation Index and Biological Abstracts, as well as the Institute for Scientific Information (ISI), the first to publish a weekly paper catalogue of new publications in 1963, called Current Contents. The advent of computerization of information has carried this indexing to its logical offshoot in the establishment of databases, such as MEDLINE and the web-based PubMed, first published by the US National Library of Medicine (NLM)[1] in 1993, and the Cochrane Collaboration,[2] published by the Cochrane Library in the UK, the purpose of which was to cope with the over one million articles published yearly in the 2000s. The rationale used by these indexing

1 NLM (National Library of Medicine), created in 1956, forms part of the National Institutes of Health (NIH). It established a retrieval system in 1965, in Bethesda, Md. USA. The website for consultable indexed citations, established first in 1986, has been available in Internet since 1993 at http://www.nlm.nih.gov/.

2 The Cochrane Collaboration established in 1993 at www.cochrane.org. after a Scottish epidemiologist named Archibald H Cochrane, is an independent library with several databases. It now has many registries of research protocols and is currently managed by the university of York in the UK at their website http://www.york.ac.uk/inst/crd/cochlib.htm/. It has many associated bodies worldwide, including the UK National Health Service (NHS).

services to classify papers is based on key words, but such descriptors have created some confusion about the characteristics of different genres for linguists and for non-native English speakers (NNES) alike. In this chapter, we will focus our attention on review articles or 'overviews' (Haynes 1992).

In the fast-moving field of medico-scientific research and technology, reviews constitute an important font of current knowledge (Lehman / Goodman 1995). Reviews indeed serve to chart known areas of research and to speculate on new and unknown areas of research (Gotti 2002: 65) in the search for evidence to deliver better medical care (Oxman / Cook / Guyatt 1994). Mulrow (1987), Haynes (1992) and Jadad *et al.* (1998) have published methodological standards and structural guidelines for assessing the scientific quality and clinical usefulness of review articles. For their part, McAlister *et al.* (1999) found that most review articles do not specify methodological standards and that their quality is thus uneven and at times not useful for clinicians.

The literature on review articles is confusing even for clinicians. Therefore, in order to improve their quality, there is a need, from a linguistic point of view, to identify the structural patterns used by author-physicians when preparing papers (Mulrow 1987). Although it is possible that no conscious or pre-determined schemata are resorted to, it is interesting to determine firstly, whether rhetorical/discursive patterns are present and, if so, to identify their communicative moves, and secondly, whether these patterns/moves are any different from the moves observed in primary research articles (RAs). The primary purpose of this chapter is then to identify the moves most frequently used in review papers, using the section-move-step pattern proposed by Swales (1990: 133-134), in two types of synoptic publications, viz., the Systematic Review (SR) and the Meta-Analysis (MA). A secondary aim of this paper is to determine whether there is any resemblance between primary and secondary RAs in biomedicine.

In order to identify these structural and discursive patterns, we must first define exactly what the medical world calls 'a systematic review' (SR) and a 'meta-analysis' (MA).

1.1. Characteristics of meta-analysis and systematic review articles according to cataloguers and publishers

Both PubMed of the NLM and the Cochrane Collaboration use a string of words and fragments called Medical Sub-Heading or MeSH terms, organized in a nested tree-structure. These additively formulated strings represent bigger branches on the 'tree'. Table 1 shows the formulation of the string of MeSH words for the type of publication called 'meta-analysis'.

MeSH Heading	Meta-Analysis
Tree Number	E05.318.780.500 investigative techniques
Tree Number	G03.850.520.445.500 environmental and public health
Tree Number	H01.770.644.728.501 natural sciences
Tree Number	N05.715.360.780.515 health care quality Health Care Quality, Access, and Evaluation [N05] Quality of Health Care [N05.715] Health Care Evaluation Mechanisms [N05.715.360] Epidemiologic Research Design [N05.715.360.780] Meta-Analysis [N05.715.360.780.515]
Scope Note	A quantitative method of combining the results of independent studies (usually drawn from the published literature) and synthesizing summaries and conclusions which may be used to evaluate therapeutic effectiveness, plan new studies, etc., with application chiefly in the areas of research and medicine.

Table 1. Showing nesting of MeSH terms for meta-analysis within the category N05.

The Centre for Reviews and Dissemination (CRD), which is run by the National Health Service (NHS) of the UK and which forms part of the Cochrane Collaboration at the University of York, defines them both as follows in its self-training guide and notes issue (2002: 2):

> A *systematic review* is a review that strives comprehensively to identify and synthesise all the literature on a given topic (sometimes called an overview). The unit of analysis is the primary study and the same scientific principles and rigour apply as for any study. If a review does not state clearly whether and how all relevant studies were identified and synthesised, it is not a systematic review.
>
> *Meta-analysis* is a statistical technique for assembling the results of several studies in a review into a single numerical estimate.

This definition was initially used to determine whether a publication in the corpus we analyzed was a SR or a MA:

> Many reviews are not systematic but are still valuable and helpful so long as the reader is aware and takes account of the fact. A systematic review can be performed on any type of scientific evidence, both *quantitative and qualitative*. Consequently not all systematic reviews contain meta-analyses. However a meta-analysis that is not a systematic review is likely to be highly biased and should be used with extreme caution or not used at all. (My italics)

Although the Cochrane Collaboration then, restricts the definition of a MA to a method or statistical technique, we followed the standard used by the NLH PubMed which conflates the statistical techniques with the genre to refer to secondary publications that use this kind of data synthesis.

To summarize, MAs and SRs fall under the category of scientific summaries or overviews dealing with health care and offer support which may be quantitative (in the case of MAs) or semi-quantitative (in the case of SRs) for their conclusions based on evidence from independent or primary studies. Thus, in agreement with Greenhalgh (1997), one of the exponents of Evidence-Based Medicine (EBM),[3] they may be considered secondary studies. The general features characterizing MAs and SRs are shown in Table 2.

---

3 EBM or Evidence-Based Medicine is a school of thought, first enunciated in Canada, which advocates searching the medical literature for the best methodological proof of procedures in order to improve patient care.

Systematic reviews

- A single well-defined question is chosen or an aim/ hypothesis of the overview is then defined.
- All the relevant published literature is identified in a reproducible manner then analysed systematically so as highlight similarities, differences and errors of procedure, results and conclusions of the publications chosen.
- This systematic approach may result in a definitive answer to the original question or hypothesis. Semi-quantitative data such as a L'Abbe plot but no hard statistical data are prepared.

Meta-analysis

- Similar to a systematic review, this type of publication is limited to answering a specific well-defined question but differs from a systematic review in that it offers a statistical synthesis of the results of various scientific or clinical studies in support of the answer or hypothesis.
- The results of a meta-analysis is often expressed in terms of statistical strength of the hypothesis in favour of or against a specific treatment by means of a Forrest plot (Fig 1).
- In a Forrest Plot, the horizontal lines can express relative or absolute risk reduction, or confidence interval (90 or 95%) and their significance (p-value) among the various research publications or treatment outcomes.
- A statistically inconclusive meta-analysis may be considered a systematic review.

Table 2. Summary of characteristics of evaluative secondary RAs. (Information based on The Cochrane Collaboration and EBM papers.)

2. Methods

2.1. Retrieval and initial evaluation

Because the medical literature is so vast, it was necessary to limit the publications to one area of medicine. Three clinical pathologies, all within internal medicine, were chosen: diabetes, kidney dysfunctions and some cardiopathologies, expressed using key words: 'heart' OR[4] 'cardiovascular', 'diabetes' and 'kidney' OR 'renal'. Searches were

4 'OR' is a Boolean operator and is used to expand a search.

thus performed using these key words as MeSH terms, and were limited to: 'systematic analyses' and 'meta-analyses' in PubMed. Only publications retrieved from core English language clinical journals[5] published between 2000 and 2004 were selected. In this way, a single corpus was retrieved with those key words catalogued as MeSH words. From this set, an electronic copy of as many publications as possible was downloaded and constituted the corpus listed in the Appendix.

2.2. Framework for moves analysis

The opinion of three independent physician-informants, familiar with the above mentioned medical topics was sought for clarification about the purpose of the text and any technical explanation of graphs and flowcharts. Because any given publication is difficult to classify, we found it helpful to use this checklist to identify MAs and SRs:

1. Clearly stated title and objectives for the review;
2. Comprehensive strategy to search for studies that address the objectives of the review (relevant studies) to include unpublished as well as published studies;
3. Explicit and justified criteria for the inclusion or exclusion of any study;
4. Comprehensive list of all studies identified;
5. Clear presentation of the characteristics of each study included and an analysis of methodological quality;
6. Comprehensive list of all studies excluded and justification for exclusion;
7. Clear analysis of the results of the eligible studies using statistical synthesis of data (meta-analysis) if appropriate and possible;
8. Sensitivity analyses of the synthesised data if appropriate and possible;

---

5 The expression 'core medical journals' refers to a set of over 100 widely-read English language journals indexed in the PubMed database.

9. Structured report of the review clearly stating the aims, describing the methods and materials and reporting the results. (From the Cochrane Collaboration at http://www.york.ac.uk/inst/crd/cochlib.htm)

This checklist was used by the three informant-physicians who were asked to read the publications of their specialty from our corpus. It is interesting to note that characteristic No. 7 above defines MAs as statistical reviews that synthesize primary studies. The Centre for Reviews and Dissemination is the only one, to our knowledge, which has published standards for the characteristics of both SRs and MAs.

Once we achieved agreement as to the composition of our corpus, we proceeded to identify the moves in each one of the fifteen papers we analyzed. We adopted three basic models from the literature on scientific RAs: 1) Swales' (1990: 140) CARS model of section-move-step originally published for article introductions 2) Hopkins / Dudley-Evans' (1988) model which identifies important and characteristic linguistic features in the discussion section and 3) the set of moves used by Nwogu (1997) in all the IMRD[6] sections in RAs. Table 3 summarizes the moves present in these three models, which we used as the basis for our moves analysis.

Swales' (1990) model	Hopkins / Dudley-Evans' model (revised by Peacock 2002)	Nwogu's model (amplified by Kanoksilapatham 2005)
Introduction **Move1. Establishing a territory** • centrality claim • topic generalisations • review items of previous research **Move 2. Establishing a niche** • counterclaim or gap or question raising or continuing a tradition	Discussion & conclusion **1. Introduction move** • information : back-ground, research aims/methodology • statement of result(numerical or graph) or finding (non-numerical) • reference to prior research	Introduction **Move 1. Presenting background** • reference to established knowledge • reference to main research problem **Move 2. Review related research** • reference to previous research • limitations of previous research

6 IMRD (also IMRaD) first used by Swales (1990) refers to the sections Introduction, Methods, Results and Discussion/Conclusion, commonly used in preparing scientific laboratory reports and primary RAs.

Move 3. Occupying the niche • outline purpose or announce present research • *announcing principal findings* indicating RA structure and features Methods : no specific moves lexical , grammatical and syntactic characteristics Results Lexical grammatical and syntactical characteristics Discussions & Conclusion 1. summarizing results 2. What results suggest with references 3. Further questions Modified version contains 8 moves (pg 172) 1. background 2. statement of results 3. (un)expected outcome 4. reference to prior research 5. explanation 6. exemplification 7. deduction & hypothesis recommendation	**2. Evaluation move** • statement of result(numerical or graph) or finding (non-numerical) • reference to prior research • claim (generalisation arising from results: contribution) **3. Conclusion move** • finding (non-numerical) • claim (generalisation arising from results: contribution) • limitation • recommendation	**Move 3. Presenting new research** • research purpose • main procedure Methods **Move 4. Data collection procedure** • source of data • data size • criteria for data collection **Move 5. Main experimental procedures** • research apparatus • recounting expt. process • criteria for success **Move 6. Describing data-analysis procedures** • defining terminologies • process of data classification • analytical instrument/procedure • modification to procedure. Results **Move 7. Indicating consistent observations** • highlighting overall observations • indicating specific observations • accounting for observations made **Move 8. Indicating non-consistent observations** Discussion & Conclusion **Move 9. Highlighting overall /main research outcome** **Move 10. Explaining specific outcome** • stating specific outcome • interpreting the outcome • indicating significance of outcome • contrasting present and previous outcome **Move 11. Stating conclusions** • research implications • promoting further research

Table 3. The three models used for moves analysis in Primary RAs.

Many researchers have studied and classified communicative moves in legal publications (Bhatia 1993), and in the medico-scientific field (Adams-Smith 1984, Hopkins / Dudley-Evans 1988, Nwogu 1997, Williams 1999, Skelton / Edwards 2000). Peacock (2002), Samraj (2005) and more recently Lorés (2004) as well as Kanoksilapatham (2005) have also identified variations in move sequences in specific sections of primary RAs from different academic disciplines. All these studies have dealt with primary research articles (RAs) or specific parts of RAs in science. To the best of our knowledge, no moves analysis of secondary RA in medicine has so far been carried out. Ruiying / Allison's (2004) research on secondary RAs in linguistics is the only study that has analyzed secondary RAs.

We adopted the procedure outlined by Peacock (2002): 1) identify sections 2) identify boundaries for each move within each section by linguistic clues and text meaning 3) assign as many sentences as possible to a move. Agreement (95%) was validated by a second coder, a language teacher and proof-reader of medical publications. Any disagreement was sorted out by discussion with the help of the physician-informants who had read the publications and who clarified the interpretation of the information that was the source of disagreement. We will describe and discuss our findings in the following section.

3. Results and discussion

3.1. Retrieval and initial evaluation

Raw data of publications retrieved are given in Table 4, using all the key words for one-year periods between 2000-2004. The data clearly shows that before 2003, secondary reviews were either not published or not indexed in PubMed.

Year	*2004*	*2003*	*2002*	*2001*	*2000*
all MeSH words, English human, core medical journals, systematic analysis or meta-analysis	1101	1469	4	0	0

Table 4. Retrieval data according to year of publication.

3.2. Move sequence

From a structural point of view, all the SRs and MAs of our corpus resemble primary research articles (RAs) in that they follow the IMRD format (Swales 1990: 134). All the publications of this corpus conformed to the standard of having the Swalesian IMRD sections and concur with the definition of Ruiying and Allison (2004: 266) that secondary studies “critically review trends in the research and professional literatures, and synthesize research carried out by others”. We will now describe the sequence of moves of each section.

3.2.1. Introduction section (moves 1, 2, 3)

A summary or abstract, usually with the IMRD sequence, is always present. The introduction to the paper itself is generally formulated according to Swales’ CARS model of 3 moves/steps. Not all the steps were present, as has been observed by others, such as Lorés (2004) who analyzed abstracts from linguistics RAs, Ruiying / Allison (2004) who examined a linguistics corpus and Kanoksilapatham (2005) who studied a biochemistry corpus of primary RAs. However, the following Swalesian moves/steps were always present in the introduction:

Move 1: Establishing a territory, e.g. centrality claim;
Move 2: Establishing a niche, e.g. indicating a gap and raising a question;
Move 3: Occupying a niche, e.g. introducing the aim or purpose of present study.

However, Swales' move3-step2 (Announcing principal findings) and step3 (Indicating RA structure and features) were not always present. Instead, we found that move 3 was either a question or a description of the way in which the aim was to be achieved. The aim of these publications is clearly defined, but there is a significant difference between them in the strength of the aim, that is, in the way the claim is to be substantiated or the hypothesis verified. Whereas in systematic reviews the claim may not always be proved or disproved, in the case of meta-analyses, the verification process is always substantiated by statistical calculation using pooled data extracted from the primary publications. Usually, the introduction ends with a recapitulation or summative statement followed by advance signaling of the methods used:

(1) We then searched for evidence from randomised controlled trials of the effects of ACE inhibitors and AIIRAs on renal outcomes and mortality in patients with diabetic nephropathy.

It is for this reason that we prefer to define this move as 'Introducing the study', and subdivide it into 2 steps – a sequence which is more in harmony with the findings of Kanoksilapatham (2005) in her study of primary biochemistry RAs.

3.2.2. Methods section (moves 4, 5)

Like primary RAs, the next section is the methods section, which describes in detail the search strategy for primary publications and the criteria used for evaluation. It must be emphasized here that while RAs observe cells or patients, systematic review and meta-analyses observe primary RAs/Randomized Clinical Trials (RCTs)[7] generally selected from a database of primary publications. Hence we find:

(2) We searched Medline (1966-September 2003) and Embase (1988-September 2003) optimally sensitive search strategies developed by the Cochrane Collaboration.

---

7 RCT stands for Randomised Clinical Trial and may be considered a clinical RA. It is usually prospective in design and may deal with different domains such as therapy, prevention or screening. Therapy aims at determining which of the competing treatments or interventions is the most effective.

We observed that the search strategy was always described with information about the search words, databases and the language of publication. Data extraction and quality assessment was also described. There were three instances (20%) of authors' disagreement on the choice of publications because of well-defined inclusion and exclusion criteria and in the way the data was to be interpreted. In these cases, consensus was achieved and a brief note appeared in the systematic review or meta-analysis as:

(3) any discrepancy between the two researchers was resolved by discussion.

Unlike the 4-move sequence proposed by Kanoksilapatham (2005) for biochemistry RAs, we observed only two main moves (4 and 5) in this section and they were always present:

Move 4: Search strategy for selection of studies.

Step 1: Identification and justification of RAs or RCTs, with inclusion and exclusion of the criteria of selection.

(4) Our search identified 694 published articles; we retrieved the full text of 69 and reviewed them to assess whether they provided information on glycosylated haemoglobin and cardiovascular risk.

Step 2: Dealing with aberrations or disagreements between researchers.

(5) Papers identified by the search strategy were reviewed for eligibility.

Step 3: Defining extraction of parameters or subgroups to be compared. This step defines what data are to be extracted and compared from the publications judged suitable. This list of outcomes to be compared furnishes the basis for the sequence of cycles seen in both the results and discussion sections.

(6) Data were extracted on symptom scales used, methods of data collection, durations of assessment, whether individual or global symptoms were used, whether reduction or absence of symptoms was the main outcome measure, the types of symptoms assessed, whether frequency and/or severity were

evaluated, and whether quality of life and patient satisfaction measures were used.

Move 5: Procedures used in data synthesis. This move is described in great detail in meta-analyses and consists of two steps:

Step 1: Extraction of data from roster of publications and researcher blinding[8] for quality control, such as in:

(7) Eligible trials underwent data extraction using a predesigned data extraction form, which was checked by a second reviewer, who did not know [...].

Step 2: Synthesis, statistical modeling and software used, as in (8):

(8) Analysis was performed as a metaregression using the trial intervention as the explanatory variable. All analyses were undertaken in STATA version 8.0 and RevMan 4.2.

While in Kanoksilapatham's biochemistry corpus, the moves of Detailing equipment (her move 6) and Describing statistical procedures (move 7) were optional, in our corpus her move 7 was always present and was often quite detailed with inclusion of computer software specification for data analysis and computer modeling and a brief description of how the results are to be represented and interpreted as in (9):

(9) The results are shown in the form of a L'Abbé plot, a technique primarily used to explore heterogeneity among trials.

In the case of one systematic review of our corpus (No. 3), a statistical synthesis of patient data was attempted but because patients' subgroups were not comparable between RAs, no statistical synthesis was possible.

(10) Reliable estimates of the unconfounded relative effects of ACE inhibitors compared with AIIRAs could not be obtained owing to small sample sizes.

---

8 Blinding means that the researcher was unaware of the opinion or choice of his/her peers.

The authors explicitly state that the inability to apply statistical modeling to the data and the consequent semi-quantitative methods used, place their publication into the category of systematic reviews and not among the meta-analyses one.

Linguistically, many of the features described by Swales were seen, such as the use of the past passive, the explicit indication of author identity (*we*) or the initials of the primary investigator. This is an unusual feature but may be related to the attribution of credits, so important in the fierce competition for grants or tenure common in many university systems. Verbs usage is limited to a restricted range, such as: *searched, identified, considered, analysed, performed, sought, collated, assessed, extracted, used* and *computed*. Inclusion or exclusion criteria were often indicated as modals, generally showing obligation, such as *had to occur*.

In agreement with Swales (1990), noun phrase stacking and nominalization of adjectives are seen and theme-rheme configuration often may be read as 'known-new' information as we can see in the examples below:

(11) Finally, we examined whether larger trials differed from smaller trials in their results, using the test described by Begg and Mazumdar which examines the rank correlation between the natural logarithm of the risk ratio and the weight of a study.

(12) The Q test is based on the chi-squared distribution, and it provides a measure of the sum of the squared differences between the results observed and the results expected in each study.

Examples 11 and 12 may appear complex but both rely on what Swales (1990:168) calls 'inferential bridging' or relying on the reader's background knowledge. They are both in fact a device used to explain procedures so as to pre-empt criticisms by potential readers.

3.2.3. Results section (move 6)

In systematic reviews, the results section is shorter than in meta-analyses, but they both contain many tables and graphs showing data synthesis. In the corpus, this type of diagram appears only in meta-analyses and indicates a statistic called 'the risk ratio'. While a description of the meaning of this statistic is outside the scope of this paper, it is important to refer to it since it is fundamental in the discussion of step 2 in the discussion section below.

In this section, we observed only one move, the purpose of which was to state the results extracted from the RAs/RCTs. This move consisted of three steps:

Step 1: Data description of tables (mainly in meta-analyses). The author's presence was very strong here with phrases beginning with *we:*

(13) We identified 31 trials that reported both absence of heartburn and healing of oesophagitis.

There were many expressions of outcomes or interventions, depending on the type of study, but in the MAs we analyzed, the most relevant data are represented by the term *pooled relative risk.*[9] This expression was not found in systematic reviews.

(14) Fig 1 presents the results of all analyses of persons with type 1 diabetes. The pooled relative risk [...] was 1.3.

Hedging expressions were very common, such as in the following examples:

(15) Sensitivity analyses indicated that all of the studies included in the pooled estimates *seemed to* contribute relatively equally to the estimate (no single study had substantial influence).

Step 2: Synthetic comment on each result or groups of results, such as in (16):

(16) There is a *paucity of information* on whether either symptom frequency or severity is the best measure of treatment in GORD. We identified *only* two trials (35 38) that reported symptom frequency, symptom severity, and oesophagitis healing. It is *unclear* [...].

---

9 Statistically, this term is a calculated number and represents the ratio of the incidence of disease or condition among subjects at risk, relative to the group which is not at risk.

The words in italics (my emphasis) indicate authorial comment. Other comments include descriptions of difficulties in harmonizing data from groups which were not comparable as in the example below:

(17) Four trials defined relapse as moderate or severe symptoms over 1-7 days; a similar proportion of patients were in remission using this definition compared with absence of oesophagitis, therefore, they have a symptom profile that is not exactly comparable with unselected GORD patients seen in primary care. This must be borne in mind when data from such cohorts are evaluated for the full range of reflux symptoms.

Step 3: Generalizing comments from the data tables. This step was often merged with the following section as is seen in the following example:

(18) These data support a moderate increase in cardiovascular risk with increasing levels of glycosylated haemoglobin in persons with diabetes mellitus.

3.2.4. Discussion section (moves 7, 8, 9)

The discussion section is discursive with many propositions. This section closely resembles that of RAs, which has been amply treated by many authors such as Skelton / Edwards (2000), Swales (1990), Berkenkotter / Huckin (1995), Hyland (1998) and Peacock (2002), and serves to legitimize any claim by justifying it with a finding. Thus, each claim and its finding are discussed separately according to the outcome measured, defined in the methods section under move4-step3. Generally a claim may be made on the basis of a finding-by-comparison. For example, in a metanalysis on symptoms assessment, the reappearance of symptoms in long-term RCTs may be compared with short-term RCTs, use with non-use of prior therapy, objective or self-reporting of symptoms and so on. This results in a complex structure of the discussion characterized by cyclic repetition of moves. In the discussion section, we observed three basic moves (moves 7, 8, 9) similar to those mentioned by Kanoksilapatham (2005) for primary RAs in biochemistry, but our findings regarding secondary RAs are slightly different.

In her study of primary RAs, Kanoksilapatham (2005) identifies move 12 (presenting generalizations, claims deductions or research gaps) but suggests that move 13 (stating selected findings and making overt claims) is optional. We found that both these moves were always present in our corpus of secondary RAs but they appear to form part of a single persuasive and conclusive move of evaluation, placed against the background of the scientific literature. Because of this, we suggest that these two moves should be incorporated into a single move 7, an evaluation, consisting of two steps:

Move 7: Evaluating the findings with respect to the scientific literature or Indicating the findings are in concordance with other authors, who may or may not be cited.

Step 1: Restating the purpose of the study and the hypothesis expected.

(19) *Trials* have shown a survival benefit of angiotensin converting enzyme (ACE) inhibitors but not of angiotensin II receptor antagonists (AIIRAs) in patients with diabetic nephropathy. The relative survival advantage of one class of antihypertensives over the other in this population is, however, still unknown because only *indirect comparisons based on small studies* are available.

Step 2: Making the claim. There were two variants of this step. In the first form, we observed in meta-analyses that authors stated the most salient observation(s) from the results with a statistical proof and put this observation into the context of other studies.

(20) One meta-analysis (citation) of adult data suggested that ODD might reduce nephrotoxicity, whereas other meta-analyses showed nonsignificant trends or no difference in nephrotoxicity outcomes. In our meta-analysis, we were not able to show any reduction since our RR [...].

Another variant was semi-quantitative or generalizing comments in systematic reviews with contextualization from other researchers.

(21) We found no evidence that these effects are related to baseline hypertension, type of diabetes, stage of diabetic nephropathy, and duration of treatment. However, there is strong evidence that AIIRAs are beneficial for renal outcomes, with *about a 22% reduction* in risk of end stage renal disease (ESRD).

Note that here "about a 22% reduction" indicates an approximation and is thus, in our opinion, a semi-quantitative authorial evaluation. There were several instances of authors proposing a new model of disease appearance or a hypothesis of disease mechanism:

(22) This meta-analysis indicates that, among children, ODD of aminoglycosides demonstrates a trend for better efficacy and shows similar low rates of nephrotoxicity and ototoxicity, compared with MDD. Also, we observed a trend toward fewer bacteriologic failures, which again was consistent with the results of adult meta-analyses.

Here we see that the authors make use of the word *trend* implying a tentative claim. Immediately, they proceed to compare this finding-claim with that or those of other researchers, as we saw in step 2.

Step 3: Indicating limitation to the claim. This step was not always present in MAs, but was more frequent in SRs.

Move 8: Clinical applications and recommendations. In this move, we see an explicit reference to the fact that the authors define the study as a Meta-Analysis and that they address the question of clinical efficacy, similar to that seen in other contexts, which are then cited.

(23) The clinical efficacy results of this meta-analysis on children are consistent with the results of several meta-analyses that addressed the same question among adults.

Again we see the possible application to treatment, formulated as a recommendation using modal auxiliaries:

(24) Thus, outside of a comparative randomised controlled trial, the class of agent with proved survival benefit, ACE inhibitors, should be used as first line treatment.

Hedging expressions using modal auxiliaries are also seen and have already been described in the medical literature by Skelton (1997), Salager-Meyer (1994), Varttala (1999) and Webber / Snelgrove / Mungra (2001).

Move 9: Limitations of the study and problem areas that indicate the need for further/better/clearer and more methodologically sound research. In (25) and (26) the word *need* appears either as a verb or as a noun. This move is similar to that seen in primary RAs/RCTs:

(25) Future research *needs* to focus on sustained interventions for weight loss and control and long-term outcomes for health and quality of life.

(26) Our findings highlight the *need* for an adequately powered comparative trial of ACE inhibitors compared with AIIRAs.

Table 5 proposes a summary of the sequence of moves-steps we observed in our corpus of secondary RAs.

Introduction section (moves 1, 2, 3)
Move 1: Establishing a territory e.g. centrality claim **Move 2:** Establishing a niche e.g. indicating a gap and raising a question **Move 3**: Occupying a niche e.g. introducing the aim or identifying the purpose of present study
Methods section (moves 4, 5)
Move 4: search strategy for selection of studies **Step 1:** identification and justification of RAs or RCTs, with inclusion & exclusion criteria of selection **Step 2:** dealing with aberrations or disagreements between researchers **Step 3:** defining extraction of parameters or subgroups to be compared **Move 5:** procedures used in data synthesis **Step 1**: extraction of data from roster of publications and researcher blinding for quality control **Step 2**: data synthesis, statistical modeling and software used
Results section (move 6)
Step 1: data description of tables (**present in MAs, absent in SRs**) **Step 2:** synthetic comment on each result or groups of results **Step 3**: generalizing comments from the data tables
Discussion section (moves 7, 8, 9)
Move 7 Evaluating the findings and/or claim, indicating whether the findings are in concordance with other authors **Step 1**: restating the purpose of the study and the hypothesis expected **Step 2**: making a claim supported by data from move 6-3. **Step 3:** indicating limitation to the claim **Move 8:** clinical applications and recommendations **Move 9**: limitations of the study and problem areas for further study

Table 5. List of moves and steps in Systematic Reviews and Meta-Analyses.

4. Conclusions

In this study, the sequence of moves and steps shown in Table 5 is similar to that observed by Ruiying / Allison (2004) in their corpus of linguistic secondary RAs. However, they found that the sequence of sections was: introduction, argumentation and conclusion. Moreover, their sections on argumentation (viz.: theoretical basis and pedagogical basis) were not seen in our corpus. In the secondary scientific RAs making up our corpus, we have seen that the IMRD structure proposed by Swales (1990) was always present. In fact, we encountered no difficulty in identifying these sections which were predominantly objective: introduction, methods, results and conclusion/discussion. A structured abstract always preceded the body of the paper.

The most common purpose of the study (move 3 of introduction) was to measure risk reduction (54%), but among the other purposes indicated by the authors, the most frequent ones were to establish best therapy (38%), outcomes (30%) and measurement standards (8%). Thus we can say that the orientation of secondary RAs in preparing RAs and MAs is mainly to furnish robust data so as to justify therapeutic choice in current treatment or in risk reduction, as is commonly seen in preventive medicine.

The introduction in secondary RAs follows closely Swales' CARS model for primary RAs. Similarly, in the methods and results sections, identification of moves and steps was similar to that of primary RAs. However, in the discussion section, we did experience some difficulty in deciding what was a step and what was a move, as has been observed by Paltridge (1994). The main reason for this difficulty was perhaps due to the cyclic nature of moves and steps, as suggested by Peacock (2002). The most common cycle seen was move7-step 2 of the discussion, followed by moves 8 then 9. This sequence is then repeated, however, in some papers, we found that moves 7-1 and 7-3 could appear after 8 or 9 in later cycles.

The reason for this may be as Peacock (2002) claims, that in the discussion section, the research question or purpose is passed through several cycles such as: summarizing result / what the research suggests / further questions.

In this chapter, we restricted our study to a small corpus in three medical disciplines but it would be interesting to examine the linguistic features of these subgenres and see what variations if any, appear in the different sections of MAs and SRs from other medical or surgical specialties. Moreover, paratextual features of overviews, though outside the scope of this paper, certainly merit investigation.

References

Adams-Smith, Diana 1984. Medical Discourse: Aspects of Author's Comment. *The ESP Journal* 3, 25-36.

Berkenkotter, Carol / Huckin, Thomas N. 1995. *Genre Knowledge in Disciplinary Communication: Cognition / Culture / Power.* Hillsdale, NJ: Erlbaum.

Bhatia, Vijay K 1993. *Analysing Genre: Language Use in Professional Settings*. London: Longman.

Cortese, Giuseppina / Riley, Philip (eds) 2002. *Domain-Specific English*. Bern: Peter Lang.

Gotti, Maurizio 2002. Development of English as a Language for Specialized Purposes. In Cortese / Riley (eds), 65-86.

Gotti, Maurizio / Dossena, Marina (eds) 2001. *Modality in Specialized Texts*. Bern: Peter Lang.

Greenhalgh, Trisha 1997. *How to Read a Paper: The Basics of Evidence-Based Medicine*. London: British Medical Journal Publishing Group.

Haynes, R. Brian 1992. Clinical Review Articles. *British Medical Journal*. 304/6823, 330-1.

Hopkins, Andy / Dudley-Evans, Tony 1988. A Genre Based Investigation of the Discussion Section in Articles and Dissertations in Three Disciplines. *English for Specific Purposes* 7/2, 113-21.

Hyland, Ken 1998. *Hedging in Scientific Research Articles.* Amsterdam: Benjamins.

Jadad, Alejandro R. *et al.* 1998. Methodology and Reports of Systematic Reviews and Meta-analyses: A Comparison of Cochrane Reviews with Articles Published in Paper-based Journals. *Journal American Medical Association* 280/3, 278-80.

Kanoksilapatham, Budsaba 2005. Rhetorical Structure of Biochemistry Research Articles. *English for Specific Purposes* 24/3, 269-92.

Lehman, Harold P. / Goodman, Steven N. 1995. Specifications for Formalizing Clinical Significance. *Medical Decision Making* 15, 424.

Lorés, Rosa 2004. On RA Abstracts: From Rhetorical Structure to Thematic Organization. *English for Specific Purposes* 23/3, 280-302.

McAlister, Finlay A. / Clark, Heather D. / van Walraven, Carl / Straus, Sharon E. / Lawson, Fiona M.E. / Moher, David / Mulrow, Cynthia D. 1999. The Medical Review Article Revisited: Has the Science Improved? *Annals of Internal Medicine* 139/12, 947-51.

Mulrow, Cynthia D. 1987. The Medical Review Article: State of the Science. *Annals of Internal Medicine* 106/3, 485-8.

Nwogu, Kevin N 1997. The Medical Research Paper: Structure and Functions. *English for Special Purposes* 16/2, 119-38.

Oxman, Andrew D. / Cook, Deborah J. / Guyatt, Gordon H. (For The Evidence-Based Medicine Working Group) 1994. Users' Guides to the Medical Literature VI: How to Use an Overview. *Journal American Medical Association* 272, 1367-71.

Paltridge, Brian 1994. Genre Analysis and the Identification of Textual Boundaries. *Applied Linguistics* 15/3, 288-99.

Peacock, Matthew 2002. Communicative Moves in the Discussion Section of Research Articles. *System* 30/4, 479-97.

Ruiying, Yang / Allison, Desmond 2004. Research Articles in Applied Linguistics: Structures from a Functional Perspective. *English for Specific Purposes* 23/3, 264-79.

Salager-Meyer, Françoise 1994. Hedges and Textual Communicative Functions in Medical English Written Discourse. *English for Specific purposes* 13/2, 149-79.

Samraj, Betty 2005. An Exploration of a Genre Set: Research Article Abstracts and Introductions in Two Disciplines *English for Specific Purposes* 24/2, 141-56.
Skelton, John 1997. The Representation of Truth in Academic Medical Writing. *Applied Linguistics* 18, 121-40.
Skelton, John R. / Edwards, Sara J.L. 2000. The Function of the Discussion Section in Academic Medical Writing. *British Medical Journal* 320, 1269-70.
Swales John 1990. *Genre Analysis: English in Academic and Research Settings.* Cambridge: Cambridge University Press.
Varttala, Teppo 1999. Remarks of the Communicative Functions of Hedging in Popular Scientific and Specialist Research Articles on Medicine. *English for Specific Purposes* 18/2, 177-200.
Webber, Pauline / Snelgrove, Huon / Mungra, Philippa 2001. The Use of Modality in Different Medical Text Genres. In Gotti / Dossena (eds), 399-416.
Williams, Ian 1999. Results Section of Medical Research Articles: Analysis of the Rhetorical Categories for Pedagogical Purposes. *English for Special Purposes* 18/4, 347-66.

Appendix: Corpus

1. Strippoli, G.F. / Craig, M. / Deeks, J.J. / Schena, F.P. / Craig, J.C. 2004. Effects of Angiotensin Converting Enzyme Inhibitors and Angiotensin II Receptor Antagonists on Mortality and Renal Outcomes in Diabetic Nephropathy: Systematic Review. *British Medical Journal* 329, 828-39.
2. Warsi, A. / Wang, P.S. / LaValley, M.P. / Avorn, J. / Solomon, D.H. 2004. Self-management Education Programs in Chronic Disease: A Systematic Review and Methodological Critique of the Literature. *Archives of Internal Medicine* 164/15, 1641-9.
3. Doust, J.A. / Glasziou, P.P. / Pietrzak, E. / Dobson, A.J. 2004. A Systematic Review of the Diagnostic Accuracy of Natriuretic

Peptides for Heart Failure. *Archives of Internal Medicine* 164/18, 1978-84.

4. Norris, S.L. / Zhang, X. / Avenell, A. *et al.* 2004. Long-term Effectiveness of Lifestyle and Behavioral Weight Loss Interventions in Adults with Type 2 Diabetes: A Meta-analysis. *American Journal of Medicine* 117/10, 762-74.
5. Williams, G. / Robertson, V. / Greenwood, K. 2004. Measuring High-level Mobility after Traumatic Brain Injury. *American Journal of Physical Medicine & Rehabilitation* 83/12, 910-20.
6. Levitan, E.B. / Song, Y. / Ford, E.S. / Liu, S. 2004. Is Nondiabetic Hyperglycemia a Risk Factor for Cardiovascular Disease? A Meta-analysis of Prospective Studies. *Archives of Internal Medicine* 164/19, 2147-55.
7. Chiquette, E. / Ramirez, G. / Defronzo, R. 2004. A Meta-analysis Comparing the Effect of Thiazolidinediones on Cardiovascular Risk Factors. *Archives of Internal Medicine* 164/19, 2097-104.
8. Selvin, E. / Marinopoulos, S. / Berkenblit, G. *et al.* 2004. Meta-analysis: Glycosylated Hemoglobin and Cardiovascular Disease in Diabetes Mellitus. *Annals of Internal Medicone* 141/6, 421-31.
9. Contopoulos-Ioannidis, D.G. / Giotis, N.D. / Baliatsa, D.V. / Ioannidis, J.P. 2004. Extended-interval Aminoglycoside Administration for Children: A Meta-analysis. *Pediatrics* 114/1, 111-8.
10. Puvimanasinghe J.P. / Takkenberg, J.J. / Edwards, M.B, / Eijkemans, M.J. / Steyerberg, E.W. / Van Herwerden, L.A. / Taylor, K.M. / Grunkemeier, G.L. / Habbema, J.D. / Bogers, A.J. 2004. Comparison of Outcomes After Aortic Valve Replacement with a Mechanical Valve or a Bioprosthesis Using Microsimulation. *Heart* 90/10, 1172-8.
11. Modi, P. / Suleiman, M.S. / Reeves, B. / Pawade, A. / Parry, A.J. / Angelini, G.D. / Caputo, M. 2004. Myocardial Metabolic Changes During Pediatric Cardiac Surgery: A Randomized Study of Three Cardioplegic Techniques. *The Journal of Thoracic and Cardiovascular Surgery* 128/1, 67-75.
12. Sharma, U.C. / Barenbrug, P. / Pokharel, S. / Dassen, W.R. / Pinto, Y.M. / Maessen, J,G. 2004. Systematic Review of the

Outcome of Aortic Valve Replacement in Patients with Aortic Stenosis. *The Annals of Thoracic Surgery* 78/1, 90-5.

13. Sharma, N. / Donnellan, C. / Preston, C. *et al.* 2004. A Systematic Review of Outcomes Used in Oesophagitis Drug Therapy Trials. *Gut* 53, 58-65.

PÄIVI PAHTA

This is Very Important: A Corpus Study of Amplifiers in Medical Writing

1. Introduction

Amplifiers, words like *very* in the title of this chapter,* are an exciting category of linguistic items.[1] As degree words by nature, they are versatile in their expressivity and communicative functions. They are a lexicogrammatical means by which speakers and writers can foreground, emphasize and scale up the meaning of their focus. They are tools to distinguish, to adjust the strength of claims or recommendations, to convey the author's attitude and involvement, and to influence the reception of the message. Apart from signalling commitment and negotiating interpersonal truth or value judgements locally in issues at hand, amplifiers also carry other semantic-functional meanings in discourse. They play a key role in social and emotional expression of speakers (see e.g. Labov 1984, Partington 1993, Lorenz 1999). They signal group membership and are a strong indicator of norms and practices in a speech community (see e.g. Ito /

---

* The research reported here, carried out during my fellowship at the Helsinki Collegium for Advanced Studies, is part of the Research Unit for Variation, Contacts and Change in English, funded in the National Centre of Excellence programme 2006-2011 by the Academy of Finland and the Universities of Helsinki and Jyväskylä. The study is also part of my joint project with Irma Taavitsainen on Scientific Thought-styles.

1 I use the term 'amplifier' in the sense of Biber *et al.* (1999: 554) to denote the semantic category of degree adverbs that increase intensity. For Biber *et al.* the term is synonymous with 'intensifier', a term that has been used in most recent studies investigating elements in this category (e.g. Lorenz 1999, Ito / Tagliamonte 2003, Méndez-Náya 2003, Swales / Burke 2003, Tagliamonte / Roberts 2005). In this study the two terms are used as synonyms.

Tagliamonte 2003). They are subject to fashion and rapid change; several studies refer to them as items that show the most rapid and the most interesting semantic developments in linguistic change (e.g. Bolinger 1972, Quirk *et al.* 1985: 590, Peters 1994: 269).

In scientific discourse, especially in scientific writing, the status of amplifiers is ambiguous. Because of their hyperbolic nature, amplifiers are often associated with colloquial usage and nonstandard varieties, shunned by academic writers. They are particularly incompatible with an earlier view which saw scientific texts as dispassionate reports by scientists "passively observing naturally occurring facts" (Myers 1990: 141), or as "channels of communicating independently existing truths" (Hyland 2000: 6). The objectivist view of science writing is now largely replaced by one that sees scientific discourse as social interaction and scientific texts and ideas as "historically situated cultural products" (Hyland 2000: 178). This approach views scientific writing "as a process of situated rhetorical action" and assigns a more active role to the writer, constructing scientific knowledge through "ideal texts with particular reading audiences in mind", seeking to "design their discursive structures" to match the relevant genre conventions and "the gradually unfolding expectancies and competencies of the readership they have in mind" (Candlin 2000: xv). This change of perspective does not seem to have affected the status of amplifiers in scientific writing. Usage guides advise against their use in academic writing, encouraging authors to avoid them or use them sparingly. Other, more subtle linguistic means of focusing, emphasizing and boosting are encouraged instead.

Despite their ambiguous status, amplifiers do occur in scientific texts. However, their use in scientific writing differs from that in other registers. The prescriptive recommendations play a role in this, as they both reflect and re-enforce established conventions, acquired in professionalization to disciplinary cultures. Some register-specific tendencies are demonstrated in the *Longman Grammar of Written and Spoken English* (Biber *et al.* 1999), based on the analysis of a large multi-register corpus of late twentieth-century British and American English. The quantitative findings show that amplifiers like *really*, *so* and *too*, common in Present-day English conversation, are rarely used in academic writing, whereas some other items, such as *extremely*, *fully* and *highly*, not frequent in other registers, are more common in academic prose (see Biber *et al.* 1999: 564-566).[2] Academic registers also vary: an analysis of the Michigan Corpus of Academic Spoken English (MICASE) indicates that in amplifier use academic speech has greater affinity to everyday conversation and casual speech than to formal academic prose (Swales / Burke 2003).

In this study, I examine amplifiers within a single discipline, i.e. medicine. The study is part of a larger research plan, aiming to provide an analysis of amplifiers and their use in medical discourse across time.[3] My interest here is on synchronic variation in amplifier use in different types of written texts within the domain, ranging from scientific discourse among professionals to popularized accounts intended for the general readership.[4] I approach the topic through quantification, which provides an overview of macrolevel tendencies and facilitates the selection of individual features for more situated microlevel analyses, viewing the issue from multiple perspectives.

The study is based on the analysis of *Medicor*, an electronic corpus of late twentieth-century American English medical writing. The carefully structured material covers a range of genres with varying audience design and functions, and thus makes it possible to analyse the interconnectedness of linguistic variation and extralinguistic factors within the domain. I introduce the corpus in more detail in Section 2, which also describes my methodological decisions in data retrieval and their implications for the results. Section 3 contains an overview of the corpus findings. Sections 4 and 5 examine amplifiers in relation to the corpus parameters of audience design and genre, with an emphasis on quantitative variation between different types of medical writing. In Section 6, I discuss amplifier use in relation to the communicative purposes of genres in their disciplinary context. Section 7 observes amplifiers in popular articles, a special site where two modes of communication meet in written representations of speech. Section 8 looks at the immediate linguistic

---

2 Cf. Fries (1940: 204-205), who in his grammar of American English divides intensifiers into "Standard", such as *very*, and "Vulgar", including e.g. *real* and *so*.

3 For a study of amplifiers in medieval medical writing, see Pahta (2006).

4 For other domain-specific comparative studies on the genres of medical writing, see e.g. Nwogu (1990) and Vihla (1999). For a discussion of studies on language and medicine, see Fleischman (2001).

context of amplifiers, focusing on their adjective collocations. Finally, Section 9 offers some concluding remarks.

2. Material and method

Medicor, on which this study is based, is a domain-specific corpus of Present-day American English medical texts, compiled in the late 1990s by Minna Vihla (University of Helsinki) to facilitate studies of generic variation within medical writing.[5] It contains c. 400,000 words of running text from a variety of American publications from 1983 to 1997. The careful design and structuring of the corpus on the basis of external criteria makes it a useful tool for a range of research purposes. My description here concentrates on those aspects of the corpus design that are relevant for this study.[6]

Medicor consists of texts discussing medical or health issues, irrespective of the author's background or the status of the intended readership. The corpus material thus cuts across the domain, ranging from scientific in-group discourse among researchers at one end of the scale to medical writing intended for laymen at the other extreme, with texts intended for practitioners and medical students between the two poles. In the corpus design, each text has been classified according to three parameters. The main classification divides the texts into two categories, professional and popular, on the basis of their audience design. This division is depicted in Table 1. Professional texts are aimed at medical professionals (researchers, practitioners and students of medicine), whereas popular texts are targeted at the general readership. All corpus texts aimed at professionals were also written by medical professionals, most of

5 For copyright reasons, *Medicor* is only available for in-house use at the Research Unit for Variation, Contacts and Change in English, Department of English, University of Helsinki, by permission of the compiler. I am grateful to Minna Vihla for permission to use the corpus.

6 A detailed description of *Medicor* is contained in Vihla (1998) and Vihla (1999: 36-41); the corpus texts are listed in Vihla (1999, Appendix 2).

them MDs, while the writers of popular texts include both medical professionals and journalists.

Genre	No of texts	No of words
Professional texts		
Research articles	33	114 682
Editorial articles	36	47 869
Textbook samples	11	104 922
Handbook samples	16	41 237
Total for professional texts	***96***	***308 710***
Popular texts		
Newspaper/magazine articles	66	79 177
Guidebook samples	17	10 076
Total for popular texts	***83***	***89 253***
Total	**179**	**397 963**

Table 1. The composition of *Medicor*, a corpus of late twentieth-century American English medical writing.

Another categorization embedded inside the audience design structure divides the corpus material into different genres of medical writing. The genres aimed at medical professionals include research articles, editorial articles, handbook samples derived from medical practitioner's manuals, and samples from scientific or clinical textbooks used in medical schools. Popularized writings consist of articles on medical issues from magazines and newspapers intended for the general public, and guidebook samples from a family medical guide organized as an alphabetical encyclopaedia.

A third categorization is possible with regard to the communicative function of the texts. Here the genres can be divided into directive, argumentative and expository writing. Directive texts provide advice on how to act, argumentative writing aims at convincing the readers, and expository texts explain or describe. This grid can be combined with the other two divisions into a three-dimensional genre classification based on text-external criteria. This classification is shown in Table 2.

	Directive	Argumentative	Expository
Professional	Handbook samples	Research articles	Scientific textbooks
	Clinical textbooks	Editorial articles	
Popular	Guidebook samples		Popular articles

Table 2. *Medicor*: three-dimensional genre classification based on audience design, genre and communicative function.

The data for analysis was extracted from *Medicor* using the Corpus Presenter software (Hickey 2003). Data retrieval was based on lexical searches through the corpus. The search items were selected from earlier literature on English amplifiers, and the search list does not aim to include all lexical items that potentially can occur as amplifiers in Present-day English. As Lorenz (1999: 37) points out in his corpus study of amplifiers in argumentative writing, because of the dynamic, inventive and potentially open-ended nature of intensification, there is no finite list of amplifiers.[7] In this study, I have relied on a pre-defined set, consisting of well-established closed-class and open-class amplifiers, familiar from grammar books and many earlier studies on intensification.[8] I specifically wanted to include amplifiers that in earlier research have been identified with different registers, i.e. both conversation-style items and items more typical of formal registers. My search list contained 32 items: *absolutely*, *awfully*, *completely*, *enormously*, *entirely*, *especially*, *exceedingly*, *extremely*, *fantastically*, *full*, *fully*, *greatly*, *highly*, *hugely*, *incredibly*, *particularly*, *perfectly*, *pretty*, *quite*, *real*, *really*, *so*, *strongly*, *superbly*, *terribly*, *terrifically*, *too*, *totally*, *tremendously*, *very*, *well*, *wonderfully*.

Several earlier studies indicate that the majority of amplifiers in Present-day English discourse occur as adjectival modifiers; some claim that this is their prototypical syntactic function (see Allerton 1987: 16, Bäcklund 1973: 279, Lorenz 1999: 144). In this study I also restrict my attention to those instances where amplifiers occur with

---

7 See also Bolinger (1972: 23), who notes that "[a]ny list of intensifiers has to be viewed as a sampling rather than a catalog, [...] because [the set of intensifiers] is too open-ended".

8 As *Medicor* is not lexicogrammatically tagged, another alternative would have been to use a data-driven method and glean all instances of amplifier-adjective pairs that occur in the data, using concordances, lexical searches and wildcard searches (see Lorenz 1999: 33-38).

adjectival heads. In *Medicor*, however, only less than 50% of the hits extracted in the corpus search contain an amplifier with an adjectival head. In more than half of the hits, the item occurs in some other syntactic function, modifying adverbs, verbs, determiners, pronouns or prepositional phrases, or as an adverbial on the clause level. This data, excluded from the present analysis, will provide interesting material for future studies on intensification in medical discourse.

3. Repertoire and frequency

Tables 3 and 4 contain the quantitative results of the corpus analysis. The absolute frequencies and proportions of individual pre-adjectival amplifiers in *Medicor* are shown in Table 3. In Table 4, the absolute frequencies have been converted into frequencies per 10,000 words, which facilitates comparisons between genres, represented by samples of different sizes (see Table 1). The results show that 20 amplifiers from the search list of 32 items occur with an adjectival head in *Medicor*. Nine of the search items do not occur at all, and three items are only recorded in other syntactic functions. The total number of pre-adjectival amplifiers in the material is 493. The overall relative frequency for the whole corpus is 12.4 per 10,000 words. Thus, the corpus contains a pre-adjectival amplifier every 812 words, which indicates that in general this is not a high-frequency linguistic feature in medical writing.

The repertoire of amplifiers in *Medicor* is a mixed bag. It contains items like *highly*, *extremely* and *fully* that have been characterized as particularly typical of academic writing. At the same time, there are items characteristic of conversational styles, such as *absolutely* and *pretty* – items that one perhaps would not expect to find in this material at all.

Amplifier	Professional genres						Popular genres				Total	%
	RA	TB	HB	EA	*Total*	%	PA	GB	*Total*	%		
Very	31	24	8	14	*77*	23.8	29	11	*40*	24.7	**117**	**23.7**
Highly	30	27	3	10	*70*	21.6	14	2	*16*	9.5	**86**	**17.4**
Well	6	16	3	10	*35*	10.8	6	2	*8*	4.7	**43**	**8.7**
Extremely	5	15	5	2	*27*	8.3	5	6	*11*	6.5	**38**	**7.7**
Quite	1	13	0	5	*19*	5.9	13	2	*15*	8.9	**34**	**6.9**
Too	1	4	1	6	*12*	3.7	16	2	*18*	10.7	**30**	**6.1**
Especially	1	12	3	2	*18*	5.6	11	0	*11*	6.5	**29**	**5.9**
Particularly	6	4	5	7	*22*	6.8	7	0	*7*	4.1	**29**	**5.9**
So	2	2	0	1	*5*	1.5	17	2	*19*	11.2	**24**	**4.9**
Entirely	1	7	0	1	*9*	2.8	5	0	*5*	3.0	**14**	**2.8**
Completely	1	4	2	2	*9*	2.8	4	0	*4*	2.4	**13**	**2.6**
Strongly	8	1	1	1	*11*	3.4	0	0	*0*	0	**11**	**2.2**
Fully	0	1	0	0	*1*	0.3	4	0	*4*	2.5	**5**	**1.0**
Greatly	0	4	0	0	*4*	1.2	0	1	*1*	0.6	**5**	**1.0**
Absolutely	0	0	3	0	*3*	0.9	1	0	*1*	0.6	**4**	**0.8**
Perfectly	0	0	0	0	*0*	0	3	0	*3*	1.8	**3**	**0.6**
Pretty	0	0	0	0	*0*	0	3	0	*3*	1.8	**3**	**0.6**
Really	0	0	0	0	*0*	0	2	0	*2*	1.2	**2**	**0.4**
Totally	0	1	0	0	*1*	0.3	0	1	*1*	0.6	**2**	**0.4**
Exceedingly	1	0	0	0	*1*	0.3	0	0	*0*	0	**1**	**0.2**
Total	**94**	**135**	**34**	**61**	***324***	100	**140**	**29**	***169***	100	**493**	**100**
%	19.4	27.8	7.0	12.6	65.7		28.9	6.0	34.3		100	

Table 3. Frequency and proportions of pre-adjectival amplifiers in *Medicor* and its subgenres. Genre labels: RA = research article, TB = textbook, HB = handbook, EA = editorial article, PA = (popular) newspaper/magazine article, GB = guidebook.

Two amplifiers, *very* and *highly*, stand out in the quantitative results. Together they cover c. 41% of all the data. The most frequent item is *very*, which holds this position in most studies on intensification in twentieth-century British and American English, based on different types of material from various registers.[9] With the total of 117 hits in

9 These include Fries (1940), Bäcklund (1973), Lorenz (1999), Paradis (2000), Ito / Tagliamonte (2003). *Really* is reported as the most common pre-

Medicor, *very* covers 24% of the amplifier data. In the whole corpus it occurs with the average of 2.9 times in every 10,000 words. The second most frequent item, *highly*, occurs 86 times in the corpus, with the average of 2.2 words per 10,000 words, covering c. 17% of the data.

Amplifier	**Professional genres**					**Popular genres**			**Total**
	RA	TB	HB	EA	***Total***	PA	GB	***Total***	
Very	2.7	2.3	1.9	2.9	*2.5*	3.7	10.9	*4.5*	**2.9**
Highly	2.6	2.6	0.7	2.1	*2.3*	1.8	2.0	*1.8*	**2.2**
Well	0.5	1.5	0.7	2.1	*1.1*	0.8	2.0	*0.9*	**1.1**
Extremely	0.4	1.4	1.2	0.4	*0.9*	0.6	6.0	*1.2*	**1.0**
Quite	0.1	1.2	0	0.1	*0.6*	1.6	2.0	*1.7*	**0.9**
Too	0.1	0.4	0.2	1.3	*0.4*	2.0	2.0	*2.0*	**0.8**
Especially	0.1	1.1	0.7	0.4	*0.6*	1.4	0	*1.2*	**0.7**
Particularly	0.5	0.4	1.2	1.5	*0.7*	0.9	0	*0.8*	**0.7**
So	0.2	0.2	0	0.2	*0.2*	2.1	2.0	*2.1*	**0.6**
Entirely	0.1	0.7	0	0.2	*0.3*	0.6	0	*0.6*	**0.4**
Completely	0.1	0.4	0.5	0.4	*0.3*	0.5	0	*0.4*	**0.3**
Strongly	0.7	0.1	0.2	0.2	*0.4*	0	0	*0.0*	**0.3**
Fully	0	0.1	0	0	*0.0*	0.5	0	*0.4*	**0.1**
Greatly	0	0.4	0	0	*0.1*	0	1.0	*0.1*	**0.1**
Absolutely	0	0	0.7	0	*0.1*	0.1	0	*0.1*	**0.1**
Perfectly	0	0	0	0	*0.0*	0.4	0	*0.3*	**0.1**
Pretty	0	0	0	0	*0.0*	0.4	0	*0.3*	**0.1**
Really	0	0	0	0	*0.0*	0.3	0	*0.2*	**0.1**
Totally	0	0.1	0	0	*0.0*	0	1.0	*0.1*	**0.1**
Exceedingly	0.1	0	0	0	*0.0*	0	0	*0.0*	**0.0**
Total	**8.2**	**12.9**	**8.0**	**11.8**	***10.5***	**17.7**	**28.9**	***18.9***	**12.4**

Table 4. Normalized frequencies of pre-adjectival amplifiers in *Medicor* and its subsections (N/10,000 words). For genre labels, see Table 3.

adjectival amplifier in several studies on spoken language, e.g. in a corpus of spoken Scottish English recorded in the late 1970s (Macaulay 1995), in the 1990s among London teenagers (Stenström 1999) and the younger generations in the city of York (Ito / Tagliamonte 2003), and in the early 2000s in Canadian English (see Tagliamonte / Roberts 2005: 283).

In the overall frequency, *very* and *highly* are followed in a descending order by *well*, *extremely*, *quite*, *too*, *especially*, *particularly* and *so*. Their frequencies are much lower, ranging from 43 to 24 (1.1 to 0.6 per 10,000 words), with proportions varying from 9 to 5% of all instances in the data. The lowest frequencies, 0.1 or less per 10,000 words, are recorded for *fully*, *greatly*, *absolutely*, *perfectly*, *pretty*, *really*, *totally* and *exceedingly*.

The frequency ranking shows that some order on the initially mixed repertoire of amplifiers from different register styles in *Medicor* can be imposed through quantification. In general, the items most characteristic of conversational style are not frequent in the data. However, the overall frequencies do not distinguish adequately between conversational and academic style amplifiers in the data, and more fine-grained contextualized distinctions are in order.

4. Audience design

When texts included in *Medicor* are divided into two categories on the basis of their audience design, the results indicate a higher overall frequency of amplifiers in texts aimed at the general audience than in texts intended for professionals. The popular genres contain 18.9 amplifiers per 10,000 words, while the average of amplifiers in the same amount of text aimed at professionals is 10.5.

Audience design also reflects on the repertoire of amplifiers. Most instances of conversation-style amplifiers occur in the macrolevel category of popular genres aimed at a general readership. *Pretty*, *really* and *totally* only occur in popularized texts. The amplifiers *so* and *too*, characterized by Biber *et al.* (1999) as more common in conversation and rarely used in academic writing, are also far more frequent in texts aimed for the general audience than in texts for professional readers. Contrary to the findings by Biber *et al.* (1999), *extremely* and *fully* are also somewhat more frequent in popular genres. *Strongly*, on the other hand, only occurs in professional texts.

The two items with highest overall frequencies behave differently in the professional/popular dichotomy. *Very* is almost twice as frequent in writings intended for the general audience (4.5/10,000) as in writings aimed at professionals (2.5/10,000). In contrast, *highly* is more common in the professional genres (2.3/10,000), where it covers almost 22% of all the hits, being almost as frequent as *very* (23.8%). In the popular genres, *highly* occurs 1.8 times per 10,000 words, covering only less than 10% of the instances (cf. *very* 24.7%). In the frequency ranking of popular texts *highly* only comes fourth, being slightly less frequent than the items *so* and *too*. In view of the academic flavour of *highly*, these results are not surprising.

The quantitative results also indicate great variation between individual genres within both macrolevel categories. Thus, audience design alone does not appear to govern the use of individual amplifiers in medical writing, even if it helps to clarify the picture. I shall now turn to the next level of analysis, and discuss the main findings from the perspective of genre distribution.

5. Genre distribution

Of the individual genres, the density of amplifiers is highest in the two genres intended for the general audience. Guidebooks contain as many as 28.9 amplifiers in every 10,000 words. The corresponding figure in popular articles, published in newspapers or magazines, is 17.7. In the professional genres, the frequencies vary from c. 12 per 10,000 words in textbooks and editorials to c. 8 in research articles and handbooks.

Individual amplifiers show varying genre patterns. *Very* is significantly more frequent in guidebooks (10.9/10,000) than in any other genres; in fact, the frequency of *very* explains to a large extent the high overall frequency of amplifiers in this genre. In popular articles *very* occurs 3.7 times per 10,000 words, while in the professional medical genres its frequencies range from 2.9 to 1.9. *Highly* shows less dramatic genre variation. It is most frequent in research articles and textbooks (2.6/10,000) and least frequent in handbooks (0.7/10,000). Its frequency in popular articles and guidebooks is around 2 per 10,000 words, which, interestingly, is almost as high as in editorial articles in professional journals (2.1/10,000).

The genre distributions of *so* and *too* are almost alike. The items are equally prominent in both popular genres (c. 2/10,000). Apart from editorial articles, where *too* occurs 1.3 times per 10,000 words, their incidence in all professional genres is low. The other amplifiers show more mixed genre patterns, although in most cases the absolute frequencies are so low that it is not possible to make any reliable conclusions about their genre tendencies. *Extremely* is an exception. It shows the widest range of variation between individual genres after *very*, ranging from 6.0 occurrences per 10,000 words in guidebooks to 0.4 in research articles and editorials.

6. Disciplinary context and the communicative functions of genres

The classification of texts into directive, argumentative and expository according to their communicative function in their domain-specific disciplinary context adds new dimensions to the patterns of variation. One such angle is the basic two-fold nature of medicine as science on the one hand and praxis on the other. At the extreme 'science' end of the genre scale is the research article, the site where new scientific knowledge in medicine is constructed through hypotheses, tested through reliable, usually statistical methods. It is an argumentative genre targeted at the in-group of professionals, aiming to convince them of the validity of the statements. In editorial articles of professional journals, also an argumentative genre, the emphasis is on interpretation and assessment of scientific findings. The 'practice' end of the scale contains directive or instructive manuals, providing recommendations on the best practices to professionals (handbooks and clinical textbooks) and advice to non-professionals (guidebooks).

The main function of expository texts, i.e. scientific textbooks and popular articles, is to distribute scientific background knowledge to members of the in-group and the out-group, respectively.[10]

The use of amplifiers in medical texts can be analyzed against the disciplinary roles of the texts. Table 5 shows the overall frequencies of amplifiers according to the communicative functions of the genres.

	Directive	**Argumentative**	**Expository**
Professional	Handbooks 8.0	Research articles 8.2	Scient. textbooks 13.6
	Clinical textbooks 8.3	Editorial articles 11.8	
Popular	Guidebooks 28.9		Popular articles 17.7

Table 5. Normalized frequencies of pre-adjectival amplifiers in *Medicor* according to the communicative function of genres (N/10,000 words).

The highest frequencies, as we have already seen, occur in the genre of medical guidebooks (28.9/10,000 words). Their main function is to provide descriptions of the possible courses of diseases and to give advice to non-professional readers, and thus it seems logical that they should employ amplifiers as a means of emphasizing distinctions or underlining advice and recommendations. A qualitative analysis of the discourse contexts confirms this. Amplifiers are frequently used to emphasize the rarity or extremity of cases or circumstances, their special or unusual nature, the seriousness of effects, or the importance of particular tests or treatments. These are illustrated in examples (1) to (4).[11]

(1) The test can be used for those people who should not have skin tests: people with *extremely sensitive* skin, *very young* children, and those individuals suspected to be *extremely sensitive* to an injected allergen. ('Allergy tests', GB)

10 For more detailed discussions of the communicative functions of the genres represented in *Medicor*, see Vihla (1999).

11 References to the corpus texts consist of the writer's surname or, in anonymous texts, the first word of the sample, followed by an abbreviation indicating the genre. For genre abbreviations, see the caption to Table 3; for corpus texts, see Appendix 2 in Vihla (1999).

(2) a useful service to children, who are *highly susceptible* to ear, nose, and throat infections. ('Tonsillitis', GB)

(3) The patient remains conscious but is *totally unaware* of the seizure. ('Epilepsy', GB)

(4) So it is *very important* for the patient to undergo a general medical examination with tests and extensive neurological and psychological studies. ('Alzheimer's disease', GB)

In argumentative genres, amplifiers can also be found in the discussion of similar issues as in directive texts, but the functional perspective is different. The linguistic choices in research articles, the cutting edge of the discipline, are guided by the process of creating new scientific knowledge and presenting it to the peer group. The authors use emphatic means to justify their research topics and methods, to highlight specific features in their experiments, and to assess their results; these functions are illustrated in examples (5) to (10). However, the argument in medical research articles relies to a great extent on experimental justification – on experiments and their results, which are analyzed using statistical methods, largely provided by the non-linguistic elements of the text, i.e. figures and diagrams (Vihla 1999: 109). The fact that linguistic devices are not the central means of argumentation is reflected in the low frequency of amplifiers in the genre (8.2/10,000 words). The highly conventionalized nature of the research article, with its tradition of aiming at objectivity and avoiding hyperbole, contributes to this effect as well.

(5) However, since the nipple and surrounding plastic are disposable, obviating the need for an *entirely new* device for each patient, the pacifier thermometer could be an appropriate and cost-effective option in low-volume ambulatory care settings. (Press / Quinn, RA)

(6) Information about the views of medicine clerkship directors would be *extremely valuable.* (Bass *et al.*, RA)

(7) Our nerve conduction findings suggest [...] that peripheral nerve responses in male participants may be *particularly susceptible* to the effects of hyperglycemia. (Allen *et al.*, RA)

(8) Expression of VCAM-1 within venules at mucosal sites, however, is *very low*, even in inflammatory bowel disease. (Briskin *et al.*, RA)

(9) However, a DFT defined by a single successful shock at the threshold energy can be a *very inaccurate* measure of defibrillation energy requirements. Accordingly, our results were analyzed based on clinical practice (i.e., that an adequate DFT is <20 J by the DFT+ method) rather than as a function of the measured threshold. (Gold *et al.*, RA)

(10) A *highly specific* monoclonal antibody was developed to identify and characterize the native PS1 protein. (Levey *et al.*, RA)

The primary purpose of expository medical genres is to distribute scientific background knowledge. This basic function is also seen in the discourse contexts where amplifiers occur in expository medical texts. As examples (11) to (15) from scientific textbooks illustrate, amplifiers are common in contexts providing descriptive information, highlighting particular characteristics of physiological processes and substances, or underlining distinctions. Descriptive uses, even though reflecting subjective judgements, seem appropriate for amplifiers in scientific writing, as the frequency of amplifiers in scientific textbooks is higher than in other genres aimed at professional readers (13.6/10,000 words).

(11) The analog of dopamine, 6-hydroxydopamine, is *extremely potent* in leading to a chemical sympathectomy. (Anthony / Graham, TB)

(12) The axons of many nerve cells have a prominent sheath of material called myelin, *highly refractile* in the fresh condition and appearing black in tissue fixed in osmium tetroxide. (Angevine, TB)

(13) Renal involvement, in particular glomerulonephritis, is *very common* and as many as 75% of patients with SLE have evidence of renal disease at autopsy. (Johnson *et al.*, TB)

(14) This loss of myelin results in an *entirely separate* process known as demyelination. (Anthony / Graham, TB)

(15) The morphology of the axon is, of course, *quite different* in the two situations. (Anthony / Graham, TB)

7. Layers of discourse: speech representation

One of the most remarkable findings in the analysis of discourse contexts in *Medicor* concerns the interface between written and spoken registers. In view of the stylistically mixed repertoire of amplifiers in the data, it is noteworthy that most amplifiers characterized as typical of spoken language and conversational style, such as *pretty*, *really* and *so*, occur in direct quotations or passages of speech reported from interviews. Thus, they in fact reflect an underlying layer of spoken language in written texts. Speech representation is particularly a feature of popular articles in newspapers and magazines intended for the general public, so common that it has a considerable impact on the frequency of amplifiers in this genre, also reflecting on the overall results. Most cases are likely to represent American English speech, where specifically the items *really* and *so* are prominent (see Tagliamonte / Roberts 2005). Examples (16) to (20) illustrate the use of conversation-style amplifiers in speech representation in popular medical articles.

(16) [...] says epidemiologist [...] of the University of North Carolina. "That's a *pretty interesting* way of doing science if you ask me." (Kluger b, PA)

(17) He had to count the furs daily. "That was *really hard* for me," he said. (Morrow, PA)

(18) "But because it's *so hard* to keep up with the scientific literature [...]." (Begley, PA)

(19) "Many parents are almost afraid to touch their kids because their skin is *so sensitive* [...]" says Dr.[...]. ('Hands-on-healing', PA)

(20) "Both extremes are wrong. [...] if we wait to deal with the problem until the proof is *absolutely solid* we have waited *too long*. [...]" (Schwartz, PA)

Direct quotations from interviews also partly account for the frequency of several other amplifiers in popular articles. Some of these are illustrated in examples (21)-(23):

(21) "The effect was clear after 10 days," [...] said. "[...] I could look forward with a *completely positive* attitude [...]." (Andrews, PA)

(22) said [...], a TB adviser for the disease-control centers. "An *extremely large* percentage were positive [...]." (Grady, PA)

(23) "Since most MDIs come in opaque aluminum canisters, it's *quite possible* to unknowingly run out of medicine at a critical time," says [...] MD, an asthma specialist. (Wolfe a, PA)

Speech representation also contributes to the high frequency of *very* in popular articles, and, consequently, to its prominence in *Medicor*. Some of the numerous examples from the data are given in (24)-(30).

(24) But the true level of risk posed by secondhand smoke will be *very difficult* to ever firmly establish, according to [...], chair of the department of health studies. (Schwartz, PA)

(25) "It's also a *very easy* way for people to keep track of how much medication they're actually taking," says Dr. [...]. (Wolfe a, PA)

(26) As [...], professor of pulmonary medicine at Imperial College, London, puts it: "The belief of the patient in the effectiveness of the treatment is *very important* [...]." (Gleick, PA)

(27) "Having been involved with some wonderful hospices and nursing homes," she says, "I'm *very impressed* with what can be achieved with relatively modest investments." (Horgan, PA)

(28) a prominent researcher in the field, says he has no doubt that [...] "has a *very interesting* phenomenon on her hands" with x-ray-induced healing. (Beardsley, PA)

(29) "It was apparent within about an hour that it was going to be *very unusual*," recalls Dr. [...]. (Gleick, PA)

(30) It was, he said, "*very upbeat*, showing 350 pounds melting into 135." (Kolata, PA)

8. Linguistic context: collocation

The importance of lexical collocation for amplifier use has been discussed in several studies (e.g. Bäcklund 1973, Lorenz 1999, Ito / Tagliamonte 2003). Altenberg (1991: 128) points out that in terms of collocation, amplifiers are an interesting category, as they are "subject to a number of syntactic, semantic, lexical and stylistic restrictions affecting their use in various ways and fostering a great deal of competition between them". The collocability of individual amplifiers varies: some have restricted collocability and only co-occur with a small set of specific lexical items, whereas others have wide collocability and appear across a broad range of types. Some observations on the collocation of amplifiers are also in order here, as it clearly is one of the factors conditioning amplifier use in *Medicor*; the issue will be discussed in more detail in a forthcoming study.

Most amplifiers have too few occurrences in the corpus to allow any conclusions on their collocability, or 'priming' (see Hoey 2005). A few amplifier/adjective pairs can be identified as habitually co-occurring lexical groups or "semi-preconstructed phrases that constitute single choices" (Sinclair 1991: 110), though they are not very frequent in the data. These are illustrated in examples (31) to (35), representing three different genres. The first three examples contain predictable combinations that can occur in a wide range of texts, while the last two examples are closer to domain- or register-specific institutional formulae, part of conventionalized language use connected with particular topics or genres (see Stubbs 2001).

(31) Investigators were also *well aware* that formation of attachments between cells and a matrix can affect the cells in any number of ways. (Horwitz, PA)

(32) Most people today are *all too familiar* with the devastating effects of HIV, the human immunodeficiency virus. (O'Brien / Dean, PA)

(33) While Hg2+ is known to bind strongly to sulfhydryl groups, it is *not entirely clear* that MeHg results in cell death through sulfhydryl binding. (Anthony / Graham, TB)

(34) Less obviously, it helps to direct both embryonic development and an array of processes in the *fully formed* organism, including blood clotting, wound healing and eradication of infection. (Horwitz, PA)

(35) The algorithm identified 2 factors, each comprised of 3 *highly correlated* parameters, as independent predictors of a high threshold. (Gold *et al.*, RA)

The collocational tendencies of *very* and *highly* (see Table 6) can be used to illustrate the influence of collocation on amplifier use in the data.

very	N	***highly***	N
low	15	*correlated*	6
important	5	*specific*	6
large	4	*effective*	4
small	4	*active*	3
young	4	*educated*	3
unusual	3	*selected*	3
		significant	3
		specialized	3
		unlikely	3

Table 6. The most frequent collocates of *very* and *highly* in *Medicor* ($N \geq 3$).

Neither *very* nor *highly* is particularly restricted in its collocability. This is reflected in their type/token ratios. The 117 instances of *very* occur with more than 60 adjectival heads, and the 86 instances of *highly* with over 50 different adjectives. A microanalysis of the collocates, however, reveals some differences between the items. Only six adjectives co-occur with both *very* and *highly* in the data. The shared collocates are *effective*, *likely*, *sensitive*, *significant*, *specific* and *successful*. *Significant* occurs with both items with reference to statistical significance; cf. examples (36) and (37):

(36) homozygosity for the deletion mutant was protective against HIV – was *highly significant* statistically. (O'Brien / Dean, PA)

(37) Prevention of foot problems starts with stressing that patients who smoke have a *very significant* reversible risk in addition to their diabetes for peripheral circulatory problems. (Wood, HB)

Specific has a greater tendency to co-occur with *highly* (6 occurrences) than with *very* (1 occurrence). Examples (38) and (39), illustrating the use of *specific*, also show that the single attestation of *very* occurs in a context implying negation.

(38) the cerebral cortex may respond to *highly specific* modes of visual stimuli to the retina. (Angevine, TB)

(39) It is important to note that brain biopsies (tissue samples taken from the brain) are not performed on individuals without *very specific* reasons. ('Alzheimer's disease', GB)

There is too little evidence to say anything conclusive about the other shared adjectives. A positive/negative dichotomy is attested also in the case of *effective* (40)-(41), but, with only single attestations from different genres, this could be coincidental.

(40) hospital admissions in Finland resemble those reported from Denmark by Rossing et al. (10) on the unchanged incidence of diabetic nephropathy in a very large and *highly effective* regional referral clinic. (Steffes, EA)

(41) They never gained much of a market because they were not *very effective*. (Kolata, PA)

The small number of shared adjectival collocates suggests that *very* and *highly* have semantically distinct collocational profiles in the material. Distinct profiles are also reflected in the most frequent collocates of the items, listed in Table 6. It shows a greater tendency for *very* to combine with adjectives associated with 'concrete' qualities like quantity or age, and a bias for *highly* to only co-occur with adjectives connected with more abstract or technical notions. A semantic analysis of all the adjectival heads occurring with *very* and *highly* confirms this tendency. The most salient distinction is seen in their co-occurrence with 'basic dimension' adjectives, i.e. adjectives depicting spatial or other physical qualities or evaluations that can be placed on opposing ends of the scale, such as *long – short* or *good – bad*. Almost 50% of the adjectives preceded by *very* in the data are basic dimension adjectives. *Highly*, on the other hand, tends to keep company with adjectives connected with abstract notions such as relevance or feasibility, and only rarely co-occurs with basic dimension adjectives. In the few cases where it does, it combines with adjectives that are more characteristic of formal language use than the collocates of *very*. Examples of *very* and *highly* with their basic dimension collocates are provided in (42) to (45).

(42) Dehydration may develop because of *very low* cabin humidity, but can be avoided by adequate intake of fluids and avoidance of alcohol. (Levinson, HB)

(43) AcHD results in *very rapid* pyrrole formation both in vitro and in vivo. (Anthony / Graham, TB)

(44) Nine subjects with BMI greater than 30 were excluded from the study because of potential methodologic concerns with the reliability of determination of fat mass by DEXA in *very obese* subjects. (Daniels *et al.*, RA)

(45) In the AD cases linked to mutations in PS1, the protein colocalized with a subset of the *highly abundant* amyloid plaques. (Levey, RA)

9. Conclusion

In this study, I have examined the use of amplifiers in medical discourse, analyzing material from *Medicor*, an electronic corpus of late twentieth-century American English medical writing. Combining quantitative and qualitative approaches to linguistic analysis, my aim has been to provide an overview of synchronic variation in amplifier use in different genres within the domain, ranging from scientific discourse among professionals to popularized accounts intended for the general readership.

The study confirms some tendencies observed in earlier research on amplifiers, including the differences in the repertoire and frequency of amplifiers in formal (academic) and less formal (popularized) register styles. Within the domain of medicine, amplifiers are more frequent in popularized medical texts intended for the general readership than in texts for the in-group of professionals. There is great variation in the repertoire and frequency of amplifiers between individual genres in both macrolevel categories. The density of amplifiers is highest in samples from a family medical guidebook, whose main domain-specific communicative function is directive, i.e. to give advice and recommendations in matters of sickness and health to non-professional readers. The lowest frequencies occur in research articles, professional handbooks and clinical textbooks. In popularized medical articles in newspapers and magazines, amplifiers are especially frequent in direct quotations or reported speech from interviews.

The discursive functions of amplifiers vary according to the domain-specific communicative purposes of genres. In directive medical texts, amplifiers are frequently used to accentuate the special, unusual or extreme nature of conditions or circumstances, or the importance of particular measures. In argumentative medical texts, writers employ amplifiers to emphasize the value of their research topics and methods, to highlight specific features in their experiments, and to scale up evaluations. In expository medical texts, amplifiers are often used to foreground details and underline distinctions between phenomena.

In the repertoire of amplifiers, *very* and *highly* stand out in terms of frequency. They cover more than 40% of the amplifier data in *Medicor*. The most frequent amplifier is *very*, recorded in this position also in other studies on twentieth-century written English. It ranks highest in all *Medicor* genres except for professional textbooks, where *highly* is slightly more common. Contrary to expectations, *highly* is almost as frequent in popularized medical writing as in more formal professional genres. The most salient differences in the use of *very* and *highly* are seen in their collocation. The semantic analysis of their adjective collocates shows that *very* most commonly occurs in the company of 'basic dimension' adjectives, i.e. adjectives depicting concrete qualities or evaluations that can be placed on opposing ends of the scale, whereas *highly* tends to co-occur with more abstract and technical adjectives.

To conclude, my corpus-based analysis of amplifiers in medical writing reveals an intricate and multifaceted pattern of variation, where the use of amplifiers is influenced by a complex web of overlapping social, situational and linguistic factors. These include the target audiences, the discipline-approved practices and genre conventions, the domain-specific communicative roles of genres, the written and spoken modes of communication and their mixtures in representations of one mode in the other, and the tendency of linguistic items to form habitually co-occurring clusters. In future studies, I hope to provide more details to the overview presented here, including an assessment of internal variation within genres, as well as a nuanced account of long-term diachronic shifts in domain-specific use of amplifiers in medical discourse.

References

Allerton, David J. 1987. English Intensifiers and their Idiosyncrasies. In Steele, Ross / Threadgold, Terry (eds) *Language Topics: Essays in Honour of Michael Halliday*. Vol. 2. Amsterdam: Benjamins, 15-31.

Altenberg, Bengt 1991. Amplifier Collocations in Spoken English. In Johansson, Stig / Stenström, Anna-Brita (eds) *English Computer Corpora: Selected Papers and Research Guide*. Berlin: Walter de Gruyter, 127-47.

Bäcklund, Ulf 1973. *The Collocation of Adverbs of Degree in English*. Uppsala: Almqvist & Wiksell.

Biber, Douglas / Johansson, Stig / Leech, Geoffrey / Conrad, Susan / Finegan, Edward 1999. *Longman Grammar of Spoken and Written English*. London: Longman.

Bolinger, Dwight 1972. *Degree Words*. The Hague: Mouton.

Candlin, Christopher N. 2000. General Editor's Preface. In Hyland, Ken *Disciplinary Discourses: Social Interactions in Academic Writing*. Harlow: Pearson Education, xv-xxi.

Fleischman, Suzanne 2001. Language and Medicine. In Schiffrin *et al.* (eds), 470-502.

Fries, Charles C. 1940. *American English Grammar*. New York: Appleton, Century, Crofts.

Hickey, Raymond 2003. *Corpus Presenter: Software for Language Analysis*. Amsterdam: Benjamins.

Hoey, Michael 2005. *Lexical Priming: A New Theory of Words and Language*. London: Routledge.

Hyland, Ken 2000. *Disciplinary Discourses: Social Interactions in Academic Writing*. Harlow: Pearson Education.

Ito, Rika / Tagliamonte, Sali 2003. *Well* Weird, *Right* Dodgy, *Very* Strange, *Really* Cool: Layering and Recycling in English Intensifiers. *Language in Society* 32, 257-79.

Labov, William 1984. Intensity. In Schiffrin, Deborah (ed.) *Meaning, Form and Use in Context: Linguistic Applications*. Washington, DC: Georgetown University Press, 43-70.

Lorenz, Gunter R. 1999. *Adjective Intensification – Learners versus Native Speakers: A Corpus Study of Argumentative Writing*. Amsterdam: Rodopi.

Macaulay, Ronald K.S. 1995. The Adverbs of Authority. *English World-wide* 16, 37-60.

Méndez-Náya, Belén 2003. On Intensifiers and Grammaticalization: The Case of *Swiþe*. *English Studies* 84, 372-91.

Myers, Greg 1990. *Writing Biology: Texts in the Social Construction of Scientific Knowledge*. Madison, WI: University of Wisconsin Press.

Nwogu, Kevin Ngozi 1990. *Discourse Variation in Medical Texts: Schema, Theme and Cohesion on Professional and Journalistic Accounts*. Nottingham: Department of English Studies, University of Nottingham.

Pahta, Päivi 2006. *Ful Holsum and Profetable for the Bodi:* Amplifiers in Medieval English Medical Texts. Dossena, Marina / Taavitsainen, Irma (eds) *Diachronic Perspectives on Domain-specific English*. Bern: Peter Lang.

Paradis, Carita 2000. *It's Well Weird*. Degree Modifiers of Adjectives Revisited: The Nineties. In Kirk, John M. (ed.) *Corpora Galore: Analyses and Techniques in Describing English*. Amsterdam: Rodopi, 147-60.

Partington, Alan 1993. Corpus Evidence of Language Change: The Case of Intensifiers. In Baker, Mona / Francis, Gill / Tognini-Bonelli, Elena (eds) *Text and Technology: In Honour of John Sinclair*. Amsterdam: Benjamins, 172-99.

Peters, Hans 1994. Degree Adverbs in Early Modern English. In Kastovsky, Dieter (ed.) *Studies in Early Modern English*. Berlin: Mouton de Gruyter, 269-88.

Quirk, Randolph / Greenbaum, Sidney / Leech, Geoffrey / Svartvik, Jan 1985. *A Comprehensive Grammar of the English Language*. London: Longman.

Schiffrin, Deborah / Tannen, Deborah / Hamilton, Heidi E. (eds) 2001. *The Handbook of Discourse Analysis*. Oxford: Blackwell.

Sinclair, John 1991. *Corpus, Concordance, Collocation*. Oxford: Oxford University Press.

Stenström, Anna-Brita 1999. *He Was Really Gormless – She's Bloody Crap*: Girls, Boys and Intensifiers. In Hasselgård, Hilde / Oksefjell, Signe (eds) *Out of Corpora: Studies in Honour of Stig Johansson*. Amsterdam: Rodopi, 69-78.

Stubbs, Michael 2001. Computer-assisted Text and Corpus Analysis. In Schiffrin *et al.* (eds), 304-20.

Swales, John M. / Burke, Ann 2003. *It's Really Fascinating Work*: Differences in Evaluative Adjectives across Academic Genres. In Leistyna, Pepi / Meyer, Charles F. (eds) *Corpus Analysis: Language Structure and Language Use*. Amsterdam: Rodopi, 1-18.

Tagliamonte, Sali / Roberts, Chris 2005. *So* Weird; *So* Cool; *So* Innovative: The Use of Intensifiers in the Television Series *Friends*. *American Speech* 80, 280-300.

Vihla, Minna 1998. *Medicor*: A Corpus of Contemporary American Medical Texts. *ICAME Journal* 22, 73-80.

Vihla, Minna 1999. *Medical Writing: Modality in Focus*. Amsterdam: Rodopi.

JORDI PIQUÉ-ANGORDANS / SANTIAGO POSTEGUILLO

Peer Positive and Negative Assessment in Medical English Written Genres

1. Introduction

1.1. Review of the literature

Medical English (ME) is a significant area of research in the wider fields of English for Specific Purposes (ESP) and English for Academic Purposes (EAP). Following general trends in ESP and EAP research, several studies have been undertaken in which authors' work is reviewed and evaluated (e.g. Manten 1973, Kiely 2004, Fagan / Martín Martín 2004). More specifically, Magnet and Carnet (2001) studied contradiction as a mode of criticism in 'Letters to the Editor' (LEs) drawn from two leading English-written biomedical journals. These same two scholars also approached medical LEs from a structural point of view (Carnet / Magnet 2002). Medical LEs and Editorials (EDs) were studied contrastively by Vázquez y del Árbol (2005). Other studies examined how criticism of fellow researchers is conveyed in ME writing, but these mostly focused on peer review for specialized medical journals (Chubin / Hackett 1990), including reviewers' training (Guilford 2001). The issue of academic conflict is also addressed in Salager-Meyer *et al.* (2003) from a cross-linguistic and cross-cultural perspective and elsewhere from a cross-generic standpoint (Salager-Meyer 2001, 2005) across major written academic medical genres, namely, case reports (CRs), research papers (RPs), review articles (RVs), and EDs.

Both positive and negative assessment in scientific discourse may be conveyed via a variety of linguistic resources, especially by means of hedging (Salager-Meyer 1994; Varttala 1999). A comprehensive analysis of all these stylistic devices in corpora of relevant medical texts would make this task unmanageable for a single chapter. This is why we focused our attention on the study of how positive and negative assessment is conveyed through the use of one of these linguistic resources, namely reporting verbs (RepVbs), across six distinct ME academic written genres, viz., book reviews (BRs), CRs, EDs, LEs, RPs, and RVs.

It should be clarified that this chapter does not focus on peer reviews,[1] but on how peers evaluate the work of colleagues in the above mentioned fundamental ME academic genres.

1.2. Aim

The aim of this research is to examine whether positive and negative assessment remains stable across genres or whether there are significant variations. If so, we will analyze how and why these variations occur.

1.3. Hypotheses

The above-mentioned objective may be unfolded through the testing of the following hypotheses:

a) Whether variation in the frequency and intensity of praise and negative assessment is to be detected in the different genres since the communicative function of each genre differs (Salager-Meyer 2001);
b) Whether variability of praise and criticism is to be found within the same genre, especially in the case of RPs, given the fact that each section in the RP has a specific communicative purpose (Swales 1990; Thomas / Hawes 1994).

---

1 Peer reviews are indeed a key genre in academic English in general and in ME in particular. However, to obtain a corpus of relevant texts in this area is specially difficult unless one is in a position to collect reviews regularly; for instance, being an editor of an international academic journal. Such research has been carried out in several disciplines by Gosden (2001) and in the area of linguistics by Hewings (2005).

2. Methodology

2.1. Corpus

In order to describe praise and criticism in medical writing we selected a corpus of texts from six distinct medical genres: BRs, CRs, EDs, LEs, RPs, and RVs. Table 1 provides a detailed description of our corpus. As can be seen, the subcorpora of RPs and RVs are larger than the rest since such articles tend to be longer than the other genres. In fact, in the specific case of BRs and LEs, we selected 30 texts instead of 15 so as to obtain a more representative number of words in these two subcorpora.

Medical genre	*Number of texts*	*Total no. of words*	*Total no. of RepVbs*	*RepVbs per 10,000 words*
Book reviews (BRs)	30	19,370	299	154.36
Case reports (CRs)	15	21,284	442	207.67
Editorials (EDs)	15	19,383	289	149.10
Letters to the editor (LEs)	30	13,945	310	222.30
Research papers (RPs)	15	48,892	944	197.08
Review articles (RVs)	15	56,626	1,076	190.02
Totals	120	179,500	3,360	

Table 1. Total number of medical texts, words, and reporting verbs. Normalization of results per 10,000 words.

Complementarily, in the case of RPs, we took advantage of the larger size of this subcorpus to look into the use of RepVbs and their positive and negative meanings across the various IMRAD sections of the papers (introduction, methods, results, and discussion sections) to test hypothesis (b) above.

The selection of materials for the composition of the corpus was randomly made on the basis of scientific representativity, diversity and availability, most of them through free online journals and journals the Universitat of València was subscribing to at the time this research was conducted.[2] Acknowledgements and references were not taken into account.

2.2. Variables

As indicated above, positive and negative assessment may be conveyed by means of a variety of linguistic resources, namely positive and factive RepVbs, as defined by Thompson and Yiyun (1991: 372). These include: a) verbs that present the information as true or correct, e.g. *accept*, *emphasize*, *invoke*, *note*, *point out*, *posit*, *reason*, among others; b) other evaluative verbs introducing positive assessment, such as *advise*, *affirm*, *applaud*, *bring out*, etc.; c) positive nouns and adjectives, such as *positive*, *valuable*, *satisfaction*, *demonstration*, etc.; and d) the use of emphatic forms, such as *do*, *does* or *indeed.*

Taking Thompson and Yiyun's (1991) classification as a starting point of reference, we classified them in three different classes: positive, negative and neutral. We considered the following specific verbs in all their possible conjugated forms.

2.2.1. Positive reporting verbs

Evaluative language has usually been approached taking into consideration different grammatical categories. For instance, Gea Valor (2000: 37-42), studying BRs, speaks of positive and negative evaluative language, either as complimenting or criticizing, but her study only examines adjectives, adverbs, verbs, and nouns. By contrast, our research focuses on RepVbs. By positive RepVbs we mean those verbs which provide *prima facie* a positive evaluative meaning in relation to the research being described, such as the following:

---

2 Throughout this chapter, the examples used from the different corpora will be indicated by the letter J and a digit, to indicate the journal, followed by issue number and year of publication, and an acronym indicating the genre. The titles of the journals are listed in the Appendix.

accept, acknowledge, advise, affirm, agree, applaud, assert, bring out, concur, develop, emphasize, encourage, excel, expect, explain, hypothesize, identify, improve, insist, invoke, maintain, note, notice, observe, outline, point out, posit, praise, prove, reason, recognize, recommend, remark, show, stress, subscribe to, substantiate, succeed, suggest, support, think, throw light on, urge.

It is obvious that with most verbs, which objectively might indicate a positive evaluative stance, the addition of an adverb will modify the positive sense initially observed.

(1) The author *excels* when describing the importance of tools and their applications. (J9-4[2005]-BR 22)

2.2.2. Negative reporting verbs

Negative RepVbs provide a critical assessment of the research, idea, method or analysis being reported, such as the following:

assume, attack, challenge, confuse, contraindicate, disagree, disappear, disappoint, discard, discontinue, dismiss, dispute, disregard, disrupt, distort, diverge from, doubt, fail, ignore, lack, misdirect, misinform, misinterpret, mislead, misrepresent, miss, mistrust, misuse, object to, oppose, overcorrect, overemphasize, overestimate, overgeneralize, overlap, overlook, override, overstate, provoke, question, reject, suspect, undercorrect, underestimate, underrepresent, understudy, undertreat, underuse, wan, wonder.

The following example illustrates the use of negative RepVbs:

(2) Outcome data for salvage debulking procedures for patients with advanced disease *are lacking*. (J7-241[2005]-RP)

2.2.3. Neutral reporting verbs

We considered the following RepVbs to be neutral since in most cases the context determines their orientation:

account, add, address, advance, argue, assert, assess, believe, claim, conclude, describe, distinguish, evaluate, examine, express, feel, find, focus on, generalize, indicate, inform, pose, present, propose, quote, recall, remind, report, retain, state, tackle, undertake, use, utilize.

The following example can be taken as an exemplification of a neutral RepVb:

(3) In an evaluation of different house staff schedules, Petersen et al. *examined* 3146 medical patients and *reported* that preventable adverse events [...]. (J7-241[2005]-RP)

2.3. Method of study

Our method of analysis was divided into several stages: firstly, the corpus was compiled from major medical journals whose issues are available electronically in the net. Secondly, the texts were edited so as to produce easily manageable documents for electronic analysis. Thirdly, the documents in each subcorpus were treated with *WordSmith Tools* (Scott 1996) to identify the various RepVbs under study. The percentage of each verbal category in each genre analyzed was calculated over the total number of RepVbs recorded in each category. Through the statistics package R (*The R Project for Statistical Computing*, version 2.2.1, 2005), the data were analyzed using a non-parametric chi square (χ^2) test for contingency tables. Alpha value was set up at $p < 0.05$. Finally, the data obtained were analyzed in context and results were compared across genres and across the different sections in the case of RPs. A quantitative approach was thus adopted in the three initial stages of the study, and a qualitative analysis was applied in the final account of the results obtained.

3. Results and discussion

Table 1 shows the distribution of our corpus along with the number of RepVbs (n = 3,360) recorded in the six medical genres studied. It also displays the normalization of these results per 10,000 words, showing an average number of RepVbs per 10,000 of 186.76 in the corpus as a whole. Figure 1 displays the main results of the analysis of the variables under study.

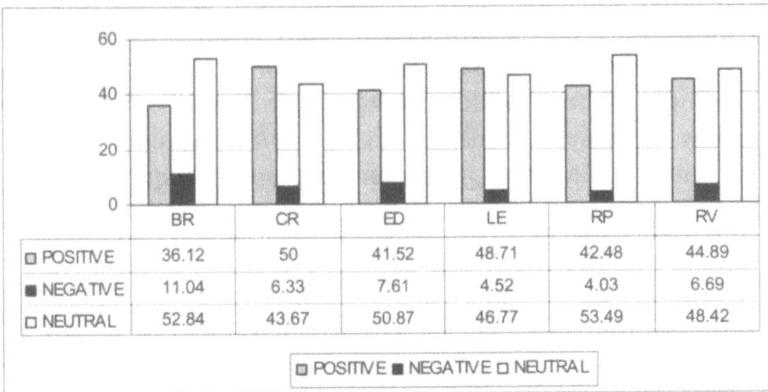

	BR	CR	ED	LE	RP	RV
POSITIVE	36.12	50	41.52	48.71	42.48	44.89
NEGATIVE	11.04	6.33	7.61	4.52	4.03	6.69
NEUTRAL	52.84	43.67	50.87	46.77	53.49	48.42

Figure 1. Percentages of positive, negative and neutral reporting items per genre in relation to the total number of RepVbs in each subcorpus.

The application of the χ^2 test to the three types of RepVbs proved to be statistically significant: $\chi^2 = 39.3603$: df = 10; p = 0.00002195. Figure 2 more specifically displays the dichotomy in the distribution of positive and negative RepVbs in the 6 ME genres examined here.

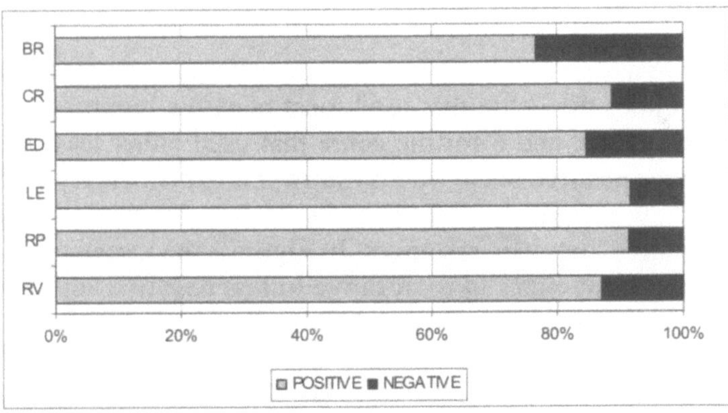

Figure 2. Positive and negative reporting items across genres in percentages.

The same χ^2 test was applied to this combination and the results obtained also proved to be significant (χ^2 = 25.6797; df = 5; p =

0.0001029). In addition, Figures 1 and 2 allow us to draw a diagram (Figure 3) that enables us to identify the genres where negative reporting items are more common, on the one hand, and the genre with less negative reporting items, on the other. It is interesting to observe that only BRs appear as the most negative and the least positive of the genres studied in terms of RepVbs. The remaining genres show complex combinations of both negative and positive RepVbs. This complexity requires complementary explanations.

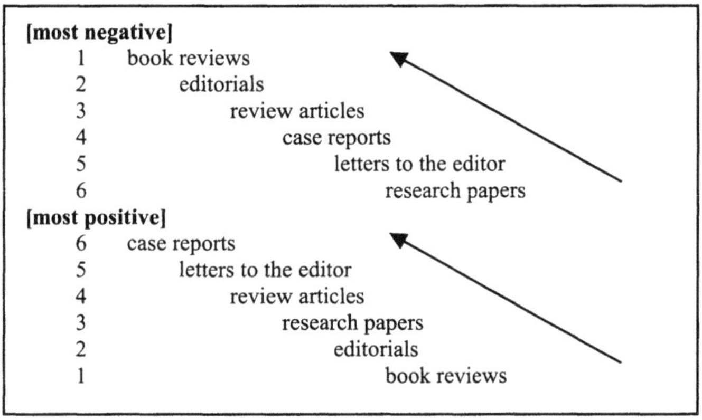

Figure 3. Most negative and most positive genres in terms of RepVb use.

In fact, if we assign a digit from 1 to 6 to each genre studied, where 1 stands for either the genre that used most negative reporting items or less positive items, and 6 for the genre that used either least negative items or more positive ones, we may draw a complementary chart that illustrates how differently each genre behaves in relation to the use of these evaluative linguistic resources. In Figure 4 the numbers stand for the gradation from either most negative to less negative and from less positive to most positive. Figure 4 shows that two genres may be identified as opposites: BRs, on the negative end, and LEs, on the positive end. In the central area, one may find RVs where positive and negative items are used in combination. EDs are close to BRs, while RPs and CRs show distinct combinations in the use of negative and positive RepVbs, as we illustrate below.

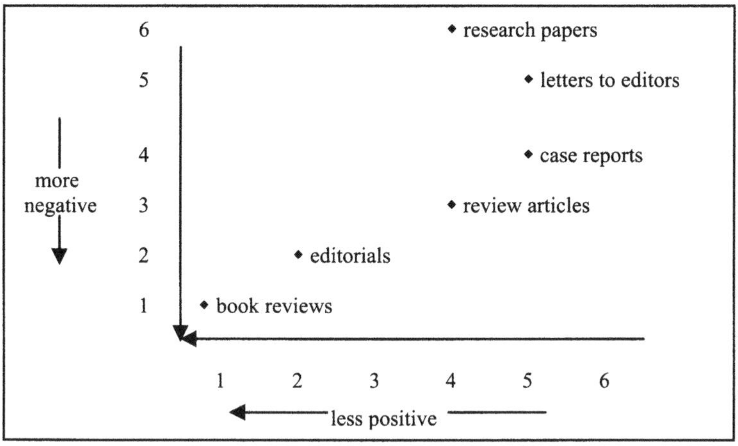

Figure 4. Visual distribution of genres according to their combined use of negative/positive reporting items.

3.1. Book reviews: the most negative

BRs play an important informative and evaluative role for researchers. Actually, as Belcher (1995: 143) pointed out, BRs "have audience as their focal point". This genre shows the lowest percentage of positive RepVbs (36.12%) and the greatest frequency of negative evaluative RepVbs (11.04%). This conforms to the intrinsic critical nature of the genre where authors have to systematically evaluate fellow researchers' publications and produce specific assessment, either positive or negative. This genre involves description, information and evaluation (Gea Valor 2000: 12).

On the one hand, we may find the positive use of RepVbs, such as *recommend*, as illustrated in sentences like "This book is an excellent resource that *is highly recommended* for clinicians" (J2-100[2005]-BR). On the negative side, we find obvious negative expressions with *disappoint*, *ignore*, or *disagree*, among others. We should point out the use of *question* as a specific verb which the authors of BR use to raise certain doubts about the veracity of the author's claims, as in (4).

(4) The concept of a medical model *has been questioned* in the past. (J2-100[2005]-BR)

A milder and subtler way to express negativity is through the use of *wonder*, as shown in (5).

(5) Chapter 13 was dedicated to thrombophilia. I *wonder* why it was included at the end of the book and not among the first 5 Chapters. I also *wonder* why Ian Jennings omits to discuss whether the decrease of fibrinolysis is (or not) a potential thrombotic risk factor. (J24-3[2005]-BR)

The results yielded through our subcorpus, however, differ from North's (1992) and Wiley's (1993) previous studies on BRs. Partly quoting North's (1992: 358) study, Wiley wrote:

> Because reviews stand on their own without accompanying commentary, and because the review will probably have more readers than the actual book, most reviewers, North says, when "forced to renounce" will "chart a cautious course." [...] It is this "faltering kindliness that makes so many reviews sound like they were written by members of a non-judgmental encounter group". (Wiley 1993)

Similarly, Belcher (1995: 146) noticed in BRs "a great deal of cautious indirectness in the expression of negative criticism in a number of disciplines". Accordingly, in this genre both extremes may be found. She further adds that "there appears to be an almost obligatory prefacing of negative commentary with positive commentary" (Belcher 1995: 146-147). This may be what prompted North (1992: 358) to say that most authors wrote "safe" reviews; our data, however, seemed to yield different results. As Hyland (2000: 61-62) puts it, this "potentially threatening genre [...] works because of the extent to which writer and reader approach the text with 'mutual co-awareness'[3] of the other". In his analysis of BR from 8 different disciplines, Hyland (2000: 49) found criticism was more frequent in philosophy and sociology book reviews, while praise was more frequent in the rest of disciplines. It could perhaps be hypothesized,

---

3 Hyland is quoting Nystrand (1987: 48), who used this expression in his discussion.

then, that this might be due to the fact that negative evaluative comments are more common in BRs than in any other genre.

In order to ascertain these apparently contradictory results, we built a control corpus of BRs from the *British Medical Journal* (*BMJ*) for comparison purposes.[4] The data obtained confirm our initial results: 170.5 RepVbs per 10,000 words (154.36 in our BR subcorpus). Table 2 shows the comparison between the two corpora. Differences between the two corpora are not statistically significant, as shown by applying the χ^2 test to the results ($p = 0.3270$), thus confirming our initial results.

	BR subcorpus		*BMJ* control corpus	
	RepVbs	%	RepVbs	%
Positive	108	36.12	62	38.51
Negative	33	11.04	24	14.91
Neutral	158	52.84	75	46.58

Table 2. Data comparison between BR subcorpus and *BMJ* control corpus.

3.2. Case reports

CRs show a complex mixture of both positive and negative RepVbs. In percentages, however, they are the most positive: 50% of the RepVbs recorded are positive (see Figure 1). Most of these positive statements are concentrated in assertions with RepVbs such as *show*, *develop*, *suggest*, or *identify*, which are used to describe progress in the cases they report. Salager-Meyer (2001) points out, however, that CRs can be considered a rather narrative genre and her results show the lowest level of scientific claim with little room for scientific argumentation. Actually, she considers CRs as "the most uncritical genre, i.e., the genre that incorporates the least number of negative appraisals" (Salager-Meyer 2005: 287). Our results, however, show that CRs combine the positive reporting forms used with a significant number of negative instances (6.33%). Interestingly, however, these instantiations of negative evaluative comments are not all addressed to

4 This corpus was made up of 15 BRs for a total of 9,441 words. These BRs were randomly chosen from recent 2005-2006 *BMJ* issues.

other fellow researchers, but most of them are used as a means to express self-criticism. This self-critical approach may be conveyed on a direct personal style, with expressions like "although questionable, our plan was" and "our lack of experience" (both from J1-48[2004]-CR), or in a more impersonal manner, as in (6):

(6) Antibiotic therapy was started and in the following days direct laryngoscopy, barium contrast esophagogram [...], but all efforts *failed* to show the site of injury. (J1-48[2004]-CR)

Occasionally, negative comments are also introduced to describe negative effects or pathological conditions, as in (7):

(7) A transthoracic echocardiography (TTE) showed severe global left ventricular (LV) dysfunction with ejection fraction (EF) of 20%. A coronary spasm *was* then *suspected* and a treatment associating [...]. (J1-48[2004]-CR)

3.3. Editorials

EDs are seldom analyzed in today's medical literature. Only a few studies have recently been published (e.g., Vázquez y del Árbol 2005). Although traditionally an ED may be understood as a message from the editor, the majority of EDs in our subcorpus are short essays on current medical issues (10 of them) that usually express the views of the editor, an invited editorialist, or the editorial staff. Some may be written as an answer to a recent publication (2), or simply an ED as a personal or institutional farewell note (1). Some of these EDs are followed by a description of the different papers in a given issue, although in our subcorpus they are seldom the main concern of the ED. Thus it may be obvious to find a certain balance in the positive/negative dichotomy of verb use. Editorialists actually refrain themselves from using either positive or negative reporting items when compared with other genre writers. The balanced position (see Figure 4) adopted by these professionals may be an indication of their effort to appear objective commentators of the current medical reality. To further substantiate this opinion, it is noticeable how often they resort to bibliographical references, as in example (8) with *improve* as the most commonly used positive RepVb.

(8) Glycolytic adenosine triphosphate (ATP) production maintains integrity of cell membranes,[16] facilitates the transport of calcium into the sarcoplasmic reticulum,[17] and *improves* membrane electrical stability. (J3-148[2004]-ED)

Exceptionally, the negativity is strengthened with the addition of a modal (*must*), or an adverb (*seriously*), through which any trace of doubt about the statement is eliminated:

(9) In view of our modern understanding of tumor biology in general and the grim prognosis of bronchial cancer in particular, the value of such extended operations *must*, however, *seriously be questioned.* (J23-128[2001]-ED)

We can also find an interesting example of negative RepVbs in the use of *lack* (10) through which, from a stance questioning whether or not "statistical feedback" is present in the literature, the editorialist answers with a conclusive "*Certainly not*", thus conveying a positive comment. Sometimes "at all" is added to emphasize the negative meaning (11):

(10) But *do we* really *lack* all statistical feedback for the selection of patients with advanced tumors for surgical intervention? *Certainly not* […]. (J23-128[2001]-ED)

(11) […] our inability to provide clear statistical evidence for treatment of such rather rare tumor situations must not be regarded as indicative that the proposed therapy necessarily *lacks* benefit *at all.* (J23-128[2001]-ED)

The results obtained in this genre partially agree with Salager-Meyer's (2001) findings, especially in the use of negative verbs (second in use after BRs; see Figure 1). She argues EDs contain almost exclusively strong criticism to papers published in the same issue of the journal. This is not confirmed in the data we obtained from our corpus, since their subject or main topic does not always correspond to describing or criticizing the papers which follow the editorial in question, as shown above, but are basically concerned with current medical issues. On some occasions, the editorialist may cite papers included in the issue being editorialized, but it is not necessarily the primary concern of the ED, and when such is the case, the ED tends to praise them.

In order to corroborate these findings, we again constructed a control corpus of EDs, also drawn from recent issues of BMJ.[5] The data obtained from this control corpus also confirmed our initial results: 160.1 RepVbs per 10,000 words, compared to 149.1 in our initial ED subcorpus. Table 3 shows the frequency of use of RepVbs and percentages:

	ED subcorpus		*BMJ* control corpus	
	RepVbs	%	RepVbs	%
Positive	120	41.52	169	44.24
Negative	22	7.61	38	9.95
Neutral	147	50.87	175	45.81

Table 3. Data comparison between EDs subcorpus and *BMJ* control corpus.

The difference was not found to be statistically significant ($p = 0.3394$).

3.4. Letters to the Editor

LEs appear at the far end in the diagram drawn in Figure 4. In other words, LEs represent the opposite genre to BRs in terms of positive and negative RepVbs. This also means that in this genre authors combine a systematic use of positive reporting items with a dramatic reduction of negative evaluative comments.

In LEs, which in the medical literature sometimes refer to published REs, RVs, CRs, etc., authors tend to use two different types of reporting expressions. On the one hand, the authors' intention for writing the LE may simply be laudatory towards a specific paper in terms of agreement ("Certainly, we *agree* with the authors", in (J21-11[2005]-LE) or congratulations ("The authors are to *be congratulated*", in (J21-11[2005]-LE).

On the other hand, and most frequently, the authors of LEs present their own case, experiment or treatment as counter reaction to some article's discussion of specific clinical cases. The letters we have

5 This control corpus consisted of 30 randomly selected EDs, from 2005-2006 issues of BMJ, for a total of 23,866 words.

gathered in our subcorpus could be said to stand between the typical letter to the editor and the letters-to-the-editor columns reporting work in progress and published in letters journals, quite common in today's scientific literature (Hyland 2000: 86). Although not critically oriented *per se*, this type of letters is often used to present just another case for comparison, as in (12):

(12) I *have* recently *suggested* that a higher level of protection (ie a full-face air-purifying respirator; FFR) is warranted,[4] because droplets under appropriate conditions may dry out and result in small airborne particles.[5] (J21-10[2004]-LE)

Moreover, LEs may confirm the veracity of the conclusions in a given paper and provide bibliographical information, also consistent with the paper's conclusions that were not mentioned by the author/s of the paper, as in (13):

(13) In the October 2004 issue of *Acta Anaesthesiologica Scandinavica*, Steffek et al.[1] provided one more piece of evidence [...]. This is consistent with the reports of others,[2,4] providing some 'words of caution' [...]. Palkar et al. reported a case of a pregnant woman who developed a sudden onset [...]. Kiczkowski and Bellars reported a case of a healthy parturient [...]. And finally, McLean et al. reported on a failure of an epidural injection [...]. (J1-49[2005]-LE)

Negative comments are reduced to a minimum (only 14 negative verbal expressions were recorded in our corpus: *fail*, three times, and *disrupt* and *suspect*, twice, as the most frequent), particularly in reference to the absence or failure of a particular treatment, as in (14):

(14) If neurological symptoms like pain or paresthesia occur, we *must suspect* knotting between the catheter and the nerve root and attempts to remove the catheter should be stopped. (J1-49[2005]-LE)

Thus, our results show a different picture of the genre when compared to Magnet and Carnet's (2001) study. These authors focus their analysis on negative statements in LEs, therefore providing a limited description of evaluative comments in the genre. Our data illustrate that LEs combine both positive and negative evaluative statements.

3.5. Research papers: a genre with internal variation

RPs constitute the most important channel for the presentation of new knowledge in today's scientific arena (Swales 1990; Hyland 2000; Salager-Meyer 2001). According to the results from our subcorpus, this "prestigious genre," as Swales (2004: 217) calls it, behaves in a fashion quite similar to that observed in the other genres analyzed here. Myers (1989), in his analysis of politeness in scientific texts, uncovered numerous face-threatening speech acts. Swales (1990) saw it reasonable, therefore, to find an implicit, sometimes explicit, critique to prior literature. Belcher (1995: 149), comparing this genre to BRs, found the criticism of prior texts in RPs to be "much more subtle and implicit". In fact, according to Swales, this subtlety might be due to consumerism and promotionalism. Indeed, authors have the audience so much in mind that the discussion section is sometimes written as if inviting applause from readers (Swales 2004: 238). As can be observed in Figure 5, these variations in the different sections of the RPs are clearly recognizable.

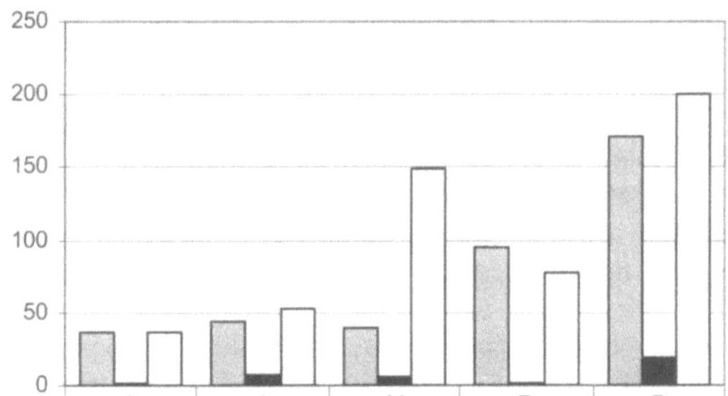

	A	I	M	R	D
Positive	37	44	39	95	171
Negative	1	7	6	2	19
Neutral	36	53	149	78	201

Figure 5. Number of instances of positive and negative RepVbs across the different sections in medical RPs.

There is a complementary relevant set of data obtained in our study of reporting expressions in this genre: it refers to the variation in the application of reporting forms across the various sections of RPs. In other words, the use of reporting items is not the same in all sections (see Figure 5). To start with, reporting items are much more frequent in the discussion section than in other sections of the RP. Our results agree with Thompson's research (1993, quoted by Swales and Feak 1994: 158) when she concludes that the discussion section abounds in commentary and propositions (see also Skelton / Edwards 2000).

As Figure 5 shows, negative reporting forms are almost completely absent in abstracts (0.002%) and in results (0.004%) sections. They are rarely used in introductions (0.014%) and methods (0.012%) sections, and they are much more frequent along with positive forms in the discussion sections (0.039%).[6] The low frequency of negative forms does not allow us to draw clear-cut conclusions. However, the analysis per section does suggest that the use of either positive or negative reporting expressions differs from one rhetorical section of RP to the other. This opens a new area for further analysis and research, since we could speculate that similar variations could be detected in other genres, especially when clearly defined sections can be determined, as in the case of RVs (cf. Mungra this volume) and CRs.

Taking a look at some of the RepVbs used, we could observe that verbs such as *develop* and *show* are used more frequently than others. Some expressions simply refer to data collected and commented on in the discussion section, as in example (15):

(15) This post-hoc retrospective analysis *shows* that use of ACE inhibitors before the onset of AF enhances acute ECV outcome but it does not improve maintenance of sinus rhythm. (J10-5[2005]-RP)

Negative forms have a rather important function in both introductions and discussions, particularly in the latter. In the introduction, where the previous research is usually evaluated, negative expressions are less frequent and less conspicuous in RPs than in EDs and RVs

6 Due to the scarcity of RepVb instances, we were unable to apply the χ^2 test to the individual analysis of the sections in RPs.

(Salager-Meyer 2001). Salager-Meyer (2005: 287) also points out how tactful RP authors are precisely because they "intend to avoid the boomerang effect of a negative appraisal of their peers' work". Both in the introduction and discussion sections, therefore, authors are very careful in their choice of words when incorporating negative comments, and when they do, they especially tend to focus on their own specific research. The following examples try to illustrate this point, as in examples (16), from an introduction, (17) and (18), from discussion sections:

(16) Studies with more generalizable target populations *are lacking*. [...] We developed indicators of hypertensive care and determined whether patients had received the indicated care [...]. (J10-5[2005]-RP)

The negative evaluation implied by the use of *lack*, in the first part of the example, is sometimes hedged by a modalized expression, as can be seen in the following:

(17) Thus, reports in the literature of nonoperative measures *may lack* details on their major complications. (J10-4[2004]-RP)

Example (18), from a discussion section, is a reflection of the authors' own experiment that did not yield the expected results:

(18) Stratification of patients into the categories of low-flow ischemia or occlusive ischemia related to an embolic event *failed* to demonstrate any clinically or statistically significant differences in presentation. (J1-5[2005]-RP)

In the methods section, usually more descriptive and less negative than other sections, writers may refer to some shortcomings in their own or in a colleague's methodology. Example (19) describes the object of the experiment:

(19) Liver lesions *were addressed* with radiofrequency ablation (RFA), hepatic resections (both anatomic and nonanatomic), or combination therapy. (J7-241[2005]-RP)

It is obvious that argumentation, whether based on conflicting or non-conflicting views, appears mainly in the discussion section of the RP, as has been seen in the above histogram (Figure 5). For example,

Fagan and Martín Martín (2004), comparing RPs in psychology and chemistry, found "academic conflict", as illustrated by the number of argumentative and counter-argumentative expressions, in both the introduction (45% in psychology and 33% in chemistry) and in the discussion sections (52% and 63%, respectively), while it is almost non-existent in the methods section in which they only recorded 5 instances (2%) in their psychology corpus and none in their chemistry corpus.

3.6. Review articles: a central genre

Although the scientific community considers RVs as extremely useful because they gather, summarize and critically assess existing literature (Salager-Meyer 2001) and provide an up-to-date account in a particular field, they can be considered as the least noticeable genre in their use of positive RepVbs. However, together with RPs and EDs, they are the most central ME genres. Their use of negative RepVbs, third runner-up to BRs, might be pointed out as significant in terms of the basic aim of RVs.

Fail is the most commonly used verb in the subcorpus of RVs with 19 instances, with *lack* and *assume* as next in use. The following examples illustrate the use of *fail* leaving no doubt as to the success or failure of a report on statistical significance (20).

(20) Most comparative studies report no difference between primary and secondary success rates (87-96% vs 84-89%, respectively).[50,55,81,89,91] One shows a higher success rate for secondary cases but *fails* to report the statistical significance.[16] Two report lower success for secondary compared with primary cases but fail to report the statistical significance.[51,92] (J11-112[2005]-RV)

One further comment deserves the use of the verb *assume* which, in principle, was interpreted as a negative RepVb. Most examples of the use of this verb appear in a negative context, such as the following:

(21) At present, there is no evidence to support this latter suggestion and groins in which sentinel modes are not found *cannot be assumed* to be clear. (J11-112[2005]-RV)

In other instances, when this verb could be understood as neutral since its meaning could go in either direction, the context confirms that the author doubts as to the feasibility of a treatment or method by using words that refer to the arbitrary use of certain techniques, therefore implying a negative report. Example (22) illustrates our point:

(22) The probabilities of observing 1-minute Apgar scores of 1, 2, 3, 4, 5 and 6 *were arbitrarily preset* at 0.3, 0.25, 0.2, 0.08, 0.05 and 0.04 for the poor outcome group and 0.04, 0.05, 0.08, 0.2, 0.25 and 0.3 for the good outcome group, representing a nearest rounded effect size (log odds ratio: R) of 1.5. In other words, it *was assumed* that most asphyxiated infants with poor outcome could have 1-minute Apgar scores of 13, whereas those with good outcome would tend to have Apgar scores ranging from 4 to 6. (J11-112[2005]-RV)

In her 2005 study, Salager-Meyer calls RVs and EDs "epicritical genres" (2005: 283). Our data would confirm this, although RVs seem to project a milder tone. RVs, as a genre "based on the meticulous and scrupulous examination" (Salager-Meyer 2005: 285) of selected studies on a given subject, are expected to be critical indeed. In fact, our results show that BRs are the most critical genre studied.

4. Conclusions and implications

4.1. Conclusions

From the above results and comments, we may draw the following conclusions:

a) the use of positive and negative reporting items is a common linguistic resource in the expression of written academic research across ME genres;
b) the use of positive and negative reporting items is not consistent across the different genres in ME;
c) BRs appear to be the genre with the most frequent use of negative reporting in combination with few positive reporting items, most likely due to the genre intrinsic critical nature;

d) LEs represent the opposite genre in terms of their use of reporting expressions;
e) RVs are a central genre in its application of a combination of both positive and negative reporting forms;
f) EDs seem to focus on current medical issues and not only on the papers they introduce, showing a fairly high level of negative comments;
g) CRs appear as a genre that presents a complex combination of many positive and negative reporting items being used concurrently;
h) The analysis of reporting expressions across the different sections within RPs suggests that the use of these linguistic items also varies depending on the paper section. Further research could confirm whether this phenomenon takes place in the remaining genres of academic ME, such as the ones analyzed in this chapter.

4.2. Implications for medical writing

Reporting expressions are a key linguistic device in the transmission of scientific medical research and are systematically used in varying degrees, in different medical genres. Accordingly, the incorporation of the teaching of the use of these forms in ME teaching settings seems quite relevant. Our analysis suggests that certain reporting expressions are more common in some genres than in others and that variation within the same genre also takes place. Medical writers could be made aware of these variations. Their increased awareness of the application of this linguistic resource, both in its positive and negative forms, might help them become more successful authors as well as more capable readers of ME texts. Nonnative English-speaking medical writers may have learned to use positive and negative reporting either intuitively or the hard way – having their papers rejected. However, more emphasis on raising junior researchers' awareness to the appropriate application of this linguistic resource in their field may ease their way to their main professional objectives: publish in mainstream scientific journals and therefore make their research visible on the international scene of scholarly communication.

References

Belcher, Diane 1995. Writing Critically across the Curriculum. In Belcher, Diane / Braine, George (eds) *Academic Writing in a Second Language. Essays on Research and Pedagogy*. Norwood: Ablex, 135-55.

Carnet, Didier / Magnet, Anne 2002. *Letters to the Editor*: strategies d'utilisation par une communauté de chercheurs francophones et tentative de caractérisation du genre. *ASp, la revue du GERAS* 35-36, 89-102.

Chubin, Daryl E. / Hackett, Edward J. 1990. *Peerless Sciences: Peer Review and U.S. Science Policy*. Albany, NY: SUNY Press.

Fagan, Anna / Martín Martín, Pedro 2004. The Use of Critical Speech Acts in Psychology and Chemistry Research Papers. *Ibérica* 8, 125-37.

Gea Valor, M. Lluïsa 2000. *A Pragmatic Approach to Politeness and Modality in Book Reviews*. Valencia: SELL Monographs 6.

Gosden, Hugh 2001. 'Thank you for your critical comments and helpful suggestions': Compliance and Conflict in Authors' Replies to Referees' Comments in Peer Reviews of Scientific Research Papers. *Ibérica* 3, 3-17.

Guilford, William H. 2001. Teaching Peer Review and the Process of Scientific Writing. *Advances in Physiology Education* 25, 167-75.

Hewings, Martin 2005. Corpus Analysis for ESP: The State of Play and Future Directions. Plenary speech, IV International AELFE Conference. Cáceres, Spain, October 3-5.

Hyland, Ken 2000. *Disciplinary Discourses: Social Interactions in Academic Writing*. London: Longman.

Kiely, Richard 2004. Learning to Critique in EAP. *Journal of English for Academic Purposes* 3, 211-27.

Magnet, Anne / Carnet, Didier 2001. Quelques aspects de la contradiction et de la remise en cause dans le genre *Letters to the Editor*. *ASp, la revue du GERAS* 31-33, 51-62.

Manten, A. A. 1973. Scientific Review Literature. *Scholarly Publishing* 5/1, 75-89.

Myers, Greg 1989. The Pragmatics of Politeness in Scientific Articles. *Applied Linguistics* 10, 1-35.
North, Stephen M. 1992. On Book Reviews in Rhetoric and Composition. *Rhetoric Review* 10, 348-62.
Nystrand, M. 1987. The Role of Context in Written Communication. In Horowitz, R. / Samuels, S. J. (eds) *Comprehending Oral and Written Language*. San Diego, CA: Academic Press, 197-214.
Salager-Meyer, Françoise 1994. Hedges and Textual Communicative Function in Medical English Written Discourse. *English for Specific Purposes* 13, 149-70.
Salager-Meyer, Françoise 2001. From Self-highlightedness to Self-effacement: A Genre-based Study of the Socio-pragmatic Function of Criticism in Medical Discourse. *LSP & Professional Communication* 1/2, 63-85.
Salager-Meyer, Françoise 2005. Dissension across Academia Genres. *Quaderns de Filologia. Estudis Lingüístics* 10, 279-92.
Salager-Meyer, Françoise / Alcaraz Ariza, María Ángeles / Zambrano, Nahirana 2003. The Scimitar, the Dagger and the Glove: Intercultural Differences in the Rhetoric of Criticism in Spanish, French and English Medical Discourse (1930-1995). *English for Specific Purposes* 22, 223-47.
Scott, Mike 1996. *WordSmith Tools*. Oxford: Oxford University Press.
Skelton, John R. / Edwards, Sarah J. L. 2000. The Function of the Discussion Section in Academic Medical Writing. *British Medical Journal* 320, 1269-70.
Swales, John M. 1990. *Genre Analysis. English in Academic and Research Settings*. Cambridge: Cambridge University Press.
Swales, John M. 2004. *Research Genres. Exploration and Applications*. Cambridge: Cambridge University Press.
Swales, John M. / Feak, Christine B. 1994. *Academic Writing for Graduate Students*. Ann Arbor, MI: The University of Michigan Press.
Thomas, Sarah / Hawes, Thomas P. 1994. Reporting Verbs in Medical Journal Articles. *English for Specific Purposes* 13, 129-48.
Thompson, Dorothea K. 1993. Arguing for Experimental 'Facts' in Science: A Study of Research Article Results Sections in Biochemistry. *Written Communication* 8, 106-28.

Thompson, Geoff / Yiyun, Ye 1991. Evaluation in the Reporting Verbs Used in Academic Papers. *Applied Linguistics* 12, 365-82.

Varttala, Teppo 1999. Remarks on the Communicative Functions of Hedging in Popular Scientific and Specialist Research Articles on Medicine. *English for Specific Purposes* 18, 177-200.

Vázquez y del Árbol, Esther 2005. A Genre-based Study of Biomedical Editorials and Letters to the Editor: A Contrastive Analysis. *Ibérica* 10, 145-60.

Wiley, Mark 1993. How to Read a Book: Reflections on the Ethics of Book Reviewing. *JAC* 13/2 (online journal).

Appendix

J1. *Acta Anaestesiologica Scandinavica*
J2. *Addiction*
J3. *American Heart Journal*
J4. *American Journal of Kidney Diseases*
J5. *An International Journal of Obstetrics & Gynaecology*
J6. *Annals of Hematology*
J7. *Annals of Surgery*
J8. *Archives of Surgery*
J9. *BioMedical Engineering OnLine*
J10. *BMC Cardiovascular Disorders*
J11. *BJOG: An International Journal of Obstetrics & Gynaecology*
J12. *Bulletin of the Medical Library*
J13. *Cancer*
J14. *Cardiovascular Ultrasound*
J15. *Current Controlled Trials in Cardiovascular Medicine*
J16. *Journal of Obstetrics and Gynaecology*
J17. *Medical Pediatric Oncology*
J18. *Respiration Physiology*
J19. *Reviews in Cardiovascular Medicine*
J20. *Surgical Practice*
J21. *The Hong Kong Medical Journal*
J22. *The Internet Journal of Cardiology*
J23. *The Journal of Thoracic and Cardiovascular Surgery*
J24. *Thrombosis Journal*

FRANÇOISE SALAGER-MEYER / MARIA ANGELES ALCARAZ ARIZA /
MARYELIS PABÓN / NAHIRANA ZAMBRANO

Paying One's Intellectual Debt: Acknowledgments in Scientific/Conventional and Complementary/Alternative Medical Research

1. Introduction

Acknowledgments (ACKs) are central to Austin's (1962) motley class of 'behabitives', which express, perfunctorily if not genuinely, certain feelings toward the hearer. These feelings and their linguistic expressions are appropriate to particular occasions, such as expressing gladness or gratitude. In Brown and Levinson's (1987) famous account of linguistic politeness, thanks and ACKs tend to produce a debt of gratitude which the listener must somehow reciprocate. This obviously concerns the domain of orality.

At the risk of stating the obvious, ACKs are by no means an exclusive feature of oral discourse. In fact, in the scholarly communication process (or marketplace of ideas, e.g. Fairclough 1995; Hyland 2000), the practice of ACK – whose purpose is to give credit to those people and/or agencies who, one way or another, provided some sort of support without being directly involved in the research – is an important social and cognitive feature which allegedly has its roots in the letters that three centuries ago used to accompany scientific papers sent to patrons and powerful benefactors (Atkinson 1999; Hyland 2004). The history of ACKs would thus date back to the time when the benevolence and generosity of those in authority were a pre-requisite for publication (Giannoni 2002).

ACKs appeared as a section as such in the 1940s, but it is only in the 1960s that they became a widespread practice and standard feature of the research article (RA), thus reflecting "the democratisation of scientific culture, just as in movie credits, where even technical advisers and electricians get acknowledged". (Gross *et al.* 2002: 181).

Apart from being present as a mandatory or non-mandatory form in RAs, ACKs are also found in books, PhD dissertations and MA theses (Hyland 2003, 2004). It has been argued that ACKs play such an important role in today's scholarly communication that they should be used conjointly with established bibliometric indicators (such as citations) in a researcher's academic audit process (Cronin 1995; Giles / Councill 2004).

1.1. Acknowledgments: a genre, a part genre, a paratext, a parking lot, a supercitation?

Certainly, ACKs belong neither to the primary genre of research papers (cf. Swales 1996) nor to secondary, more pedagogic genres, nor to Swales' "occluded genres" (Swales 1996, 2004). ACKs, which in Hyland's parlance (2003: 253) form part of "the paraphernalia of today's research articles", have received various names. Hyland himself opines that they are a "Cinderella genre"[1] in the sense that they are a taken-for-granted part of the background, "a practice of unrecognised and disregarded value" (Hyland 2003: 242) "whose importance to research students has been overlooked in the literature" (Hyland 2004: 306). Along the same lines, Giannoni (2002: 9) refers to ACKs as a "minor and largely overlooked academic genre" and Cronin *et al.* (1992: 122) as "a long neglected textual artifact" that belongs to the "academic auditors' armamentarium" (Cronin 1995: 38).

ACKs have also been called a "paratext", alongside titles, headings, prefaces, illustrations and dedications (Genette 1997, cited in Giannoni 2002: 8), or a "part genre" (Swales 2004: 31) that reflects, on the one hand, sub-author collaboration and, on the other, the distributive cognition of science writing, thus highlighting trends in collaboration beyond co-authorship. For his part, Caesar (1992: 87), more specifically referring to ACKs in academic books, labels them

1 Hyland (2004) provides powerful reasons for considering the ACK section in PhD and MA theses as a genre in its own right.

"a consoling gesture whereby the book, no matter how scholarly, demonstrates its accountability as a social product".

For information and social scientists, ACKs are rather viewed as "exchange of gifts" (McCain 1991: 495), "expressions of solidarity" characteristic of schools organised as mentoring systems (Ben-Ari 1987: 137), "supercitations" (Edge 1979: 118), "sub-authorship collaboration" (Patel 1973: 81), "trusted assessorship in action" (Mullins 1973: 32, cited in Cronin 2005: 56) or in a vivid metaphor as "a parking lot for miscellaneous contributions" (Cronin 2005: 56), whether social, cognitive and/or technical, which typically fall short of meeting generally accepted criteria for awarding co-authorship.[2]

Social scientists have also documented the social significance of ACK practices in a variety of disciplines: e.g. Heffner (1979) in biology, psychology, political science and chemistry; McCain (1991) in genetics; Cronin (1995) in information science, psychology, history, philosophy and sociology; Laband / Tollison (2000) in biology and economics, and Giles / Councill (2004) in computer science. All these in depth-studies show that ACKs are certainly no trivial flourish of academic life, but that, like citations, they respond to social expectations. Unlike citations, however, they do not entail intellectual accountability and legal liability for an article's content. These studies have also indicated that ACKs define a variety of cognitive and social relationships among researchers within and across disciplines and can thus be used to map networks of influence to help better understand the context of scientific research.

Whichever the label adopted, Hyland (2003) pertinently observes that ACKs are perhaps the most explicitly interactional genre of the academy, in the sense that they form a bridge between the personal and the public, the social and the professional, the academic and the lay. A bridge, indeed, and a rhetorical collegial space where authors repay their "intellectual indebtedness" (Davis / Cronin 1993: 591).

---

2 The dividing line between authorship and acknowledgment is not always very clear today, and the concept of authorship in contemporary science is an increasingly problematic construct, especially in the biomedical sciences (Rennie *et al.* 1997).

As far as we know, only two applied linguists have addressed the issue of ACKs in academic writing. On the one hand, Hyland's research on the generic move structure of ACKs in PhD and MA theses (Hyland 2003, 2004; Hyland / Tse 2004), and, on the other, Giannoni's (1998, 2002) cross-linguistic study of ACKs in Italian- and English-written research articles, and in academic books (Giannoni 2006). These studies underline, inter alia, the dialogic nature of the ACKs section by positing that it is the only part of the research article which reflects the contingency of scientific research.

From this review of the literature, it seems to us abundantly clear first of all that ACKs are a well-established facet of the scholar's rhetorical repertoire and a more or less institutionalised practice across scientific fields and, secondly, that their importance in scholarly communication is now well documented by scholars from a variety of different disciplines. Nonetheless, as Hyland (2003) observes, much work remains to be done on ACKs and research needs to be extended to several disciplines and languages.

This is why, in order to deepen our knowledge and understanding of ACKs' sociopragmatic features, we would like to present here the results of a research on the content of ACKs in two different medical corpora published between 2004 and 2005, viz. a corpus made up of 'scientific/conventional medicine'[3] RAs (published between 2004 and 2005 in reputable, top-ranking scientific medical journals) and a comparable corpus of complementary/alternative medicine (CAM) RAs (see §1.2).[4] Our research thus adopts a genre-based approach, drawing on "the most developed and comprehensive

---

3 This kind of medicine is also indistinctly called regular/organized medicine (Studdert *et al.* 1998), academic medicine (Delbanco 1998), biomedicine, Western or mainstream medicine (Fontanarosa / Lundberg 1998), scientifically-proven, evidence-based medicine (Fontanarosa / Lundberg 1998) or Western allopathic medicine (Eskinazi 1998). Jonas (1998) refers to scientific medicine with the following expressions: mainstream, official, scientific, orthodox, conventional, mainstream and/or modern medicine.

4 In spite of the fact that both adjectives (*complementary* and *alternative*) are frequently used interchangeably, they should not be confused (Udani 1998). *Complementary* means 'adjunct to' (not 'in place of') conventional western medicine, whereas *alternative* means 'in place of', 'instead'. For a more detailed definition of CAM, see Salager-Meyer *et al.* (2006).

rhetorical theory to address writing in recent times" (Dias *et al.* 1999, cited in Swales 2004).

1.2. Why complementary and alternative medicine (CAM)?

Before presenting our corpus and the method followed to analyse it, we would like to briefly explain why we decided to focus on a genre of medical research (CAM research) which, in spite of its increasing worldwide popularity, has not so far been the object of any discourse analysis, whereas written and oral scientific/conventional (SC) discourse has been studied quite extensively.

In the early 20th century, scientific medicine emerged as the dominant model for health care in the West. Yet, despite its success, people have continued to seek treatment outside mainstream services. Today, in the United Kingdom, for example, about 1 in 10 of the adult population consults a CAM practitioner every year (Thompson / Feder 2005a). In the 1990s, the US population made an estimated 425 million visits to providers of unconventional therapies, a number that exceeded the number of visits (388 million) to all primary care physicians (Eisenberg *et al.* 1993). Moroever, it is estimated that the market for CAM therapies has surged 69% since 1989 and that it is growing as fast as 30% annually (Studdert *et al.* 1998).

CAM's popularity is growing along with the call for its integration into the National Health Service (Thompson / Feder 2005b). This has been accompanied by a growth not only in the number of CAM journals (Brodin / Danell 2005),[5] but also in the number of CAM-related papers published in mainstream internal medicine journals, precisely because the worldwide success of CAM is urging the conventional as well as the unconventional medical world to submit CAM-related products and practices to randomized

5 Most CAM journals were launched between 1970 and 1990, but it is the year 1996 that marked off a period of dramatic expansion for CAM as a scientific field. Today, according to Shekelle *et al.* (2005), there are at least 10 databases specialized in CAM, covering a total of 695 different CAM journals.

controlled trials in order to prove their claims of efficacy and safety (Thompson / Feder 2005a).

Because of this increasing popularity and because there is so much passion in the debate between mainstream medicine and CAM advocates, we thought it would be interesting to investigate in what ways, if any, CAM research and discourse differentiate themselves from their orthodox, scientific medicine counterparts. We thus designed a wide research project on the discourse of CAM, the first results of which are chronicled here. To our knowledge, this is the first paper that deals with CAM discourse from a pragmalinguistic perspective.

2. Corpus

This study presents the findings of a content and linguistic analysis of the textual space of ACKs drawn from 50 randomly selected English-written medical RAs, distributed as follows:

1) 25 RAs dealing with SC medicine issues published in leading mainstream scientific medical journals, referred to as the SC sample.
2) 25 RAs concerned with CAM-related issues published in CAM journals, referred to hereafter as the CAM sample.

The 25 SC papers represent a broad cross-section of medical practice and were drawn from four large-circulation US and UK medical journals of persistence and pedigree, viz., *The Journal of the American Medical Association (JAMA), Annals of Internal Medicine, The Lancet* and *The New England Journal of Medicine*. The 25 CAM papers also represent a broad section of CAM practice, i.e. the so-called 'big five': homeopathy, acupuncture, chiropractic, herbal medicine and osteopathy (Thompson / Feder 2005a: 856). They too were drawn from the two most reputable and highly regarded (refereed and indexed) CAM research journals, viz. the *Journal of Complementary and Alternative Medicine* and *BMC (Bio Med Central) Complementary and Alternative Medicine*. British and

American texts were grouped together because we were not concerned with language varieties. It is important to mention here that the guidelines for authors of all six journals explicitly require not only a clear ACK statement including, inter alia, the exact identification of funding sources, but also a detailed explanation of financial disclosures, financial and non-financial conflict of interest and the funding organizations' or sponsors' involvement in the research being reported.

In studies of this kind, it is recommended to draw the sample texts from top-ranking journals because, as Connor (2004) argues, their articles have undergone strict peer review and editorial scrutiny. This ensures that the articles published in these journals are fairly representative of the journal genre in content and style or, in Bazerman's words (1994: 23), that the texts are "situationally effective" and are the result of "expert performance" (Bazerman 1994: 131). Because the papers analysed in both medical research types were drawn from highly regarded journals in terms of importance and multiyear impact factor, we can safely assume that our two sub-corpora are comparable.

3. Methods

3.1. Methods used and variables analysed

We first of all recorded some demographic data regarding each of the 50 papers, i.e. the number of authors per paper and their institutional affiliation data. The number of funded and unfunded research projects as well as the number of funding sources in each paper was also recorded. All selected papers were scrutinized to discover any ACK set apart at either the beginning or end of the RA. Medical journals indeed have different editorial policies regarding the presentation of ACKs, and although most of these are generally found in clearly identifiable article-ending sections, they are not always labelled.

Regarding their etiquette, ACKs may be "compound entities" (Cronin *et al.* 2004: 162) where authors in one breath thank peers for ideas, federal or industrial funding bodies for financial support and colleagues for moral support. Funding agencies, however, are sometimes thanked/mentioned in a separate textual space preceded by the heading 'Fundings'. In cases where the funding support formed part of a textual space in its own right, we counted both paratexts (ACK and Fundings) together. The total number of running words making up the ACKs and funding spaces was then calculated. The number of acknowledged individuals mentioned by name and the unnamed entities credited were also recorded in each article.

Apart from the length of such texts, we also looked for any mention of financial disclosure, sponsor involvement and conflict of interest.

3.2. Detailed content analysis of ACKs and their rationale

The next step consisted in the analysis of the motivations that underpin the ACKs in each paper. Because ACKs embody a wide range of relationships between people, agencies, institutions and research, we classified all ACKs using a seven-part typology which is a somewhat modified version of Cronin (1995), Hyland (2003) and Giles / Councill (2004):

1) Moral support: e.g. thanking someone for his/her enthusiasm, encouragement, wisdom.
2) Instrumental / technical support, e.g. providing access to tools, facilities, specimen samples, technologies and infrastructural resources; offering technical expertise such as CPR (cardio-pulmonary resuscitation), help in data collection/entry/ management, sample preparation, etc.
3) Financial support, i.e. recognition of external and/or intra-mural funding from national and/or international private and/or public educational institutions, federal/governmental research agencies and/or industrial (pharmaceutical industry) sources/sponsors. Our classification of financial sources is a modified version of Giles / Councill (2004).

4) Conceptual support, also called "academic support" (Hyland 2003) or "peer-interactive communication (PIC)" (McCain 1991: 512), includes thanks for advice and discussion, comments on the manuscript, critical insights, intellectual guidance, valuable suggestions, assessment of the study's soundness, etc.
5) Clerical support, i.e. secretarial services.
6) Editorial/linguistic support, i.e. editing, proofreading or translating the manuscript.
7) Unclassifiable, when it proved impossible to categorize an ACK according to any of the above categories, whether because of inherent ambiguity, vagueness or lack of contextual clues.

The frequency of each ACK category was calculated for each text and then for each subcorpus. A sample of ten ACKs was analysed independently by the team members who then compared their respective interpretations and rationale for classification. There was a high degree of agreement, and in the few cases of disagreement, a specialist informant acted as referee.

4. Results

4.1. Authorship and institutional affiliation

Table 1 shows that the mean number of authors per paper is double in SC compared to CAM, and that authors working in Anglophone countries are also much more numerous in the SC corpus than they are in its CAM counterpart.[6] Indeed, 84% of the SC papers were written by researchers working in an Anglophone context (USA, Canada, UK, Australia), and mostly (52%) by Anglophone researchers alone. By contrast, only 13 CAM papers (52%) were written by Anglophone researchers. Of the remaining 12 CAM papers, 9 (36%) were the work of Asian authors (India, China, Taiwan and Vietnam), while 3 (12%)

6 For the sake of simplicity, we will refer to authors working in English-speaking countries as 'Anglophone writers or researchers', although their mother tongue might not be English.

were written by European scientists from France, Germany, Denmark and the Netherlands, which are the countries where CAM therapies are indeed today most popular (Hanssen *et al.* 2005).

1. AUTHORS	**CAM**	**SC**
Mean No. of authors/paper	4.8	9.12
Anglophone authors only	12 (48%)	12 (52%)
Anglophone authors + others	1 (4%)	8 (32%)
Anglophone authors (Total) **	13 **(52%)**	20 **(84%)**
Non-Anglophone authors (Europe) ***	3 (12%)	4 (16%)
Non Anglophone authors (Asia) □	9 (36%)	---------
Non-Anglophone authors (Total)	12 **(48%)**	4 **(12%)**
2. ACKNOWLEDGMENT (ACK)		
Total No. of papers with ACKs	22 (88%)	25 (100%)
Total No. of ACK speech acts	66	125
Mean length of ACK (in No. of words)	54.22	82.59
Total No. of named acknowledgees *	46	119
Mean No. of named acknowledgees/paper	1.8	5.6
3. FUNDING		
Total no. of papers funded	15 (60%)	24 (96%)
Total no. of funding bodies	28 (over 15 papers)	74 (over 24 papers)
Average No. of funding bodies/paper	1.8	3
4. SPONSOR INVOLVEMENT		
No. of papers in which authors personally received funds from sponsors	--------	9 (36%)
No. of papers in which sponsors were directly involved in the study's design, manuscript review, etc.	--------	4 (16%)
5. CONFLICT OF INTEREST (CoI)		
Total No. of papers mentioning a CoI	1 (4%)	6 (24%)

Table 1. General demographic data about the Complementary/Alternative (CAM) and scientific medicine (SC) samples. (* A named acknowledgee is a person who is clearly identified by his/her surname. ** Canada, Australia, USA, UK. *** France, Germany, Netherlands, Denmark. □ India, China, Taiwan, Vietnam).

4.2. ACK frequency and length

Table 1 also shows that ACKs are present in almost all the papers in both categories: 88% in the CAM category, in spite of the fact that the guidelines to both journals require that ACKs be clearly mentioned (see §2), and 100% in its SC counterpart. The total number of ACK speech acts in the SC sample was double that recorded in its CAM counterpart. This explains why the average length of ACKs is almost twice as long in SC, as compared to CAM. Admittedly, the length of ACKs in SC papers is in fact much greater than that, since we did not take into account four texts in which the list of acknowledgees was given in an appendix at the end of the paper because of its length: two of these had a one page-long list of credited persons (over 100 individuals) and in the other two, the list was over two pages long. Interestingly enough, these four papers were multicentered clinical trials reporting drug-related research sponsored by pharmaceutical laboratories.

4.3. Number of named acknowledgees

Table 1 also indicates that the number of credited individuals was much greater in SC than in CAM. It should be mentioned, however, that the number of named acknowledgees is in fact much higher in the SC papers because, as explained above, four papers are typical examples of hyperauthored 'Big Science' articles crediting over 100 individuals each.

4.4. Unnamed acknowledgees

The types of unnamed acknowledgees are roughly identical in both subcorpora (nursing staff and paramedics, patients and their families, facilities, residents, volunteers, hospitals/clinics/universities, etc), except in one hypotherapy (equine-assisted therapy) CAM paper where horses were thanked for their contribution to the study. It is finally interesting to mention that only non-native English speakers (NNESs) from developing countries thanked their institutions for providing facilities to carry out the reported study. Surprisingly, and contrary to what was observed in philosophy and sociology papers (Cronin *et al.* 2003), not a single anonymous reviewer was thanked in either sub-corpus.

4.5. Funding

Table 1 also shows that all but one paper in the SC category (96%) received some sort of funding, vs. only 60% in CAM articles. The total number of funding bodies was also much greater in the SC sample than in CAM. The average is four funding bodies per paper in the SC articles vs. 1.6 in their CAM counterparts.

4.6. Sponsor involvement and conflict of interest

Nine SC papers mentioned that the contributors received funds directly from sponsors, and four declared direct involvement of sponsors in the study's design or conduct and in manuscript drafting, review and submission. By way of contrast, not a single author in the CAM sample declared having received funds from sponsors or disclosed any sponsor's involvement in the conduct of their research. Likewise, mention of a conflict of interest was present in six SC papers. One paper only in the CAM category declared the presence of such a conflict.

4.7. Breakdown of categories by speech act motivation

It is interesting to note (Table 2) that although the frequency of each of the seven ACK motivation categories differs from one type of medicine to the other, it basically follows the same overall pattern in both medical research types. Indeed, financial, technical and conceptual/academic support are the three most frequently mentioned categories across the corpus, making up 92.8% of the total of ACK speech acts in the SC sample and 84.8% of those in the CAM sample.

ACK rationale	*CAM*	*SC*
1. Financial	**28 (42.4%)**	**74 (59.2%)**
2. Instrumental/technical	**19 (28.8%)**	**30 (24%)**
3. Conceptual/academic/PIC*	**9 (13.6%)**	**12 (9.6%)**
4. Moral	3 (4.5%)	3 (2.4%)
5. Editorial/linguistic	3 (4.5%)	2 (1.6%)
6. Unclassifiable	3 (4.5%)	2 (1.6%)
7. Secretarial/clerical	1 (1.5%)	2 (1.6%)
TOTAL	**66 (100%)**	**125 (100%)**

Table 2. Content analysis of acknowledgments in the Complementary/Alternative (CAM) and scientific medicine (SC) sub-corpora. (The total number of ACK statements in each medical research type is > 25, because papers usually provide more than one reason for acknowledging: a funding agency, a mentor, technical/instrumental/ moral support, etc. – *PIC: peer-interactive communication (McCain 1991))

Moreover, almost 60% of the speech acts in the SC papers refer to financial support, about a quarter (24%) to technical/instrumental support and only 9.6% to conceptual support. Financial support is also the most frequently acknowledged category in CAM research articles (although they account for only 42% of the total number of ACK speech acts recorded in that sample), followed by technical/ instrumental support (28.8%) and, in third position, by conceptual support (13.6%). Editorial and moral support, though much less frequent than the previous three categories, is nonetheless more frequently acknowledged in CAM than in SC.

4.8. Funding bodies

In both medical research types, financial support mostly comes from funding agencies (see Table 3). The percentage is higher, however, in the CAM category than in its SC counterpart. What is particularly interesting (but not surprising) is the role played by the pharmaceutical industry, which sponsored research in SC but not in CAM articles. Educational institutions played a much more important role as sponsors in CAM research than in SC research.

Funding Bodies	*CAM*	*SC*
1. Research agencies	**23 (82.1%)**	**46 (62.1%)**
2. Educational institutions	5 (17.8%)	7 (9.4%)
3. Pharmaceutical industry	--------	**21(28.3%)**
TOTAL	**28 (100%)**	**74 (100%)**

Table 3. Number of funding bodies acknowledged in the Complementary/ Alternative (CAM) and the scientific medicine (SC) sub-corpora.

5. Discussion

We will now discuss the findings of this investigation first by explaining in which ways CAM and SC research resemble each other (§§ 5.1, 5.2, 5.3) and, secondly, how they differ (§§ 5.4 and 5.5).

5.1. Frequency of ACK

Our quantitative data disclosed that the frequency of ACKs is quite similar in both medical research types. This should not come as a surprise since, as we explained above, the guidelines of the seven journals covered in the present study clearly require that whoever has made some sort of contribution to the preparation of the manuscript but does not qualify for authorship, should not only be named in the ACKs but also have agreed in writing to be named.

The very high frequency of ACKs in both samples is consistent with previous studies of ACKs in other 'hard' scientific fields such as genetics (McCain 1991), chemistry (Cronin *et al.* 2004), computer science (Giles / Councill 2004), but also in some 'soft sciences' such as psychology and sociology (Cronin 1995). Cross-disciplinary studies of ACKs (Cronin *et al.* 1992; Cronin 1995) have shown that philosophers and historians are much less assiduous in crediting the multifarious contributions of behind-the-scene actors. Cronin (1995) rightly argues that the cross-disciplinary differences observed in ACK frequency could suggest a gradation from soft to hard subject matters. Biomedicine certainly aligns itself with the hard disciplines, at least as revealed in the ACK sections of papers published in the top ranking journals we examined (see § 5.5).

5.2. Category breakdown or pattern of ACK

Our research also shows that of all the ACK discourse recorded, it is financial support that is most frequently acknowledged in both medical research types. Such a "ritualised genuflection" (Cronin 1995: 14) towards funding bodies corroborates other researchers' results in the hard sciences (Cronin *et al.* 2004).

The second most frequently acknowledged type of support in our study was technical/instrumental support, a clear reflection of the technical and equipment-intensive nature of biomedical research, and of the fact that research in the medical field (as most research in the hard and some soft sciences today) is an enterprise that involves peer interdependence, teamwork and frequent material collaboration among peers. It is not surprising to find a greater frequency of linguistic/editorial support in the CAM category than in its SC counterpart because, as was stated above, half of the CAM papers were written by NNESs who resorted to some sort of linguistic support (proofreading/editing or translating).

What is surprising, though, is the very low frequency of ACKs aimed at conceptual or academic support in both medical research types. This is known to be the most frequently acknowledged type of intellectual debt in several fields: astronomy (Verner 1994, reported in Cronin 1995: 34), library and information science (Cronin *et al.* 1993) and computer science (Gilles / Councill 2004), to the point that some researchers have even considered it to be at least as valuable as citations (Edge 1979; McCain 1991; Cronin *et al.* 1993). In 'softer' fields, such as history, sociology, philosophy and psychology (Cronin 1995; Cronin *et al.* 2003) and in PhD dissertations and MA theses (Hyland 2003) across a range of hard and soft disciplines, conceptual support or academic assistance also predominates.

5.3. Collaboration and interdependence

As we pointed out in Section 1, modern scholarship is per se collaborative. Such collaboration naturally leads to multi-authored papers, especially in biomedicine, where extreme cases of mass authorship have been reported (e.g. Satyanarayana 1987; Medline 2001; Meadows 2005; Cronin 1995, 2005). Other fields, though they may differ in degree, do not differ in process (Hunt 2003). As a matter of fact, the worldwide trend towards multi-authorship, a phenomenon also referred to as "author inflation" (Sobal / Ferentz 1990), is now very well documented in almost any field of enquiry, especially in the hard sciences, but is also on the increase in the social sciences. This "hyperauthorship" (Epstein 2000) is partially driven by the increasing division of labour in research tasks that involve multiple specialists (epidemiologists, statisticians, etc.), all of whom may expect authorship.[7]

What is interesting about the quantitative findings reported here is not so much that they corroborate the strongly collaborative character of present Anglo-American scientific medical research (which hardly needs to be corroborated), but that they point out striking differences in the way SC and CAM research is conducted. Indeed, all the figures in Table 1 (to the exception of the frequency of ACK in both medical research types) suggest convincingly that CAM research is no doubt collaborative, but certainly not to the extent of SC medical research. Indeed, not only are CAM articles written by a much lower number of contributors/co-authors, but they also acknowledge a much lower number of named individuals, hence the greater average length of the ACK space in 'Big Science' SC papers. In fact, the average length of ACK in CAM papers is very similar to the one reported by Giannoni (2002) in linguistics articles.

All this underscores the fact that the CAM scientific network is not as firmly established as that in SC medicine or other old fields of scientific enquiry. As we said before, the first CAM scientific journals appeared in the 1970s. CAM is thus a relatively new field of scientific

---

7 Sometimes the list of contributors (or co-authors in biomedical research) is so long that the reader is referred to the journal's website (e.g. bmj.com) to inspect their names.

inquiry; as a consequence, its sociotechnical and sociocognitive networks are much less elaborated than they are in SC medical research, which as a field of scientific enquiry is over a century old. All the quantitative data reported above underline this recency. What is more, multispecialities concerning health problems do not exist in the traditional medicine on which CAM is founded. They do however exist in SC, especially since the mid 20th century.

5.4. Funding

As for the funding of research, the fact that 60% of papers in the CAM category and all but one (96%) of those in the SC category mention some sort of financial support, shows that this type of support is crucial in today's biomedical activities. Nonetheless, our findings not only disclose that CAM research receives far less funding than SC research, but also reveal that the sources of funding differ from one type of medicine to the other, with the pharmaceutical industry sponsoring about a quarter of the SC papers we examined[8] but not a single CAM paper. This is not surprising, in view of the fact that the pharmaceutical industry is not particularly interested in the efficacy of herbal treatments, acupuncture or homeopathy.[9]

It is worthwhile mentioning here that the role of the pharmacological industry has been harshly criticized over the last ten years or so by scientific medical journal editors and researchers (e.g. Bodenheimer 2000; Lancet Editorial 2002; Blumenthal 2004; Rothman / Stephen 2005, among many others) who denounce the fact that scientific medicine has become heavily and damagingly tainted by commercial interests and conflicts. "We are becoming, willingly or unwillingly, agents of big pharma, prescribing a pill for each ill",

8 Had we examined randomized clinical trials only, the proportion of industry-funded research would have been much greater.

9 In the USA alone, the pharmaceutical industry financed over 62% of biomedical research in 2000 (Bekelman / Gross 2003), i.e. about US$30 billion. The proportion of industry-funded research has increased in most countries while government funding has declined: in the USA the proportion of industry-funded medical research has almost doubled since 1980 (Henry / Lexchin 2002)

writes Peter Davies (2002: 1168), adding that consultants and journal editors who accept money from big pharma are losing any possibility of maintaining objectivity, perspective and impartiality. Richard Smith (2005), former editor of the *British Medical Journal*, recently went a step further by proposing a radical solution in which medical journals should no longer publish commercially sponsored clinical trials but rather serve to critique them.

5.5. Limitations of the study

A fuller understanding of ACKs in the biomedical literature will obviously require more extensive and varied data gathering and analysis. Indeed, the data presented here are limited in scope and number. First of all, the corpus examined is quite small, especially if we compare it to the corpora analysed in previous ACK research. We do however believe that the features found are sufficiently numerous to yield some insight into the issues at hand (cf. Mauranen 1993; Banks 2005; Flowerdew 2005; Webber 2005, on the value of working with small corpora in genre analysis studies). The second limitation of the research has to do with the kind of journals we deliberately consulted (see § 2), i.e. top-ranking journals that are expected to publish only well written, properly formatted and socially validated research that meets community standards, however these are defined. It may well be that the style and practice of ACK behaviour differ in less prestigious journals and/or that the tendency to acknowledge others' contributions is more fully observed and detailed in 'pedigreed' journals than it is in lower status journals.

6. Conclusions

We have examined the frequency and content of the ACK paratext in two different types of English-written medical research papers: scientific research papers published in scientific medical journals, on the one hand, and CAM research papers published in CAM journals, on the other. Our findings first of all corroborate the view that the ACK space is the only place in a research paper where science is portrayed as a dialogic process that reveals the complex web of interpersonal debts implicit in the construction of knowledge. Our findings also indicate that there are important differences between the CAM and SC modalities of acknowledgment; these underline the recency of CAM as a field of scientific inquiry, as shown by the shorter ACK space, the much lower number of contributors, acknowledgees and sources of funding in CAM research, when compared to the 'Big science' SC research papers. The motivations underlying ACKs are however similar in both research types, with the most frequent ones being financial and instrumental/conceptual.

The differences observed should not come as a surprise, because we are dealing with two different kinds of medical research (both in their principles and their praxis), but the similarities observed indicate that CAM is becoming a 'modernized, westernised' kind of medicine that resorts to research methods officially recognized as valid in the SC Western world.

Diachronic, cross-linguistic and cross-generic ACK research (including the analysis of commercially-sponsored drug related research vs. basic research) would nicely complement the findings reported here and provide valuable historical and experimental data on ACK behaviour and its etiquette.

References

Atkinson, Dwight 1999. *Scientific Discourse in Sociohistorical Context: The Philosophical Transactions of the Royal Society of London. 1675-1975.* Mahwah, NJ: Erlbaum.

Austin, John L. 1962. *How to Do Things with Words*. Cambridge, Mass.: Harvard University Press.

Banks, David 2005. The Case of Perrin and Thomson: An Example of the Use of a Mini-corpus. *English for Specific Purposes* 24/2, 201-11.

Bazerman, Charles 1994. *Constructing Experience*. Carbondale: Southern Illinois University Press.

Bekelman, Justin E. / Gross, Cary P. 2003. Scope and Impact of Financial Conflicts of Interest in Biomedical Research: A Systematic Review. *JAMA (Journal of the American Medical Association)* 289, 454-65.

Ben-Ari, Eyal 1987. On Acknowledgments in Ethnographies. *Journal of Anthropological Research* 43/1, 63-84. Reprinted in J. van Maanen (ed.) *Representation in Ethnography*. Thousand Oaks, CA: Sage, 1995, 130-64.

Blumenthal, David 2004. Doctors and Drug Companies. *The New England Journal of Medicine* 351/18, 1885-90.

Bodenheimer, Thomas 2000. Uneasy Alliance: Clinical Investigators and the Pharmaceutical Industry. *The New England Journal of Medicine* 342/20, 1539-43.

Brodin, Jenny-Ann / Danell, Rickard 2005. Spiritualised Medicine? A Bibliometric Study of Complementary and Alternative Medicine. 4S & EASST Conference, Paris, 26-28/8/2004.

Brown, Penelope / Levinson, Stephen C. 1987. *Politeness. Some Universals in Language Usage*. Cambridge. Cambridge University Press.

Caesar, Terry 1992. On Acknowledgments. *New Orleans Review*. 19/1, 85-94.

Connor, Ulla 2004. Intercultural Rhetoric Research: Beyond Texts. *Journal of English for Academic Purposes* 3/4, 291-305.

Cronin, Blaise 1995. *The Scholar's Courtesy. The Role of Acknowledgments in the Primary Communication Process*. London: Taylor Graham.

Cronin, Blaise 2005. *The Hand of Science*. Lanham, MD: Scarecrow Press.

Cronin, Blaise / McKenzie, Gail / Stiffler, Michael 1992. Patterns of Acknowledgments. *Journal of Documentation* 48/2, 107-22.

Cronin, Blaise / McKenzie, Gail / Rubio, Lourdes 1993. The Norms of Acknowledgments in Four Humanities and Social Sciences Disciplines. *Journal of Documentation* 49/1, 29-43.

Cronin, Blaise / Shaw, Debora / La Barre, Kathryn 2003. A Cast of Thousands: Co-authorship and Subauthorship Collaboration in the 20th Century as Manifested in the Scholarly Journal Literature of Psychology and Philosophy. *Journal of the American Society for Information Science and Technology* 54/9, 855-71.

Cronin, Blaise / Shaw, Debora / La Barre, Kathryn 2004. Visible, Less Visible and Invisible: Patterns of Collaboration in 20th Century Chemistry. *Journal of the American Society for Information Science and Technology* 55/2, 160-8.

Davies, Peter 2002. Letter to the Editor. *The Lancet* 359/9319, 1168.

Davis, Charles. H. / Cronin, Blaise 1993. Acknowledgments and Intellectual Indebtedness: A Bibliometric Conjecture. *Journal of the American Society for Information Science* 44/10, 590-2.

Delbanco, Thomas L. 1998. Leeches, Spiders and Astrology: Predilections and Predictions. *JAMA* 280/18, 1560-2.

Edge, David 1979. Quantitative Measures of Communication in Science. *History of Science* 19, 102-34.

Eisenberg, David M. / Kessler, Ronald C. / Foster, Cindy / Norlock, Frances E. / Calkins, David R. / Delbanco, Thomas L. 1993. Unconventional Medicine in the United States. *New England Journal of Medicine* 328, 246-52.

Epstein, Mikhail 2000. Hyper-authorship: The Case of Araki Yasusada. *Rhizomes* 1. Available at www.rhizomes.net/Issue1/toc.html.

Eskinazi, Daniel P. 1998. Factors that Shape Alternative Medicine. *JAMA* 280/18, 1621-3.

Fairclough, Norman 1995. *Critical Discourse Analysis*. London: Longman.

Flowerdew, Lynne 2005. An Integration of Corpus-based and Genre-based Approaches to Text Analysis in EAP/ESP: Countering Criticisms against Corpus-based Methodologies. *English for Specific Purposes* 24/3, 321-32.

Fontanarosa, Phil B. / Lundberg, George D. 1998. Alternative Medicine Meets Science. *JAMA* 280/18, 1618-9.

Genette, Gérard 1997. *Palimpsests: Literature in the Second Degree*. Lincoln: University of Nebraska Press.

Giannoni, Davide S. 1998. The Genre of Journal Acknowledgments: Findings of a Cross-disciplinary Investigation. *Linguistica e Filología* 6, 61-84.

Giannoni, Davide S. 2002. Worlds of Gratitude: A Contrastive Study of Acknowledgement Texts in English and Italian Research Articles. *Applied Linguistics* 23/1, 1-31.

Giannoni, Davide S. 2006. Evidence of Generic Tension in Academic Book Acknowledgements. In Bhatia, Vijay K. / Gotti, Maurizio (eds) *Explorations in Specialized Genres*. Bern: Peter Lang, 21-42.

Giles, C. Lee / Councill, Isaac G. 2004. Who Gets Acknowledged: Measuring Scientific Contributions through Automatic Acknowledgment Indexing. *PNAS* 101/51, 17599-604.

Gross, Alan G. / Harmon, Joseph E. / Reidy, Michael S. 2002. *Communicating Science: The Scientific Article from the 17th Century to the Present*. Oxford: Oxford University Press.

Hanssen, B. / Grimsgaard, S. / Launso, L. / Fonnebo, V. / Falkenberg, T. / Rasmussen, N. 2005. Use of Complementary and Alternative Medicine in the Scandinavian Countries. *Scandinavian Journal of Primary Health Care* 23/1, 57-62.

Heffner, Alan G. 1979. Authorship Recognition of Subordinates in Collaborative Research. *Social Studies of Science* 12, 535-58.

Henry, David / Lexchin, Joel 2002. The Pharmaceutical Industry as a Medicines Provider. *The Lancet* 360, 1590-5.

Hunt, Roderick 2003. Scientific Authorship. *Science Editor's Handbook*. European Association of Science Editors.

Hyland, Ken 2000. *Disciplinary Discourses: Social Interactions in Academic Writing*. London: Pearson Education.

Hyland, Ken 2003. Dissertation Acknowledgments: The Anatomy of a Cinderella Genre. *Written Communication* 20/3, 242-68.

Hyland, Ken 2004. Graduates' Gratitude: The Generic Structure of Dissertation Acknowledgments. *English for Specific Purposes* 23/3, 303-24.

Hyland, Ken / Tse, Polly 2004. "I would like to thank my supervisor": Acknowledgments in Graduate Dissertations. *International Journal of Applied Linguistics* 14/2, 259-75.

Jonas, Wayne B. 1988. Alternative Medicine: Learning from the Past, Examining the Present, Advancing the Future. *JAMA* 280/18, 1616-7.

Laband, David N. / Tollison, Robert D. 2000. On Scientific Appraisal. *Quarterly Journal of Austrian Economics* 3/1, 43-8.

Lancet Editorial 2002. Just how Tainted has Medicine Become? *The Lancet* 359/9313, 1167.

Mauranen, Anna 1993. *Cultural Differences in Academic Rhetoric: A Text Linguistic Study*. Frankfurt/M.: Peter Lang.

McCain, Katherine W. 1991. Communication, Competition and Secrecy: The Production and Dissemination of Research-related Information on Genetics. *Science, Technologies and Human Values* 16/4, 491-516.

Meadows, Jack 2005. Differences between the Sciences in their Handling of the Research Literature. *European Science Editing* 31/4, 113-6.

Mullins, Nicholas C. 1973. *Theories and Theory Groups in Contemporary American Sociology*. London: Harper and Row.

Patel, Narsi 1973. Collaboration in the Professional Growth of American Sociology. *Social Science Information* 12/6, 77-92.

Rennie, Drummond / Yank, Veronica / Emmanuel, L. 1997. When Authorship Fails: A Proposal to Make Contributions Accountable. *JAMA* 278/7, 579-85.

Rothman, Kenneth J. / Evans, Stephen 2005. Extra Scrutiny for Industry Funded Trials. *British Medical Journal* 331, 1350-1.

Salager-Meyer, Françoise / Alcaraz-Ariza, María Á. / Pabón, Maryelis 2006. Complementary and Alternative Medicine (CAM): Why it is Time for the Linguistic Community to Turn its Attention to CAM Discourse. *Revista Canaria de Estudios Ingleses*. In press.

Satyanarayana, Karuturi 1987. Whose Names and How Many Names should be on a Scientific Paper? *European Science Editing* 30, 3-5.

Shekelle, Paul G. / Morton, Sally C. / Suttorp, Marika J. / Buscemi, Nina / Friesen, Carol 2005. Challenges in Systematic Reviews of Complementary and Alternative Medicine. *Annals of Internal Medicine* 142/12, 1042-9.

Smith, Richard 2005. Medical Journals are the Extension of the Marketing Arm of Pharmaceutical Companies. *PLoS Med* 2/5, 138.

Sobal, Jeffrey / Ferentz, Kevin S. 1990. Abstract Creep and Author Inflation. *The New England Journal of Medicine*. 323/7, 488-9.

Studdert, David A. / Eisenberg, David M. / Miller, Frances H. / Curto, Daniel A. / Kaptchuk, Ted J. / Brennan, Troyen A. 1998. Medical Malpractice Implications of Alternative Medicine. *JAMA* 280/18, 1610-5.

Swales, John 1996. Occluded Genres in the Academy: The Case of the Submission Letter. In Ventola, Eija / Mauranen, Anna (eds) *Academic Writing: Intercultural and Textual Issues*. Amsterdam: Benjamins. 45-8.

Swales, John 2004. *Research Genres: Exploration and Applications*. Cambridge: Cambridge University Press.

Thompson, Trevor / Feder, Gene 2005a. Complementary Therapies and the NHS. *British Medical Journal* 331, 856-7.

Thompson, Trevor / Feder, Gene 2005b. CAM before the Storm: Authors' Reply. *British Medical Journal* 331, 1205.

Udani, Jay 1998. Integrating Alternative Medicine into Practice. *JAMA* 280/18, 1620.

Verner, Dima A. 1994. Astronomy Acknowledgment Index 1992. *Messenger* 71, 59.

Webber, Pauline 2005. Interactive Features in Medical Conference Monologue. *English for Specific Purposes* 24/2, 157-81.

Irma Taavitsainen

Audience Guidance and Learned Medical Writing in Late Medieval English

1. Introduction

Metadiscourse is a pragmatic and rhetorical language phenomenon involving strategic language use in text production and communication. In recent studies on modern scientific writing, metadiscourse has been recognised as an important component and a social practice in negotiating meaning. Yet the scope of metadiscourse has been defined in various ways and the methodology is still under development. The historical dimension poses a special challenge in tracing the formation of conventions and establishing a method of assessment that would best reveal the diachronic developments. The continuum of medical writing reaches back to the Late Medieval period. My earlier study on the pilot version of the Middle English part of our project corpus showed that surgical writings and specialised texts were at the top of the frequency list of metadiscourse features (Taavitsainen 2000). In the present study I shall have a closer look at early medical writing with a bottom-up empirical method. The practices deviate from modern conventions and classifications of modern metadiscourse do not apply as such.

My aim in this study is to probe into the earliest phase of metadiscursive practices in English medical writing in the Late Medieval period by combining corpus linguistic methodology with discourse analysis. Corpus-based analysis tends to reduce the role of context, and according to the present views on metadiscourse, contextual assessment is the way in which metadiscourse can be discerned and qualitative semantic analysis is needed. In my earlier study I focused on metadiscourse as comments about the evolving text in which the author intrudes in some way to direct readers' reception

(Taavitsainen 2000; Gläser 1995; Swales 1990). My present study continues on the same basis with modifications according to Hyland's (2000, 2005) and Ifantidou's (2005) views (see section 4). In the following assessment, I shall focus on overt expressions of textual guidance and on comments about the evolving text in order to discuss the social practices of discourse in early scientific writing. My earlier study made a difference between textual and interpersonal metacomments.[1] Textual comments make the organization of the discourse explicit and help the reader to focus on important points. Interpersonal comments may be pleas or reader-centred phrases and instructive passages with overt guidance on how to act upon the text. Both kinds can be realised either by personal or impersonal means, relating to involved versus detached styles of writing. Prefatory materials consist of metadiscourse and the genre of prefaces is metadiscursive in itself (see below). The function of the genre is to guide readers' perceptions and including such passages in texts constitutes a developing social practice in Middle English. Prefaces increase towards the end of the period and some show an eloquent and polished diction usually attributed to Renaissance texts (Taavitsainen 2002a). I shall focus on contextual assessment to discover to what extent and how the features that may work on the metatextual level are used, and whether any patterns can be discerned. I shall discuss these problems and relate my findings to the larger patterns of scholastic thought-style. I shall take the learned tradition of writing and individual texts as my starting point in this assessment and define characteristics of metadiscourse of spearhead medical and scientific writing. My focus is on the unfolding discourse and on the contexts and *loci* of metadiscoursal features.

My theoretical point of departure is the variationist model of language and language change and the basic assumption of 'orderly heterogeneity', conditioned by linguistic and extralinguistic factors (Weinreich / Labov / Herzog 1968; Samuels 1972; Milroy 1992; Labov 1994; Rissanen *et al.* 1997). All language use consists of choices from options available at the time of writing, and the

---

1 In Hyland / Tse (2004: 161), textual metadiscourse is subsumed under interpersonal as it takes account of the reader's knowledge, textual experiences, and processing needs. See below, section 4.

realisations of texts are influenced by several factors, including the author, the audience, and the situation. Levels of education and competence vary, and it is often impossible to locate early anonymous texts on the scale from learned to 'popular'. The variationist model of language change has mostly been applied to the levels of phonology, morphology and syntax, but it is possible to apply it to changes in discourse features and styles of writing (Schiffrin 1994: 314; Taavitsainen 1997). Genres unfold in different ways and have their own linguistic co-occurrence patterns (Biber 1988). Variation is always present and changes are taking place, but there are more stable phases and periods of rapid change.

2. Thought-styles and language change

The Scientific Thought-styles project[2] aims at explaining how and why the linguistic realisation of medical texts has changed over a period of six hundred years. It is possible to achieve new precision by using a large number of medical texts with a broad coverage of genres, combining the methodologies of corpus linguistics with insights from discourse and genre analysis. The underlying intellectual commitments of science influence thought-styles and reflect on the linguistic repertoire of language features in texts. Scientific conceptions, objects of inquiry, methods, evaluations, and intellectual commitments are mediated through language, both its microlevel linguistic features and argumentative structures. In a diachronic perspective, the central question is what continued and what changed

---

2 The Scientific Thought-styles project aims at describing stylistic changes in medical English in a long diachronic perspective in a multifaceted sociohistorical framework. The project is now part of the Research Unit for Variation, Contacts and Change of the English departments at Helsinki and Jyväskylä Universities (see http://www.eng.helsinki.fi/varieng). Corpus compilation for research material belongs to our project plan. Middle English Medical Texts is now finished (see below), and Early Modern Medical Texts is under way. The current project members are Irma Taavitsainen, Päivi Pahta, Martti Mäkinen, Turo Hiltunen, Maura Ratia, Carla Suhr and Jukka Tyrkkö.

through different historical contexts (Crombie 1994, 1995). In the field of science, medicine acted as the spearhead in vernacularization. It was both a science and a craft, combining theory and practice (Crisciani 2000; French 2001: 68-75), and this is reflected in medieval medical writing (see Taavitsainen 2004a). The language of science was Latin, but texts of all kinds started to be translated, compiled or composed in the vernacular; this was a pan-European phenomenon in the fourteenth and fifteenth centuries. By the end of the medieval period texts on scientific and technological subjects were becoming increasingly common. Vernacularisation poses several problems, e.g. the target audience and purpose of writing changed when the texts were taken out of their original institutional context. In the translation process, features of the source language were transferred to the target language, and the underlying thought-styles influence all levels of discourse including the ways in which the author places himself in the discourse and how the audience is taken into account in the text. Interpersonal expressions and the presence of interactive features of communication, like first and second person pronouns, address terms and direct questions, contribute to social engagement and involvement in texts. The absence of such features and the presence of depersonalised phrases and the passive voice have a contrary effect as they create detachment (Biber 1988). Scholastic science was logocentric and relied on 'hearsay' as the source of knowledge; in texts this is manifested in frequent use of speech act verbs of reporting to indicate whose sayings are referred to (Taavitsainen / Pahta 1998). Scholasticism reached its peak at the centres of learning and medicine in Italy in the twelfth century. Innovations started to take place in medical science from the twelfth century onwards, as e.g. methods of medical teaching underwent changes at universities (Siraisi 1990: 13, 48).

Evidentiality and modality are essential features of scientific writing. Evidentiality relates to the reliability of knowledge and mode of knowing, what was considered the appropriate sources of knowledge and how the processes of 'doing science' were recorded in different periods. These are core issues in the history of scientific writing, and are at the heart of thought-styles.[3] Scholasticism is associated with deduction as the mode of reasoning and authorities and axioms as the source of knowledge. In contrast, empiricism relies on induction, and the source of knowledge is observation. The coding conventions vary: scholastic writings rely on authorities and deal with their sayings with reliance; knowledge is based on hearsay and reflects absolute certainty with prescriptive impersonal constructions and deontic modality. In contrast, empiricism displays a cautious and tentative attitude to new findings, e.g. in Royal Society texts, written with subjective epistemic judgements, cautiously discussing the possible implications of observation (Taavitsainen 1994, 2001b, 2002b). Features of evidentiality and modality serve to distinguish between different underlying thought-styles in spearhead writings. They are important for styles of scientific writing and it is possible to achieve new knowledge of the developments with more refined research tools like the electronic corpus *Middle English Medical Texts* (see below).

3. Models of metadiscourse and historical texts

Metadiscourse has been considered an open-ended category in the sense that authors can add items to the repertoire of metadiscursive features, innovating and renewing language use (Hyland 2005: 37). This view is in accordance with the variationist approach to language

3 Chafe (1986) distinguishes four major components of evidentiality: the reliability of knowledge, the mode of knowing, the source of knowledge, and the matching of knowledge against verbal resources or expectations. His view gave us inspiration to develop our own charts of the source of knowledge and the degree of certainty attached to it through different periods of medical writing (Taavitsainen / Pahta 1998: 162; Vihla 1999; Taavitsainen 2001b: 27). Close concepts include *stance* (Biber / Finegan 1989; Conrad / Biber 2000), and *appraisal* for the semantic resources to negotiate emotions, judgements, and evaluations, and the resources for amplifying and engaging the readers (Martin 2000: 145). Other related concepts include e.g. hedges and affect; for a discussion see Hunston / Thompson (2000).

change: in a diachronic perspective paradigms gain new variants, old ones fall out of use, and the proportions vary according to sociolinguistic, situational and generic facts. Metadiscourse reveals the writer's awareness of the reader, including elaboration, clarification, guidance and interaction.[4] Hyland (2005) gives an overview of modern theories and presents his own model for distinguishing metadiscursive uses from other uses of the same linguistic features; his model has recently been challenged from the Relevance Theory point of view (Ifantidou 2005).

The features of metadiscourse vary in scope from narrow to almost all-encompassing assessments of linguistic features. There is a fuzzy area where distinctions are impossible to make. In historical texts, this grey zone is necessarily wider as we do not know the facts, and the means for expressing abstract ideas in vernacular writing had not developed. It is not possible to apply modern models of metadiscourse to early stages of medical writing without modifications; interpretations according to the modern ways of thinking are often misleading, and sociohistorical facts sometimes give evidence which is contrary to expectations. In general, groupings and classifications vary in the literature. Hyland's (2005: 43-44) main categories are interactive, including code glosses, endophoric markers, evidentials, frame markers and transition markers, and interactional with attitude markers, boosters, self-mention and engagement. He defines interactive resources as the ways writers signal the arrangement of their texts based on their appreciation of the reader's likely knowledge and understanding. Interactional resources are more personal and involve the reader collaboratively in the development of the text. The difference between the two categories does not work in early medical writing, and consequently the distinction is not made in the present assessment. Semantic distinctions are often too minute, and we do not know enough of the background of these early texts, e.g. the target audience remains at the level of educated guesses with

---

4 Several different definitions of metadiscourse have been offered, e.g. most recently by Hyland / Tse (2004) and (Hyland 2005), where it is described as "self-reflective expressions used to negotiate interactional meanings in a text, assisting the writer (or speaker) to express a viewpoint and engage with readers as members of a particular community" (Hyland 2005: 37).

only a few exceptions. Early translators and authors had difficulties in expressing complicated relations and ideas in natural philosophy. The illocutions of the author and translator remain obscure at several places and confused passages are common. The use of pronouns is problematic in several texts as it is impossible to know who the 'I' or the 'he' in the text are (see below). The material poses its own restrictions and it is sometimes difficult to know what the exact meaning is.

4. Material of the study

Middle English Medical Texts (MEMT hereafter) is an electronic resource of about half a million words of running text from c. 1375 to c. 1500, and an Appendix from c. 1330. In compiling the corpus, our aim was to cover the broadening field of vernacular medical writing as comprehensively as possible, from the top-level theoretical treatises transmitting specialised knowledge through learned surgical and anatomical texts to simple recipes for practical use. The texts vary in length, as short texts are included *in toto*, but for copyright reasons many longer texts are represented by extracts. The texts have been classified into three categories labelled 'Surgical texts', 'Specialised texts', and 'Remedies and *materia medica*'.[5] Some texts in the first category represent the highest academic level of writing, being derived from university texts. They consist of expository passages

5 The exact word counts are: *Middle English Medical Texts* (MEMT) 495,322 words; surgical texts 136,527 words; specialised treatises 87,259 words; and remedies and *materia medica* 216,270 words. Most texts are written in prose, but we have also included verse (31,797 words) and an Appendix of trilingual texts from c. 1330, covering 23,469 words. The MEMT CD contains a catalogue with background information on the texts and an introduction that places medical writing in Late Medieval English in its sociohistorical context. *Medical and Scientific Writing in Late Medieval English* (Taavitsainen / Pahta 2004) contains articles based on MEMT, and one of its chapters (Pahta / Taavitsainen 2004) places vernacularisation in its sociohistorical context. Taavitsainen, Pahta and Mäkinen (2006) discuss the uses of MEMT in detail.

with frequent definitions of terms, but some include more instructive sections as well. Academic and surgical treatises were totally new in the vernacular, and fourteenth- and early fifteenth-century translations include both surgical writings by famous surgeons and anonymous texts. Most are direct translations from Latin, and the well-established Greco-Roman conventions of scientific writing served as their model; the influence of the underlying Latin prose is conspicuous. Most surgical texts are known by the name of the original Latin author and the translations are anonymous, with the exception of John Trevisa's translation of Bartholomaeus Anglicus's learned thirteenth-century Latin encyclopaedia *De proprietatibus rerum* from 1397/8. The earliest originals of surgical writings are perhaps Lanfrank's texts, written at the end of the thirteenth and turn of the fourteenth century. John Arderne (1307-c.1377) wrote in Latin, though he was an English surgeon. Chauliac's more technical Latin treatises were translated several times into English. The original audience was highly learned, but it is not known who the actual readers of the vernacular versions were. The books have the air of expensive display objects and show little wear (Taavitsainen 2004b). MEMT contains extracts from five different editions and manuscripts. Probably the most original Middle English surgical text is *Chirurgie de 1392,* a compilation from various sources (Rawcliffe 1995: 132). Most specialised texts are anonymous. Some carry the name of the original author, but even these texts have undergone considerable changes in the vernacularisation process. Some specialised texts are connected with the long and complicated tradition of classical Greek texts transmitted through various versions and pseudo-versions in Latin. The third category 'Remedies and *materia medica*' contains heterogeneous materials including recipes, prognostications and herbals, but it also contains texts with more theoretical parts and references to learned doctrines, e.g. the *secreta secretorum* tradition has long roots in wisdom literature. Some of these treatises have prefaces and metatextual comments and these are included in my assessment as well.

5. Qualitative analysis of metadiscourse in Late Medieval medical writing

My method of assessment in the following is qualitative reading aided and supported by computerised searches in our electronic corpus. This bottom-up analysis reveals that the levels of metadiscourse vary: some work at the macrolevel of discourse to arouse the audience's interest in the text and convince the readers, some work more locally at the microlevel. Scholastic thought-style is explicit with the authoritative phrases, deontic modality with absolute certainty in logocentric concerns.

(1) And **it is to witte þat** in all vlcerie3 beyng wiþin þe lure, or moiste ragadiis puttyng out quitour or blode, þis **I sey þat** þe vlcere3 be no3t bubones, i. e. owles, **of whiche it shal be seid aftirward**, for þai be al vncurable: þat if a leche may no3t wiþoute grete anguissh, als wele of hymself as of þe pacient, opne þe lure of þe pacient wiþ tonges, **as it is seide afore, þan owe þe leche** oonly putte in of tapsimell [...]. (Arderne, Fistula: 36)

The realizations of metatextual passages are often mixed, combining the impersonal and the personal mode of writing. Both impersonal and personal metacomments are found intertwined in early medical writing. The focus in the following assessment is on the way audience guidance is realised in unfolding discourse, and I shall also discuss how linguistic features associated with metatext are connected with the underlying text types and work at the macrolevel to enhance the efficacy of the healing methods and cures presented in the treatise.[6]

6 Exposition, instruction and narration are especially relevant here. Text types are categories established by linguists according to the occurrences of linguistic features (see Werlich 1982). Thus they are different from genres that can be defined according to text-external parameters. Traditions of writing are a third grouping of texts (see Taavitsainen 2001a).

5.1. Macrolevel metadiscourse

Macrolevel metadiscourse includes the genre of prefaces and other prefatory materials: they are metadiscursive by definition in relation to their main texts, as they include information about its provenance, a dedication to the patron, and an address to the intended audience and guidance on how the text should be understood or acted upon. All these components are seldom present in Late Medieval prefaces. Macrolevel metatext can also be found in the genre of case reports, embedded in the main text; in these cases the narrative passages enhance the credibility of the contents and serve the efficacy function. I have also included typical discourse *loci* and the enumerative text strategy in my assessment of macrolevel features.

5.1.1. Prefatory materials

A typical locus for the use of the first person singular is in prefatory materials. In general, Late Medieval texts do not have separate prefaces but short preambles and explanations of the provenance of the text. Dedications to patrons are present in some texts, but not very commonly; this was an incipient social practice that became the rule in the sixteenth century. A fairly long preface is found in *Chirurgie de 1392.* The text opens with a prayer, an embedded genre, serving an interpersonal aim and reflecting the importance of religion in the medieval world. Pious wishes conform to the decorum of eloquence, and the author continues explaining the provenance of the text. The compiler was a London surgeon, possibly also a physician, narrating his personal experience:

(2) graunte 3ou gr=a=ce þa=t= þis compilacioun schal haue so forto vsen & disposen þe fruyt of medicyns & of worchinge in it conteyned, **þa=t= it turne specialy to þe worschipeof god, & profi3t of þe peple.** The which compilacioun of sirurgie **I haue compilid & drawen** aftir þe discr=e=t auctorite of my moost worschipful maistris [...]. þa=t= **I haue assaied & proued** in my tyme. (Chirurgie de 1392: 1a)

A lengthy metatextual passage about the disposition of the treatise follows. This is explicit guidance as the organization of the treatise is discussed for the benefit of the reader. The personal touch of the compiler is noticeable:

(3) The which compilacioun **I haue departid** in þre parties, to euery partie ordeyned a certeyne distinccioun wiþ her chapitris **In þe firste partie I haue ordeyned**: þe anothamye of a man; & þe.iiij. complexiouns [...] **In þe.ij. partie I haue putt** þe diffinicioun of a sirurgian, [...] **In þe þridde partie I haue putt** an antidotarie of sirurgie wiþ watris, [...]; wherfor **I praie & counseile 3ou** þat vsen þe worchinge in þis doctr=i=ne [...]And also þat **3e seien for his soule þat compilide þis tretis,** & for alle þo þat helpide þerto & for alle cristen, a pater noster & an aue marie. And þou3 it be so þat **y, sumtyme addynge & sumtyme wiþdrawynge, haue transposid** þe **ordynaunce of þes myn aforseid maistris,** & so by-causeof ignoraunce haue fallen oþirwhile into errour, **I biseche 3ou tendirly** þat it schal reden or heren or vndirstonden **þat 3e haue me excusid**, & **þat 3e adden & fulfillen benygly þe defautis in it conteyned**, aftir þe decre of þe worschipful Galien [...]. And if þer failen onyþing, it schal ben bi hem benygly fulfillid. (Chirurgie de 1392: 1a)

The author employs modesty formulae and interpersonal pleas. The passage shows that rhetorical conventions often attributed to Renaissance rhetorics of the sixteenth century were already established in the vernacular. The other prefatory passages are not as elegantly polished, but show similar features. The prologue of Lanfrank's *Chirurgia Parva* is addressed to "Leve frende Bernard", and explains the purpose of writing. In speech act terms, a promise finishes the passage as the end shifts the focus to profit and gain:

(4) **I 3it will make A booke** in which **I will take** by þe grace of god a full lore þat fallithe to þe instrument of Surgery. **ne I thynke not** in this wark **to rehersse bot short**, fewe and sad medycinis. nertheles for gret nede **I ne hold** hem not feble, but to hem **þou myght fully trust**. for **I set aftir thi biddyng** assayed cures and a short maner of curyng of woundes, postumes, bylis, cankers, festers, and som curys of eyen, and of Algebra **A littill after that skyll taught me to werke And thorowe experience** by long tyme by me confermyd. **I trust so** muche to þe sotilte of **thi witt that by this fewe þou shalt com to A gret werk and thorow that thow shalt haue þe name of a gret leche.** (Lanfrank, Chirurgia Parva: 66)

Lanfrank's longer text has a very short prefatory note. It combines the impersonal mode with the first-person singular and the exclusive *we*:

(5) Now þese chapitles of þis book ben y-ordeyned, **I wole fulfille my purpos** pursuynge **ech chapitle bi ordre, & confermynge my I haue longe tywordis aftir þe auctorite of myn auctouris and wiþ experiment** þat me vsed wiþ þe help of god. (Lanfrank, Chirurgia magna: 7)

Mondeville's treatise begins in the same traditional way:

(6) In þe name of þe trinite, [{þr{]e personys & oo god, [{fa{]dir & sone & holy g[{oos{]t, **I þinke** wi=t=h þe gr[{ac{]e of god to drawe out þe general rulis of surgerie þa=t= **ben moost nedeful** to a surgian to knowe, þat wole be of þe parfit science of helynge [...]. (Mondeville: 275a)

Specialised treatises have prefatory passages as well, e.g. the following is a highly learned and abstract preamble with an address by name and attributes that show that the author and addressee are of the same standing. The pronoun of the third person singular *he* probably refers to the original author, as the translation brings an additional layer to the text and shows that the language had not fully developed to express the abstract ideas of expository prose at this stage.[7]

(7) **In þis book bene vii chapitres contened** and **in þe first he putteþ** vnder what þing out of kynde a sekenes is conteyned}] *Ri3t dere frende Nero* as **it acordeþ þe significaciouns of wyrchyng for to be considered** of þe essencion or beyng of kynde and of þe sekenes so **it is nedeful** þat þe science or þe connyng of þe þings with w<h>ich curacioun or helyng schal be giffen for **to be perceyued** of þe same essencion or beyng. **It is no3t profitable** forsoþe þat þe significacions of helyng or curyng [...]. Bot for þat al men bene acorded in þis **it is no3t nedeful þat we dispute of þam** siþen it is no gret þing [...]. (Galen, De ingenio sanitatis: 183)

The remedybook tradition contains prefaces as well. Texts in this category range from simple lists to treatises with complicated transmission like *secreta secretorum* texts. The opening of the second book of *Secrete of Secretes* serves as an efficacy assertion and there is a reference to the theoretical basis of medical knowledge, the balance of humours as the prerequisite for health:

---

7 A similar transfer is found in e.g. Benvenutus Grassus and in some learned commentaries, and shows the difficulties of transferring learned genres into the vernacular (see Taavitsainen 2004a).

(8) **For sothe now Y wille teche the** medycynes and other privitees that shall be **sufficient y-now** to the conservacion of **thy** helthe, so that **thow shalt nede none other leche**, the which conservacion of sanyte and of helthe is **better and precioser** than any medecyne, and **they ben full necessarie to the**, and to the gouernaill of the worlde. Of conservancie of helthe. **And vnderstonde wele** that ther is no way to do no thyng by, neyther to gete no thynge by, but only by myght and potencie [...]. (Secrete of secretis: 48)

5.1.2. Efficacy: Case reports and promises of profit and gain

There is a high frequency of first person singular pronouns in Arderne's texts. A closer scrutiny shows that 75% of them in Arderne's *Fistula* and more than 90% in *Clysters* occur with past tense action verbs in narrative passages and in case reports. The identity of the narrator is emphatically expressed in the opening of the text:

(9) [{I, I{]ohn Arderne fro the first pestilence that was in the 3ere of oure lord 1349 duellid in Newerk in [...] ther I helid [...] At last I, forseid Iohn Arderne, y-sou3t and couenant y-made, come to hym and did my cure [...] I helid hym perfitely [...] ffor whiche cure I gatte myche honour and louyng [...] (Arderne, Fistula: 1)

Some of the case reports are given in more detail; for example, the following is found in *Clysters*. The first-person narrative of the doctor is intertwined with the third-person narrative of the patients.

(10) Þis oyntment, forsoþ, luffed I mych: with þis medicyne cured I a fischer at london, [...] Wherfore he was almost dede, what of akyng, bolnyng, and brynnyng, and what of þe vncouenable cure of a barbour þat putte in þe wounde scharpe tente3 of lynne cloþe, and putte aboue diaquilon. His cure, forsoþ, remoued away, I putte to about euensang-tyme of þe forseid valence with anoyntyng of oile of roses, And bifore cokcrow þe pacient was delyuered of akyng and þe arme biganne for to swage, and in the mornyng he sleped wele, and þe arme was purged of quitour by the wounde. Bot witte þou þat I putte no tent in þe forseid wounde, bot al-only with 3ettyng in of oile and puttyng aboue of þe valence without any-þing atuix I cured hym finaly; wherfor I gatte mych honour. At nothyngham, forsoþ, I cured anoþer perfitely with þe forseid medicyne, þat was smyten in þe arme, bot no3t þorow, with a knyfe; of whos life men despaired for akyng and anguysch of þe pacient. (Arderne, Clysters: 100)

This is very much in praise of the narrator himself, to prove that his methods of curing were successful; in speech act terms this is boasting. Interpersonal pleas are inserted in the text to convince and engage the reader, e.g. *witte þou, God knoweth that I lye not.* The whole narrative works as a metatext on the efficacy of the cures.

First person narrative is found in other treatises as well, but not to the same extent. The following passage emphasises the value of experience and observation as the source of knowledge:

(11) But truly **I haue goon** to alle þe grettiste charnellis þat beþ aboute londoun, where þat beþ scolle bonys, wiþoute noumbre, for to prouen by experience þe verri soþe, & haue handlid, seen, & asserchid euery boon of þe heed, bi himsilf; **wher-fore y seie aftir þat I sau3, and felde**, þat by myn vndirstondynge, þer beþ sixe principal bonys of þe heed; (Chirurgie 1392: 19)

Such assertions are common, and often the texts finish with promises of profit and gain. The ethical rules of conduct given in Arderne's text contain some passages with metatextual reflections and assurance of the profit that the application will bring to the reader:

(12) Many þinges, forsoþe, bene to be kepte of a leche, wiþoute **þese þat ar seid afore**, þat **may no3t be noted here** for ouer moche occupying. But **it is no3t to dout** þat if þe **forseid** be wele kepte þat-ne **þai shal giffe a gracious going to þe vser to þe hi3te of worship and of wynnyng;** (Arderne, Fistula: 8)

This is an efficacy passage, a promise of profit and gain to those who adhere to the rules. Such passages are common in medieval medical texts, including recipes (Jones 1998). This kind of metatext with first-person narrative and impersonal phrases working in the direction of efficacy seems to be typical of the early period but has fallen out of use in the course of time.

5.1.3. Discourse loci

Metacomments in textual organization can be thought of as a net of references imposed upon the text to guide the reader through discourse, adjusting the text according to the addressee or the target group. Metatextual passages are typically found at the opening position of treatises and in topic shifts.

(13) **To trete of þe propertees of mannes body** and of þe parties þerof, **we schul first biginne** to trete of þe qualitees of þe elementis and of þe humoures of whiche þe body is maad. (Trevisa 2: 129)

(14) **Off þe nature of wommen is for to speke. Fyrst we sal be gynne** of þe preuy partees of hem þat is her stones be þe wheche spermat is mynystered by. (Nature of Wommen: 85)

Phrases of impersonal prescriptive use are combined with interpersonal pleas, and personal comments (see below). Chauliac's texts provide the most explicit examples of writing conventions. The passage below is argumentative, discussing the importance of the contents of the treatise to follow. A clear pattern can be distinguished, and it is made absolutely clear for the reader why it is necessary to study the text and act accordingly:

(15) And if þat is profitable to phisiciens, moche more forsoþe **it is necessarie** to cirurgiens, [...]. But **þou, konnynge þe kynde of eueriche lyme, 3it forsoþe þow schalt knowe** [...] Þus ledeþ Henry of Hermondavilla by resoun in þe firste book of his Cyrurgie: Euery werkman is iholden to knowe þe subiecte in þe whiche he wircheþ, and ellis he erreþ in wirchynge. But **a cirurgien is a werkman of þe helþe of manis body; þerfore he is holden to konne þe kynde of composicioun of it**. And by þis manere resoun, he is holden to konne anothomye. [...] **It folweþ þerfore þat it is nedefulle** to leches, and namely to cirurgiens, to konne anothomye [...]. (Chauliac, Cyrurgie: 27)

Audience guidance is important in topic shifts. A typical metatextual passage in such positions consists of an anaphoric part and a cataphoric reference:

(16) [...] **of which it is seid aboue**. And also þer passeþ an holowe veyne ascendyng, **of which it shal be seid with-in**, boþe passyng bi diafragma. (Chauliac, Anatomy: 114)

An interesting Latinate feature is *Þise y-seye*, an impersonal text-organizing phrase modelled after the Latin ablativus absolutus.

(17) **Þise y-seye, it is to go** to þe partie3 contened with-yn þe wombe, wher first comeþ to 3irbus. þat of G is seid omentum. (Chauliac, Anatomy: 118)

Passages with topic shifts vary in detail from brief comments to long lists of items to be dealt with:

(18) Also fro þe selfe lyuer goþ oute propre weyes & colatorie3. beryng þe superfluitee3 of þe **forsaid** digestioun to þair propre places, **which shal be seid. Of which is shewed þe acte, þe posicioun, þe substaunce, þe colligance, & oþer þinge3, which bene inquired in þe lyuer as in oþer membre3.** (Chauliac, Anatomy: 128)

The above example displays a common pattern: an anaphoric reference to the preceding text serves as a short summary of the previous section, and reference to the preceding text is made specific with cohesive ties like *foreseid. Now* is often used as a discourse marker to signify topic shift, and other proximal deictic features like *this, present, here*, are also used as text-anchoring devices to engage the reader. Similar passages are found in all learned texts, especially at the opening positions of sections, but topic shifts and new sections can also be marked with similar means in remedybooks, e.g. in Cophon's collection, a new recipe is introduced by the same means:

(19) **Now it is to know** whan þe fleumatik is mengyd wiþ þe colerik and comyng in to þe face and makeþ þare whelks. (Cophon's Experymentes: 25)

5.1.4. Enumerative text strategy

A structurally important feature in learned scholastic texts is the enumerative text strategy. This is a structural device, created with the help of metatext. It has a dual function, as it provides a text-organizing device and at the same time it helps the reader by pointing out constituents of a whole. In learned texts the enumerated items often consist of abstract ideas in order of importance:

(20) FOr after Galien, þe Lanterne of Leches, in þe 17 book [...] **foure profites beeþ**, or condiciouns, of þe science of anothomye: **Oone,** forsoþe and þe moste, is to þe mervayle of Goddes power. The **secounde** [...] The **þridde** is [...] But **it is so necessarie** to þe helynge of sikenessis **and profitable** to eueriche leche to knowe tofore þilke anothomye [...] (Chauliac , Cyrurgie: 26)

As discussed above, passages containing metatext combine a variety of features working in the same direction. The following *secreta secretorum* passage shows a concentration of metadiscursive features at the beginning of a passage "In how many maners is helthe conserved". It begins with a direct address, uses superlatives to enhance the importance of the contents and the enumerative strategy to make the structure explicit, repetitions in other words explain the contents, and appeals to the reader's cognitive processes are also present:

(21) **O Alexandre**, in medecynes is conteyned **the most certeyn and most veray techyng**, that the conseruance of helth standeth **principally in 2 thynges**. **First** that a man vse convenient metes accordyng to his age, to the seson [...] **that is to sey**, that he vse such metes and [...] the which confermed his nature, **þat is to say**, that accordeth with his complexion. **Secondly,** that he be purged of all superfluous and corruptif humours. And **vnderstande wele** that the bodies of men, [...] (Secrete of secretes: 50)

5.2. Microlevel metadiscourse

Rather than entire passages of inserted genres and larger structures that form the backbone of the text, microlevel metadiscourse works more locally. It may consist of phrases and pleas, or pronouns. Together these features contribute to the overall style of writing, and the co-occurrence patterns are important for further conclusions.

5.2.1. Grammatical constructions and scholastic phrases

Deontic modality with frequent use of prescriptive phrases is connected with scholasticism, and these phrases may serve as a distinguishing feature between various levels of learnedness in Late Medieval medical and scientific texts (Taavitsainen / Pahta 1998). Semantic groups of verbs are important here. The category *It is to* + verb illustrates the point: it is commonly found with verbs of cognition in texts of the most learned kind. Public verbs of saying are frequent especially in Chauliac's works and Mondeville's text. The construction is typically used in metatextual comments to emphasise the importance of the topic and to catch the reader's attention.

Chauliac's texts have the highest frequencies of the phrase *it is to* + V. In Anatomy the most frequent metatextual phrase is *it is to be seid* (5); other verbs are *sewe, go, begynne, speed*. The Interpolated version has *speke, wete, knowen, sene*; Cyryrgie *goo, knowe, be seide/saide, come, be seyn, wete/wite, saye/say* and *see*; Wounds *take hede, wite/wete* (7), *understonde, bide, be treted*; and Ulcers has *recourse, hafe recouse, take hede*. The construction *it is to* occurs seven times in Arderne's *Fistula*, once with *procede, vnderstand, turne agayne* and *witte*, and once it is found in a warning *it is to be-war*. In Clysters *it is to witte* is found twice. Mondeville's text has *witen/wite* (9), *knowen*, and *noten*; Chirurgie 1392 has *wite* (2), Lanfrank *speke* and Surgery *understand*.[8]

In specialised texts cognitive verbs are even more conspicuous. De spermate has *noted* (6), *wist (and knowen)* (8), *seen, kepen, vnderstonde*; De xii portis *wist* (9), *be seen*; Phlebotomy *wyt/wete* (13), *eschewe, sei*; Canutus *wete, eschewe, be drede, vnderstande, beware*; Benvenutus *vnderstonde, leue, be noted, be merkyd*; De humana natura, *be seide*. When the moon is in Aries has *wytte*, but it could be a stylistic loan from more learned texts.[9]

In the remedybook and *materia medica* category, *Secreta secretorum* tradition texts contain *it is to be doughted* and *it is to be knowen*; Governayle of Health has *it is to witt* (2) and Caxton's Gouernayle of helthe has *it is to wete* (3); Reynes Bloodletting has the same phrase once, and Cophon's Experimentes has the phrase with *know* (2) and with *touch*. Other instances in these texts give advice about concrete actions and are not metatextual: *ete, vse hot metys, aryse erlye*, etc. An interesting feature is the occurrence in the remedybook tradition of the brief form *I wis, iwis*, which it is not used in surgical or specialised texts. This phrase seems to have become grammaticalised into an amplifier or a line filler, used in verse to provide a rhyme; *I seye* is used in the same way. Similar passages occur in other verse treatises.

8 Some of the occurrences are not metatextual. In Chauliac, *it is to be bounden and no3t to be kutte* and *it is to wirch* refer to actions of surgery. In Arderne the construction is found twice with the verb *labour*.

9 It may well be that the phrase was so conventionalised in learned prose that the authors and translators could revert to it as a stock phrase of scientific writing when needed (cf. below).

(22) Y=e= bokys tellyn, for sothe **I wys**,
Y=e= hoote dropesye yat it is;
And qwa~ne it comyth to y=e= herte **I seye**
But 3if he hawe helpe sone schal he deye. (Stockholm verse recipes: 360)

5.2.2. Personal pronouns: author's position and audience guidance

Personal pronouns are used in several ways in these texts. Traditions of medical writing differ in this respect (cf. also case reports, above). The frequency of personal pronouns is usually interpreted as a sign of involvement, but in early scientific writing personal pronouns do not always contribute to involvement but can serve other functions. The use of the authorial *we* is a case in point: the tone is highly authoritative and in line with the impersonal phrases discussed above. This is the 'exclusive' use of *we* [-vocative] (Wales 1996: 58). It is the rule in early learned texts, as e.g. in the opening of Book 5 of Trevisa's translation on human anatomy, in combination with impersonal phrases:

(23) For **we** haue ispoken of þe propirtees of humoures, **now it fallip to speke** somwhat of þe disposicioun of membres þat ben imaad and componed of þe **forseid** humours. And **first of þe propirtees þerof we schal speke** in general, **and þanne** of eueryche somwhat in special. (Trevisa 1: 163).

Direct guidance to the reader occurs in several treatises with the second-person singular pronoun and reference to cognitive processes:[10]

(24) And somme beþ iliche, þat Constantyn clepiþ omiomerata, þat is 'symple and of one kynde wiþ þe parties þerof', **as to oure knoweinge**. For eueryche par[{t{]ye of fatnes is fatnes, and so of oþir. **þanne gedre þou hereof** þat membres of kynde i-ordeined to craft makeþ þe souled body parfite, and takeþ of þe soule þe influens of vertue. (Trevisa 1: 165)

Second person guidance with cognitive verbs is very common in some texts, e.g. the phrase *wite þou* occurs in Arderne's texts 37 times. Prototypically second-person singular pronouns occur in instructive passages, e.g. in the following with frequent use of imperative forms.

10 For the overall view of Late Medieval practices of personal pronouns in address, see Burnley (2003).

This kind of instruction is typical of the remedybook tradition of the period, reflected in the frequency of *þou* in recipes (see Taavitsainen 2001c; Mäkinen 2002; Grund 2003; Carroll 2004).

(25) Ane emplastre þat is called Nerbone is made þus: **Recipe** diaquilon, and [...] **resolue** it vpon þe cole3, and **boile** it alwaie3 with a spatulre vnto it bigynne to wex blak. And **if þou wil haue it** ri3t blak boile it langer, and **if þou wilt haue** broune **boile** it lesse. ffor whi [...] And after þat **þou wilt haue** it hard or softe be added þerto [...] When it haþ boiled ynou3 **sette** it fro þe fire and **late** it stande stille without mouyng by þe space of a 'pater noster'- & 'aue maria', þat þe litarge of þe lede [...] and þan **moue** it with a spature strongly vnto þat it be colded. When, forsoþ, it is cold þat it may be malaxed, **enforme** þerof trocistes vpon a table in quantite as it pleseþ þe, and **kepe it to þine vse**. Þis emplastre is called Noirbone, for þof-al it be blak neþerlesse it is gode, for it heleþ wele [...]. (Arderne, Clysters: 91)

A second person *3e/3our* polite address is found in a case report in a passage consisting of instruction to doctors on how to treat their patients; the choice of the pronoun here is in accordance with the high status of the supposed patient. The passage provides a model of polite speech, probably to be learnt by heart:

(26) þan sey þe lech þus to þe pacient, reward yhadde to þe person of þe pacient **'Witte 3our gentilnes and 3our hi3nes, and also 3our godehertynes**, þat þe gracious perfeccion of þis cure ow not only to be recced as now to þe possibilite **of my gode bisynes**, bot also to **3our gode and abydyng pacience** [...]. (Arderne, Fistula: 22)

6. Metadiscourse and the repertoire of linguistic features

In this chapter I have focused on the use of metatext in unfolding discourse and on its audience-guiding function. Metatextual expressions have an important role in textual organization and the reception by emphasising important passages and focusing the reader's attention. The *loci* of such comments seem to be regular, and it is natural that the opening position is the most prominent point, whether the opening of the whole treatise, a section or a new topic. A distinct prefatory part is found in some texts, but full prefaces are not very common. There are some examples with eloquent patterns and politeness formulas that show how conventions and social practices in non-literary prose were taking shape already in the late fourteenth century.

The two alternative ways of expressing metacomments in early English medical writing, the impersonal and the personal, are intertwined in the discourse of the Late Medieval period. The key phrase in scholastic thought-styles seems to be the impersonal phrase *it is to* with a cognitive verb, most often *it is to wit,* reflecting deontic modality and absolute certainty. An interesting feature is the occurrence of the abbreviated form *I wys, iwis*, in verse, but not in prose.[11] Imperative forms appealing to the addressee directly, *witte thou,* are common, but individual texts vary a great deal in this respect. Surgical texts are ahead of others in the formation of conventions and in their ability to express complicated relations and abstract ideas. Impersonal metatext is commonly combined with authorial, exclusive *we*, and the tone is authoritative, in accordance with the original Latin texts. The prevailing mode is detached, but personal pronouns show high frequencies in some texts. E.g. Arderne employs second-person pleas and first-person narratives in case reports, where the overall effect is added efficacy and the mode is very different from the cautious first-person narratives with epistemic modality in Royal Society reports. Prefaces show a different, interpersonal style in a polished and eloquent form, in imitation of Latin. A diversified picture emerges: individual texts vary, and the author's role is constructed in different ways. All texts display absolute certainty and reliance on received learning.

Metadiscourse has a long history in English medical writing. The early phases of vernacular writing follow the model of Latin scientific texts. The categories discussed in this article have been defined by a bottom-up assessment of a large computerised database. As a lead to locating the phrases and passages I used corpus searches of linguistic features that commonly serve metadiscursive functions

---

11 Prose was a more sophisticated means of expression in the Late Medieval period than practical verse, which provided rhymes to aid the memory and simple rules on health issues.

and express the author's place and audience involvement in texts. The bottom-up method led to a different categorization from modern assessments. This chapter provides a starting point and one step forward towards a more ambitious goal of charting the changing thought-styles, i.e. what changed and what remained constant in the underlying commitments and modes of knowing.

Primary sources

Middle English Medical Texts 2005. Compiled by Irma Taavitsainen, Päivi Pahta and Martti Mäkinen, with MEMT Presenter Software by Raymond Hickey. Amsterdam: Benjamins. Its text catalogue gives bibliographical information on the source texts.

References

Biber, Douglas 1988. *Variation Across Speech and Writing.* Cambridge: Cambridge University Press.

Biber, Douglas / Finegan, Edward 1989. Styles of Stance in English: Lexical and Grammatical Marking of Evidentiality and Affect. *Text* 9/1, 93-124.

Burnley, David 2003. The T/V Pronouns in Later Middle English Literature. In Taavitsainen, Irma / Jucker, Andreas H. (eds) *Diachronic Perspectives on Address Term Systems.* Amsterdam / Philadelphia: Benjamins, 27-45.

Carroll, Ruth 2004. Middle English Recipes: Vernacularisation of a Text-type. In Taavitsainen / Pahta (eds), 174-91.

Chafe, Wallace 1986. Evidentiality in English Conversation and Academic Writing. In Chafe, Wallace / Nichols, Johanna (eds) *Evidentiality: The Linguistic Coding of Epistemology.* Norwood: Ablex, 261-312.

Conrad, Susan / Biber, Douglas 2000. Adverbial Marking of Stance in Speech and Writing. In Hunston / Thompson (eds), 56-73.

Crisciani, Chiara 2000. Teachers and Learners of Scholastic Medicine: Some Images and Metaphors. *History of Universities* 15, 75-101.

Crombie, Alistair C. 1994. *Styles of Scientific Thinking in the European Tradition*. 3 vols. London: Duckworth.

Crombie, Alistair C. 1995. Commitments and Styles of European Scientific Thinking. *History of Science* 33, 225-238.

French, Roger 2001. *Canonical Medicine: Gentile da Foligno and Scholasticism*. Leiden: Brill.

Gläser, Rosemary 1995. *Linguistic Features and Genre Profiles of Scientific English*. Frankfurt am Main: Peter Lang.

Grund, Peter 2003. The Golden Formulas: Genre Convention of Alchemical Recipes in the Middle English Period. *Neuphilologische Mitteilungen* 104/4, 455-75.

Hunston, Susan / Thompson, Geoff (eds) 2000. *Evaluation in Text: Authorial Stance and the Construction of Discourse.* Oxford: Oxford University Press.

Hyland, Ken 2000. *Disciplinary Discourses: Social Interactions in Academic Writing*. Harlow: Pearson Education.

Hyland, Ken 2005. *Metadiscourse.* London: Continuum.

Hyland, Ken / Tse, Polly 2004. Metadiscourse in Academic Writing: A Reappraisal. *Applied Linguistics* 25/2, 156-77.

Ifantidou, Elly 2005. The Semantics and Pragmatics of Metadiscourse. *Journal of Pragmatics* 37, 1325-53.

Jones, Claire 1998. Formula and Formulation: 'Efficacy Phrases' in Medieval English Medical Manuscripts. *Neuphilologische Mitteilungen* 99, 199-209.

Labov, William 1994. *Principles of Linguistic Change*, Vol. 1: *Internal Factors*. Oxford: Blackwell.

Mäkinen, Martti 2002. On Interaction in Herbals from ME to EModE. *Journal of Historical Pragmatics* 3, 229-51.

Martin, James R. 2000. Beyond Exchange: APPRAISAL System in English. In Hunston / Thompson (eds), 142-75.

Milroy, James 1992. *Linguistic Variation and Change. On the Historical Sociolinguistics of English.* Oxford: Blackwell.

Pahta, Päivi / Taavitsainen, Irma 2004. Vernacularization of Scientific and Medical Writing in its Sociohistorical Context. In Taavitsainen / Pahta (eds), 1-18.

Rawcliffe, Carole 1995. *Medicine and Society in Later Medieval England.* Stroud: Alan Sutton.

Rissanen, Matti / Kilpiö, Matti / Kytö, Merja / Meurman-Solin, Anneli / Nevanlinna, Saara / Pahta, Päivi / Taavitsainen, Irma 1997. Introduction. In Rissanen / Kytö / Heikkonen (eds), 1-15.

Rissanen, Matti / Kytö, Merja / Heikkonen, Kirsi (eds) 1997. *English in Transition: Corpus-based Studies in Linguistic Variation and Genre Styles*. Berlin: Mouton de Gruyter.

Samuels, Michael L. 1972. *Linguistic Evolution.* Cambridge: Cambridge University Press.

Schiffrin, Deborah 1994. *Approaches to Discourse.* Oxford: Blackwell.

Siraisi, Nancy G. 1990. *Medieval and Early Renaissance Medicine.* Chicago: University of Chicago Press.

Swales, John M. 1990. *Genre Analysis: English in Academic and Research Settings*. Cambridge: Cambridge University Press.

Taavitsainen, Irma 1994. On the Evolution of Scientific Writings from 1375 to 1675: Repertoire of Emotive Features. In Fernandez, Francisco / Fuster, Miguel / Calvo, Juan José (eds) *English Historical Linguistics 1992*. Amsterdam: Benjamins, 329-42.

Taavitsainen, Irma 1997. Genre Conventions: Personal Affect in Fiction and Non-fiction in Early Modern English. In Rissanen / Kytö / Heikkonen (eds), 185-266.

Taavitsainen, Irma 2000. Metadiscursive Comments and the Evolution of Early English Medical Writing 1375-1550. In Kirk, John M. (ed.) *Corpora Galore: Analyses and Techniques in Describing English.* Amsterdam: Rodopi, 191-207.

Taavitsainen, Irma 2001a. Changing Conventions of Writing: The Dynamics of Genres, Text Types, and Text Traditions. *European Journal of English Studies*, Special issue, ed. by Lilo Moessner, 139-50.

Taavitsainen, Irma 2001b. Evidentiality and Scientific Thought-styles: English Medical Writing in Late Middle English and Early Modern English. In Gotti, Maurizio / Dossena, Marina (eds) *Modality in Specialized Texts*. Bern: Peter Lang, 21-52.

Taavitsainen, Irma 2001c. Middle English Recipes: Genre Characteristics, Text Type Features and Underlying Traditions of Writing. *Journal of Historical Pragmatics* 2, 85-113.

Taavitsainen, Irma 2002a. Historical Discourse Analysis: Scientific Language and Changing Thought-styles. In Fanego, Teresa / Méndez-Naya, Belén / Seoane, Elena (eds) *Sounds, Words, Texts, Change: Selected Papers from the Eleventh International Conference on English Historical Linguistics*. Amsterdam: Benjamins, 201-26.

Taavitsainen, Irma 2002b. Variation and Formularity: Prefatory Materials in Early Scientific Writing. In Lentz, Katja / Möhlig, Ruth (eds) *Of Dyuersite & Chaunge of Langage: Essays Presented to Manfred Görlach on the Occasion of his 65th Birthday*. Heidelberg: C. Winter Universitätsverlag, 290-304.

Taavitsainen, Irma 2004a. Transferring Classical Discourse Conventions into the Vernacular. In Taavitsainen / Pahta (eds), 37-72.

Taavitsainen, Irma 2004b. Scriptorial 'House-styles' and Discourse Communities. In Taavitsainen / Pahta (eds), 209-40.

Taavitsainen, Irma / Pahta, Päivi 1998. Vernacularization of Medical Writing in English: A Corpus-Based Study of Scholasticism. *Early Science and Medicine* 3, 157-85.

Taavitsainen, Irma / Pahta, Päivi (eds) 2004. *Medical and Scientific Writing in Late Medieval English*. Cambridge: Cambridge University Press.

Taavitsainen, Irma / Pahta, Päivi / Mäkinen, Martti 2006. Towards a Corpus-based History of Specialized Languages: *Middle English Medical Texts*. In Facchinetti, Roberta / Rissanen, Matti (eds) *Corpus-based Studies of Diachronic English*. Bern: Peter Lang, 79-94.

Vihla, Minna 1999. *Medical Writing: Modality in Focus*. Amsterdam: Rodopi.

Wales, Katie 1996. *Pronouns in Present-day English*. Cambridge: Cambridge University Press.

Weinreich, Uriel / Labov, William / Herzog, Marvin 1968. Empirical Foundations for a Theory of Language Change. In Lehmann, W.P. / Malkiel, Y. (eds) *Directions for Historical Linguistics*. Austin: University of Texas Press, 95-195.

Werlich, Egon 1982. *A Text Grammar of English*. Heidelberg: Quelle & Meyer.

LAURA WRIGHT

On the Global Dissemination of Medical Writing: Medicines Required by a Sea-surgeon in 1715

On 15 November 1715 a copy of a request for medical supplies to be sent to the Island of St Helena from London was entered into the island's *Consultation Book*. At the time, St Helena was of great strategic importance to the European sea powers. Situated in the middle of the South Atlantic, it was valuable to shipping as a source of fresh water and Vitamin C-bearing fruit for sailors on board vessels bound for and returning from the Spice Islands. St Helena had long been contested by the Portuguese, Dutch, French, and English, when in 1673 the English took it for the final time. The island was then granted by the reigning monarch to the British East India Company in London (known as 'the Honourable Company'), to hold in perpetuity. The Honourable Company set up the island infrastructure, including the keeping of records in the *St Helena Consultation Books*, one copy of which is now kept in the India and Oriental Office at the British Library in London. The *St Helena Consultation Books* are mainly written in the English of the day, but the invoice or list under consideration here is written in Medieval Latin and English, in the kind of abbreviated and suspended form that was typical of medical writing.

Our doctor's list shows the drugs, herbs and equipment that he deemed essential or desirable in treating the Island's population, which consisted of the Island administrators, free planters, freed slaves, East India Company soldiers and slaves from many countries. The doctor also wanted "to make essays on mineral stones", perhaps indicating that he was keen to perform experiments on his new surroundings.

My initial question was to wonder where he got his medical nomenclature from, because although his usage of medical symbols and abbreviation and suspension symbols is unremarkable, some of the items on his list are for pre-prepared drugs, such as *Aqua Regulata* 'Our Eye Water', sold in London by William Salmon for a shilling per ounce, or *Aqua Epidemica* 'The London Plague-water'. The answer, in these and other cases, lies in the London Royal College of Physicians' *Pharmacopoeia Londinensis; or, the New London Dispensatory* of 1685,[1] which was heavily supplemented by William Salmon.[2] It seems likely that our island doctor (who hailed from Cannon Street, a short walk away from Salmon's London residence) used this volume, as much of what he wrote in abbreviated or suspended form can be found treated in full therein. I suggest, therefore, that the medical language as written by our sea-faring doctor (and surely by other ship's surgeons) was conditioned by the publications of William Salmon. I highlight Salmon's role because his reputation hitherto has not been of the highest. The *Oxford Dictionary of National Biography* notes that he was apprenticed to a mountebank: "indeed there is little evidence that he made any original contribution to medical knowledge", and academic papers label him a quack.[3] Nevertheless Salmon was a prolific author and many of his works would have been read and used by doctors of the age, so whilst his actual contribution to medical knowledge might not have been large, his role in the global dissemination of medical writing must have been considerable.

In what follows I shall firstly present what I have been able to discover about the island doctor, Thomas Price, and then give the text of his invoice. After this follows a translation and a brief discussion of terms.

---

1 I record my gratitude to the British Library, and to Ian Murray, Archivist of the Company of Barber-Surgeons. Many thanks also to Martti Mäkinen and Paivi Pahta.

2 William Salmon, 1644-1713, medical empiric and author, first set up a medical practice near the Smithfield gate of St Bartholomew's Hospital, then at the Red Balls tavern in Salisbury Court off Fleet Street; then in George Yard near Broken Wharf, at the Blue Balcony by the ditch side near Holborn Bridge; and finally in 1698 at the Great House by Black Friars Stairs.

3 E.g. The title of Geshwind's (1995) article: 'William Salmon, Quack-doctor and Writer of Seventeenth-century London'.

1. The 1715 St Helena Doctor: Thomas Price, Surgeon

Thomas Price is first mentioned in the Barber-Surgeons' *Apprentice Bindings* for the year 1697.[4] Usually apprentices were fourteen years of age when they were bound to their masters, which would give him a birth-date of 1683. We learn that on 2 November 1697, Thomas Price, son of Thomas Price of Cannon St., victualler, put himself as apprentice to Richard Lee, Surgeon, for seven years to the given day. Apprentices usually worked for seven years for their master whilst they learnt their trade, and then applied for the freedom of the company as a qualification to practice. The *Register of Admissions to the Freedom* of the Company of Barber-Surgeons for 7 November 1704 records Thomas Price's admission to the Company, although his master is given as Edward, rather than Richard, Lee.[5] Thomas Price is next mentioned in the Company of Barber-Surgeons' records as a sea-surgeon.[6] Three years after gaining his freedom of the Company he worked on board the *Rupert* for two years and four months, and then on the prizeship (meaning that it had been captured from an enemy nation) *Salisbury* for the winter of 1710-11. He boarded the *Russell* the very next day and worked at sea for nine months, but is then unaccounted for, perhaps working on land, for 1712. He was working again in 1713 at sea on the *Success* for a year and five months. His whereabouts during the winter of 1714 are unknown, but by Spring 1714 he was at sea again on the sloop *Drake*. By this time he would have been about 31 or 32 years of age. Unfortunately the journals of sea surgeons' practice have not survived, although the Company of Barber-Surgeons required sea surgeons to keep two copies of their journals.

During this period Thomas Price was examined by the Company of Barber-Surgeons in order to assign him a rank, and to

4 Company of Barber-Surgeons MS 5266/2, *Apprentice Bindings* 1672-1707, p. 364.

5 Guildhall Library Microfilm MS 5265/3 *Admissions to Freedom of Barber-Surgeons* 1694-1707, p. 89.

6 Company of Barber-Surgeons MS 5264, E1, *Lists of Certificates to Navy Surgeons* 1709 to 1744, unfoliated and not in date order.

determine the size of ship on which he could work.[7] He was deemed to be of the rank of third mate of a ship classed as a second-rater in 1709, and was promoted to second mate of a smaller ship, a third-rater, in 1711. Unfortunately, his next appearance in the Company of Barber-Surgeons' records at a court held on 10 June 1715 was to be superannuated.[8] The Rough Minute Book for this date survives, and we learn that he was rendered incapable of further service due to defect of sight.[9]

Thomas Price was examined in London on 10th June 1715 and considered to be unfit due to his sight defect, yet he travelled to the Island of St Helena by 15th November 1715, where he appears to have resumed working. In fact, we learn that he was able to do so only with help, as he wrote a letter back to the East India Company in London (in the third person), fearing "that twill be impossible [...] to undergo the fatigue & daily trouble that happens not only at the Fort & in the Country & [...] being often indispos'd & of weakly constitution w^{ch}: renders him incapable of walking up & down the Hills so of't as business requires, humbly represents that the surg^{ns}. Mate of the ship S^{t}: George is very willing to Enter himself in the Honble: Compa^{s}: service as assistant or Mate".[10] We learn from the same source that William Beale of the St George did apply for the post, although I have not traced a reply giving him the appointment. It seems that Thomas Price then spent two years on St Helena, where he must have recovered from his affliction sufficiently to be able to practice.

The Company of Barber-Surgeons' *Quarterage Books* for 1717-1739 subsequently show that Thomas Price returned to London and was resident and practicing in Romford in Essex, apparently hale and hearty, until the age of about 56 or 57. The volume for 1740 is missing, and he does not appear in the volume for 1741.

---

7 Company of Barber-Surgeons MS B/2/1 *Court of Examiners Rough Minute Book*.

8 Guildhall Library Microfilm MS 5257/7, *Company of Barber-Surgeons Court Minute Book* 1707-1731, fo 128.

9 Company of Barber-Surgeons MS B/2/2, *Rough Minute Book*, no foliation.

10 British Library, India and Oriental Office, *St Helena Consultation* G/32/5 1711-1717, unpaginated.

2. Text

London, British Library, India and Oriental Office, MS *St Helena Consultation* G/32/5 1711-1717, unpaginated.

15 November 1715
Copy of the Docters Indent. (vizt.) An Invoice of Medicines Drugs &c. desired to be sent to St. Helena for the use of the Honble. Comp^{as}. servants,
Thos. Price Surgeon

Imp:^{rs}	Aq.	Stip^{t}. Rega^{l}.		§[11]	iiij	
		Theriac	ll	xij		
		Epidem		xij		
		Paon Comp			xij	
Sp^{t}:		Vini Rect			xvj	
		Minthae			ij	
		Lavend: Comp.				ij
		Cochler			ij	
		Nitr. Dulc.				j
		C.C. p^{r}. cc				j
		Sal volat Oleos				ij
		Croci				j
Tinct^{r}		Castor				ss[12]
		Antimony				ij
		Myrrh & Aloes				ij
		Aqua Fortis			ll	xij
		Quick Silv^{r}			50^{l}	L
		To make Essays on Mineral Stones				
Syr.		Balsam			ll	xij
		Espin Ceru				x
		De Althee				viij
		Cariophilor				viij
		Rosar				viij
Cons^{r}.		Ros. Rub^{r}.				viij
		Absinth			iv	

11 In this chapter the paragraph mark is used to indicate the symbol for 'ounce'.
12 In this chapter the 'ss' mark is used to indicate the symbol for 'semi'.

	Prunettor		iv	
	Cynosbity			iv
Elect.	Diascord		vj	
	Philo Persic.			vj
	Ther: Venet			vj
	Ther: Londinens		vj	
Emp	Diac: cum Gum:	ll	viij	
	Epispatic		vj	
	Adherniu			ij
	Mucilagiu			iv
	De sapon			iv
Ung	Alb: Camp.			x
	Linement Arce			vj
	Desicative Rub.		vj	
	Nutrit			vj
	Diapompha:			vj
Troc	Alb. Ras	§	vj	
Pul	Astring		ll	j
	Bol ver			j
	Liquorit		j	
	C.C.C.			xx
	Jalap			j
	C. C. Rasur			xij
	Lap. Tutae			ss
	Calamin		ss	
	Itamit			ss
	Crem: Tart			iv
Ol.	Rosar			viij
	Terebinth			viij
	Chamama			iij
	Sambuc.		vj	
Ol. Chym	Anisi			ss
	Succini		ss	
	Carriophil		§	ij
	Juniper			ij
	Vitrioli			viij
	Minthae		ij	
	Cinamomij			j

Sal	Tarter		ll	ss
	Vitriol			ss
	Absinth		ss	
	Cathartic Amar			viij
	Emetic			ss
Sem	Lini		ll	iv
	Fenugr			ij
	Suc: Liquor.			ij
	Camphor	§	vj	
	Fenecul, Dulc		ll	vi
	Carua			vj
	Coriand		vj	
	Anisi			vj
Rad	Ipecacuan			j
	Granator		viij	
	Hord. Gallic:			x
	Peruvian		j	
	serpint. virg[a].			ij
	Althaea		ij	
	Sant Rubr			iij
	Torment		ij	
	Flor: senna			vj
	Rhubarb		ij	
Bals.	Lucatell		vj	
	Terebinth		§	viij
	Anisat			viij (the symbol for 'sulphur' in margin)
	Capiua		ll	ss
Herb	pr Fotu. M			C
	pr Pectorall			C
	pr Enemat			C
Herb:	pr decoct: Amar:		C	
	Centaurius			C
	Card. Benedict			CC
Flor	Rosar Rubr:		ll	iv
	Chemama			iv
	Croc: Ang:			iv
	Cochinella		§	iv
Sem	4°. Frigd Maj:		ll	iv

	Anisi		ll	ij
	Cariu			ij
	Cymini			ij
	Bac: Lauri			iv
	Juneperi		iv	
Gum:	Gum Aloes			j
	Myrrha	ll	j	
	Sang: Dracon			ss
	Gambog.	§	vj	
	Vini Benedict		ll	iv
	Lixiu Capatal			ij
Lap:	Contayerve			ss
pulo	Gasconic	§	iv	
Oc: 69 p p[l]			ll	ss

2	hair sives
2	Lawn Ditto
6	Cupping glases
6	skins white Leathr.
6	Red ditto
2	Gross Violls in sorts
2	nests Pill boxes
4	books party Gold
1	Doz. Bladders
	Gallipotts
3	Gross Violl Corks
1	Large spunge

Wee are in great want of a small Allembick still w[ch] I desire may be sent & a sett of Apothecarys Potts & boxes, would save trouble & their Value by saveing the Medicines from decay.
(Sign'd) Tho[s]. Price Surgeon

3. Treatment of terms

In this section, the terms in Price's inventory are listed as headwords. Information is taken from the various sources listed under *References* at the end of this chapter. I have mainly used sources that could have been available to Price in the early 1700s, occasionally supplemented by later work. In particular, William Salmon's works have been consulted, and also those of John Woodall, Surgeon General of the East India Company. Although multiple ills are claimed to be cured by each medicine, I have only listed a selected few in each case.

Imp.:^{rs} *Aq. Stip*^{t}*. Regal. §iiij*
Imprimis 'firstly' 4 ounces of *Aqua Styptica* 'styptick water of vitriol' Salmon (1685: 375): stops all fluxes of blood, gives recipe. Woodall (1703: 136, 600) gives a recipe for 'The Royal Styptick'; and *Aqua Regulata* 'our eye water' Salmon (1703: 364); Salmon (1698: 363, 364). Salmon gives recipe and advertises *Aqua Regulata* at 1 shilling per ounce.

Theriac lb xij
12 pounds of *Aqua Theriacalis* 'treacle water', against plague and fevers. Salmon (1685: 445) gives recipe.

Epidem xij
12 pounds of *Aqua Epidemica* 'the London plague-water' Salmon (1685: 429), also good for measles and smallpox, with recipe.

Paon Comp xij
12 pounds of *Aqua Poeniae Composita* 'Peony Water Compound' (Salmon 1685: 442): good for falling sickness, convulsions, palsies, clears the sight, helps a bad memory, with recipe.

Sp^{t}*: Vini Rect xvj*
16 pounds of *Spiritus Vini* 'rectified spirit of wine' (Woodall 1655: 45): "Spirit of wine of all vegetables is the most precious thing, it is the truest of all Cordials". Salmon (1707: 182) gives recipe.

Minthae ij
2 pounds of *Spiritus Menthae* 'spirit of mint'. Salmon (1705) advertised preparations of mint at half a crown an ounce. Mints "do profit the stomack, appease the hickok, stop vomiting" (Woodall 1655: 80).

Lavend: Comp. ij
2 pounds of *Spiritus Lavendulae Compositus Mattiae* 'spirit of lavender compound' (Salmon 1685: 440): against falling sickness, barrenness, convulsions, apoplexy, loss of memory, dimness of sight, with recipe. "This is a troublesome medicament to be made, nor can it be done in a short time". Salmon (1705) advertised preparations of lavender at 18d an ounce.

Cochler ij
2 pounds of *Spiritus Cochleariae Compositus* 'spirit of scurvy-grass compound' (Salmon 1688: 426): for cold diseases, against palsy, apoplexy, lethargy. Salmon (1705: IV, XI) sold '*Spiritus Cochlearis*: Spirit of Scurvy-grass' at 12d an ounce.

Nitr. Dulc. j
1 pound of *Spiritus Nitri* 'spirit of niter' (Salmon 1707: 70): opens the bowels, cures pleurisies and fevers, gives recipe.

C.C. p^r. cc j
1 pound of *Spiritus Cornu Cervi per se* 'spirit of harts-horn per se' (Theobald 1761: 52); ingredient in a medicine for freeing the lungs. Salmon (1685: 207): the horns are "Sudorifick, Alexipharmick, and Analeptick, cephalick and Hysterick." Woodall (1655: 65) "it is given in want of Unicorns horn [...] it comforteth the heart, is good against poyson, provoketh urine".

Sal volat Oleos ij
2 pounds of *Sal volatile Oleosum* 'Our Volatile Oily Salt', sold by Salmon (1705: III, III) at 5 shillings an ounce. *Sal volatile* 'ammonia' (Forsyth 1826).

Croci j
1 pound of *Spiritus Croci* 'spirit of saffron' (Salmon 1688: 429): facilitates birth and after-birth.

Tinct^r Castor ss
Half a pound of *Tinctura Castorei composita* 'tincture of castor compound' (Salmon 1689: 441), gives recipe. Against vapours, heart qualms, faintings, hysterick fits, stinging of hornets and scorpions, mad dogs. *Tinctura* "a Tincture, or Elixir, is the Extraction of the Colour, Quality, and Strength of any thing" (Blancard 1684: 282).

Antimony ij
2 pounds of *Tinctura Antimonij* 'tincture of antimony' (Salmon 1698: 381): attenuates slime; against palsy, apoplexy, epilepsy, leprosy, smallpox; gives recipe. Salmon (1698: 363) advertised *Tinctura Antimonij* at 5 shillings per ounce.

Myrrh & Aloes ij
2 pounds of *Tinctura Myrrha cum Aloes* 'myrrh with aloes'. *Myrrha* 'myrrh' (Salmon 1685: 166): "It is a gummy Rosin, from an Arabian tree, the bark being cut; Expels wind, opens obstructions of the lungs, Bowels and Womb". *Aloe* (Salmon 1685: 154): "Purges the bowels well. Good against Putrefaction, it cleanses wounds, and suddenly heals them."

Aqua Fortis lb xij
12 pounds of '*Aqua Fortis,* or dissolvent of Silver' (Salmon 1707: 371), gives recipe: oil of vitriol and saltpetre. *Aqua Fortis* 'strong water' (Woodall 1655: 43): "but for

myself, I see no reason for it, nor do I know any Chirurgical use it hath, which is not much better performed by oyl of vitriol".

Quick Silv[r] *50*[l] *L*
50 pounds of quicksilver. Salmon (1705) sold preparations of mercury at ten shillings an ounce.

Syr. Balsam lb xij
12 pounds of *Syrupus Balsamicus* 'balsamic syrup' (Theobald 1761: 106, 161): Linctus for a Hoarseness; gives recipe. *Balsamus*, "or *balsanum*; the Word *Balsame* is used very differently in the Shops. 1. It signifies a certain sort of Perfume, of somewhat a thick Consistence, like an Ointment; and this is its most usual signification; as for instance, Balsame of Roses, Apoplectic, and the like. 2. There are a sort of Liquors distilled from Gum, and resinous Substances, with spirit of Wine, which are anointed outwardly, and these are called Balsams too; as Nervous Balsam, Sciatic, &c. 3. It signifies a Liquor that is anointed into the Body, thicker than Oyl, and more Liquid than an Ointment. 4. Salt things funded and melted, are called Balsame, as the Balsame of Salt of Jewels. 5. There are a sort of particular preparations called Balsams, as the Balsam of Sulphur, &c. 6. and Lastly, some Gums of Trees are called Balsams." (Blancard 1684: 38).

Espin Ceru x
10 pounds of *Syrupus de Spina Cervina* 'syrup of buckthorn, or purging thorn'. A purge of universal tendency (Salmon 1685: 604), gives recipe.

De Althee viij
8 pounds of *Syrupus de Althaea* 'syrup of marshmallows' (Salmon 1685: 589), gives recipe. Expels the stone, heals dysentery.

Cariophilor viij
8 pounds of *Syrupus infusionis florum Caryophillorum* 'syrup of clove-gillyflowers' (Salmon 1685: 589), gives recipe. A pectoral and cordial. Salmon (1705) advertised preparations of cloves at half a crown an ounce.

Rosar viij
8 pounds of *Syrupus Rosarum simplex* 'syrup of roses' (Woodall 1655: 54): "doth quench thirst, especially in fevers".

Cons[r]*. Ros. Rub*[r]*. viij*
8 pounds of *Conserva Rosarum Rubrarum* 'red rose conserve' (Woodall 1655: 55): "Conserve of Red-roses is good for the heart and head." *Conserva* "a *Conserve*, is a Composition of Flowers or Herbs beat together, to every pound whereof, if they be dry, are added three pounds of Sugar; if moister, two pounds, so that they may be kepts several years". (Blancard 1684: 75).

Absinth iv
4 pounds of wormwood conserve. Woodall (1655: 53) lists *Syrupus Absinthii* 'syrup of wormwood' which does "cause an appetite, open the veins, move urine". *Absinthe* "wormwood, Artemisia absinthium, a vermifuge, tonic, and stomachic" (Fortune 2001: 208).

Prunettor iv
4 pounds of *Conserva Prunellorum* 'conserve of sloes' (Woodall 1655: 55): "Conserve of sloes is of a comforting stiptick force."

Cynosbity iv
4 pounds of *Cynosbati* 'canker-rose, wild rose' conserve (Salmon 1685: 121): "They are of the nature of the Garden-rose, but bind much more, and therefore are very good to stop the terms and whites in women." *Cynosbatos* 'brier' (Browne 1685: 97).

Elect. Diascord vj
6 pounds of *Electuary Diascordium* 'confect of Scordium or water-germander' (Salmon 1685: 658): against plague, poison, fevers; gives recipe. "*Electuarium* is a Confection of Simple Ingredients, Paps or Piths, Gums mixed with Syrup, or Honey, of a Consistence like a Conserve; and it is either *Simple*, or *Compound*; the *Simple* consists onely of the Pith of Cassia, Tamarinds, or Pruines; but the *Compound*, for the most part of several *Simple* Ingredients, Pulps, condensated Juices, Gumms, &c. made up with Honey or Syrup. *Electuaries* are Digestive, Loosning, Purging, Strengthning, Alexipharmic, &c." (Blancard 1684: 108). *Diascordium* "a medicine made of the dried leaves of *Teucrium Scordium*, and many other herbs". (*OED*)

Philo Persic. vj
6 pounds of *Electuary Philonium Persicum* "a Persian confect, causing rest and sleep" (Salmon 1685: 659), gives recipe. Prevents miscarriage, against cholick. *Philonium Persicum* "against the abundance of blood of women's monthly terms" (Woodall 1655: 60).

Ther: Venet vj
6 pounds of *Theriaca Andromachi* 'electuary of Venice treacle' (Salmon 1685: 660), gives recipe.

Ther: Londinens vj
6 pounds of *Theriaca Londinensis* 'London treacle' (Salmon 1685: 661), gives recipe. "Not so strong as Venice Treacle. Against poison, plague and pestilential fevers." Salmon (1698: 363, 441) gives a recipe containing opium for *Theriaca Londinensis nostra* 'our new London Treacle', which was used as a cure for the plague of 1665 and which sold at 5 shillings per ounce.

Emp Diac: cum Gum: lb viij
8 pounds of *Emplastrum Diachylon Magnum cum Gummi* 'emplaster of mucilages the great, with gums' (Salmon 1685: 779): resolves tumours and swellings, gives recipe. *Diachilon magnum cum gummis* (Woodall 1655: 27): "This Emplaister dissolveth, maturateth, and mollifieth hardnesses."

Epispatic vj
6 pounds of *Emplastrum Epispaticum* 'the blistering emplaster' (Salmon 1685: 781): used to draw blisters; gives recipe.

Adherniu ij
2 pounds of *Emplastrum ad Herniam* 'an emplaster for ruptures' (Salmon 1685: 782) gives recipe: comforts a weak back and reins, fortifies the womb, prevents abortion.

Mucilagiu iv
4 pounds of *Emplastrum Mucilagium* 'emplaster of mucilage'. *Mucilagio*, "the same as *Mucago*. *Mucago* is a viscous Extraction, made of Seeds, Gums, Roots, &c. with Water". (Blancard 1684: 202). See also Salmon (1707: 761) *Unguentum de Mucilaginibus* 'Oyntment of Mucilages', "good to Ripen and break Tumors"; with recipe.

De sapon iv
4 pounds of *Emplastrum de Sapone* 'emplaster of soap' (Salmon 1685: 788): against gout, sciatica. Gives recipe.

Ung Alb: Camp. x
10 pounds of *Unguentum album Camphoratum* "very good to cool and heal any hot moist pustles: it cureth excoriations of the skin in any place, but chiefly in the yard betwixt *glans* and *praeputium*" (Woodall 1655: 32). *Unguentum* "an Ointment, is a Medicine outwardly applied, of a Consistence something thicker than a Linimentum: It is called also *Unguen*". (Blancard 1684: 297)

Linement Arce vj
6 pounds of *Linamentum Arcei* a 'precious plain Linament' (Woodall 1655: 35): "A Balm for new wounds, especially in the head."

Desicative Rub. vj
6 pounds of *Unguentum rubrum Dessicativum* 'The Red Drying Ointment' (Salmon 1707: 754): "heals and skins Sores"; gives recipe.

Nutrit vj
6 pounds of *Unguentum Nutritum, seu Tripharmacum* 'Ointment of three things'. "Good against Inflammations, Burnings, and Scaldings. Cures Scabs, Tettars, Ringworms". (Salmon 1707: 753), gives recipe. *Unguentum Tripharmacon, or*

Nutritum. Against "excoriation or bladderings of the skin; such also as are termed *Shingles*" (Woodall 1655: 32-33).

Diapompha vj
6 pounds of *Unguentum Diapompholigos siue Nihil* 'Ointment of Pompholix, or nothing' (Salmon 1707: 751): Cures ulcers, stops the Hemorrhoids; gives recipe. *Unguentum Diapompholigos* "for gunpowder burns to the face" (Woodall 1628: 17). "Good to heal painful ulcers [...] especially of the yard" (Woodall 1655: 32).

Troc Alb. Ras §vj
6 ounces of *Trochisi albi Rhasis* 'white trochees of Rhasis' (Salmon 1707: 705). "Good against many affects of the Eyes, parts inflamed, pain and heat of Urine. Soreness and ulceration of the Yard"; gives recipe. "*Trochies*, are round marked things made of Pouders, mixed with viscous Extracts and made up into Paste, and then into round little Bodies, which are to be dried up in the Shade: They are also called *Pastilli*." (Blancard 1684: 285)

Pul Astring lb j
1 pound of *Pulvis Astringens* 'a powder stopping blood' (Salmon 1688: 639): to stop blood in wounds; gives recipe.

Bol ver j
1 pound of *Bolas Armenicae vel Orientali verus* "helping the Catarrhe, Dysentery, and ulcers of the mouth" (Woodall 1655: 75). *Bolus* 'a morsel, or Clod' (Browne 1685 67).

Liquorit j
1 pound of *Liquiritia* 'powdered liquorice root'. "Rotteth flegme, moveth expectoration, cureth the cough." (Woodall 1655: 67). Salmon (1685: 10): "Outwardly the powder put into the eye, helps in a special manner the Pin and Web." Salmon (1707: 10): cures diseases of the lung and windpipe.

C.C.C. xx
20 pounds of 'powder of burnt harts-horn' (Theobald 1761: 98, 134), gives recipe, for fevers. Salmon (1685: 207) gives recipe; stops fluxes, resists poyson and is a good thing for children. Woodall (1655: 65) "And being burned, the powder thereof is very good against the bloody, or any other fluxes of the belly."

Jalap j
1 pound of powdered root of *Jalapae* (Salmon 1685: 11), or *Jalapae Resina factitia* 'Rosin of Jalap' Salmon (1685: 164): "It purgeth strongly all bad humors"; Theobald (1761: 39): "The Jalap-Root is one of the best Purges we have." "From Spanish *purga de Jalapa*, from *Jalapa*, a city of Mexico. A purgative drug obtained from the tuberous roots of *Exogonium* (*Ipomoaea*) *Purga* and some other convolvulaceous plants." (*OED*)

C. C. Rasur xij
12 pounds of *Rasurae Cornu Cervi* 'shavings of harts-horn' (Salmon 1685: 207) gives recipe, and uses raspings in Gelly of Harts-horn: "It restores in Consumptions."

Lap. Tutae ss
6 pounds of tutty stone. Salmon (1707: 755) lists tutty as an ointment: *Unguentum Tutiae* 'Ointment of Tutty', for sore eyes, and gives recipe. "Tutty, Pompholix, or Spodium, is a thin Volatile Ash, which sticks to the upper part of the Furnace when Brass is melted."; "the best of all drying Medicines, exceeding good in all malignant and cancerous Ulcers." Salmon (1707: 355). Woodall (1655: 77): *Tutia* "It is the Scum of brasse in boiling"; "Good against the distillations of the eyes".

Calamin ss
3 pounds of powder *Diacalminthe simples* 'species of calamint simple' (Salmon 1685: 633): against the stone, provokes urine, expels wind, provokes the terms; gives recipe.

Itamit ss
3 pounds of *Itamit*. I have not been able to trace this item.

Crem: Tart iv
4 pounds of *Cremor Tartari* 'powdered cream of tartar' (Salmon 1707: 175): "Opens all obstructions of the stomach, liver, spleen, Bowels, Reins, and Bladder"; gives recipe.

Ol. Rosar viij
8 pounds of *Oleum seu Spiritus Rosarum* 'oil or spirit of roses' (Salmon 1685: 465): "Quickens the senses and revives the heart. Exhilarates the mind and expels melancholy"; gives recipe.

Terebinth viij
8 pounds of *Oleum Terebinthinae* 'oyl of turpentine' (Salmon 1685: 471): "Opens all obstructions of the reins and passages of the seed"; gives recipe. Woodall (1655: 52) *Oleum Terebinthinae* "for shortnesse of breath".

Chamama iij
3 pounds of *Oleum Chamomelinum* 'oyl of Chamomil' (Woodall 1655: 48): "Good for the Collick, stone, wearinesse." "Very convenient in Glisters for all gripings and tortians of the guts."

Sambuc. vj
6 pounds of *Oleum Sambucinum* 'oyle of Elder-flowers' (Woodall 1655: 49): "Oyle of Elder-flowers doth lenifie and purge the skin, is good for the obstructions of the liver."

Ol. Chym Anisi ss
3 pounds of *Oleum Anisi Chimice*, *Oleum ex semine Anisi* 'chemical oil of aniseed' (Salmon 1685: 465): "Cures most diseases of the breast and lungs, coughs, colds, asthma, windiness of the stomack"; gives recipe. Woodall (1655: 52) *Oleum Anisi* "against the Tympany, inflation, and crudity of the stomack; against the gripings and the cryings of the intestines." Salmon (1705) advertised preparations of aniseed at 12d an ounce.

Succini ss
3 pounds of *Oleum Succini Chimice* 'chemical oil of amber' (Salmon 1685: 474): "against fits of the mother, epilepsy, palsy, lameness, wounds of the nerves, numbness"; gives recipe. Salmon (1705) sold preparations of amber at 12d an ounce. *Oleum Succini Chimice* "helpeth the pain in the head, resolution of the sinews and falling evil" (Woodall 1655: 53).

Carriophil §ij
2 ounces of *Oleum Caryophyllorum Chimice* 'chemical oil of cloves' (Salmon 1685: 466): cures vertigoes, megrims, dropsy, yellow jaundice; gives recipe.

Juniper ij
2 ounces of *Oleum ex Ligno Juniperi* 'oyl of juniper wood', or *Oleum Baccarum Juniperi* 'oyl of juniper berries' (Salmon 1685: 468, 470). Gives recipes. The wood oil cures diseases of the brain and nerves, the berry oil cures stone in the reins, pains of the yard, gonorrhoea, expels wind out of the body, urine, gravel, and the Terms. Salmon (1705) sold preparations of juniper at 18d an ounce. *Oleum Juniperinum* "for the cure of the morphew of the skin" (Woodall 1655: 52).

Vitrioli viij
8 ounces of *Oleum Vitrioli Chimice* 'chemical oil of vitriol'. Woodall (1655: 51): "freeth obstrucitons, recreateth the bowels". Oil of Vitriol "one or more of the inorganic sulphates of metals, particularly iron, copper or zinc" (Fortune 2001: 209).

Minthae ij
2 ounces of *Oleum Menthae Chimice* 'chemical oil of mint'. See *spirit of mint* above.

Cinamomij j
1 ounce of *Oleum Cinnamomi Chimice* 'chemical oil of cinnamon' (Salmon 1685: 466). Gives recipe. Provokes terms, brings away birth and afterbirth, cures consumptions.

Sal Tarter lb ss
Half a pound of *Sal Tartari, seu Sal Regis* 'the salt of tartar or wine lees' (Woodall 1655: 259; Browne 1685: 221). Salmon (1707: 176) gives recipe: "It is an excellent thing in the Stone, provokes Urine."

Vitriol ss
Half a pound of *Sal Vitrioli* 'salt of vitriol'. Salmon (1685: 375) gives recipe: "So very a gentle Emetick that it may be given to children." "Snufft up the Nostrils it gently purges the brain by sneezing."

Absinth ss
Half a pound of salt of wormwood. Woodall (1655: 50) lists absinth as an oil rather than a salt: *Oleum Absinthii* 'oyl of wormwood' "raiseth an appetite [...] Dissipateth and disperseth wind, killeth worms".

Cathartic Amar viij
8 pounds of *Catharticum Amarum* 'bitter cathartic'. *Catharticum* "is a purging Medicine, which cleanses the Stomach, the Guts, and whatsoever is vitious and *heterogenous* in the Blood, and throws it into the Common-shore of the Guts". (Blancard 1684: 54). Salmon (1685: 465) lists *Pulvis Catharticus universalis* 'universal purging Pouder'.

Emetic ss
4 pounds of emetic salt. Salmon (1705: IV.X) sold "Emeticon: or, Our Vomiting Powder at 2 shillings a seal, each seal containing 2 papers".

Sem Lini lb iv
4 pounds of *Semina Lini* 'linseed' (Salmon 1685: 148): "Good for coughs, pleurisies, consumptions. Ripens tumors." Woodall (1655: 49) lists oil of linseed, which "cureth convulsions, mitigateth the hardnesse of the arteries, muscles and nerves". Woodall (1655: 68) *Semen lini* "draweth out thornes sticking in the body".

Fenugr ij
2 pounds of *Semina Foenugraeci* 'fenugreek seeds' (Salmon 1685: 147): "These dissolve hard swellings, help hard Spleens, expel all evil Humors." Woodall (1655: 68) *Semen Fenigraeci*: cures gout in the feet.

Suc: Liquor. ij
2 pounds of *Succus Liquoritiae* 'liquorice juice'. Salmon (1685: 163) gives recipe: "This is absolutely the greatest of all Vegetable Pectorals, and performs all that the Root will."

Camphor §vj
6 ounces of camphor. Salmon (1685: 160) lists camphor as a gum: *Camphora* 'camphir'. "It is a Resinous Gum flowing from a tall tree. The Bornean Camphir is best; the other comes from China. Abates lust and vigour, hinders conception, causes Barrenness." Woodall (1655: 75): "Camphura cureth St Anthonies fire, is effectual against the Gonorraea, the white flowers of women, bleeding of the nose."

Fenecul, Dulc lb vi
6 pounds of *Semina Foeniculi* 'sweet fennel seed' (Salmon 1685: 147). These have the same qualities as aniseed.

Carua vj
6 pounds of *Semina Carui* 'caraway seed' (Salmon 1685: 144): "These hasten the Birth, ease the Colick and all pains in the Reins and Ureters." Salmon (1705) sold preparations of caraway at 12d an ounce.

Coriand vj
6 pounds of *Semina Coriandri* 'coriander seed' (Salmon 1685: 145): "Helps digestion, stops vomiting, kills worms, stops all fluxes. After meat it closes the mouth of the Stomack, and suppresses Vapours that would hurt the Head."

Anisi vj
6 pounds of *Semina Anisi* 'aniseeds' (Salmon 1685: 143): "Aniseeds provoke lust, encrease milk, sweeten the breath, and bring down swollen bellies."

Rad Ipecacuan j
1 pound of *Ipecacuantae Radicis Pulveris* 'powdered ipecacuanha root' (Pereira 1824). "The root of *Cephaëlis Ipecacuanha*, N.O. *Cinchonaceæ*, a South American small shrubby plant, which possesses emetic, diaphoretic, and purgative properties; also popularly applied to various forms in which the drug is employed." (*OED*). Theobald (1761: 97) gives a recipe for *Bolus ex Ipecacoanha.*

Granator viij
8 pounds of pomegranate root. Salmon (1707: 21) lists this as a peel rather than a root: *Ganatorum immaturorum Malicorium* "Of Pomegranates: the peel cools and binds in an extram manner; Fastens loose Teeth."

Hord. Gallic: x
10 pounds of *Hordeum Gallicum* 'French barley'. "Good for inflammations, excelleth against the sorenesse of the throat." (Woodall 1655: 67)

Peruvian j
1 pound of Peruvian root. Salmon (1685: 157) lists this as a balsam: *Balsamum Peruanum* 'balm of Peru'. "It is a sweet-scented Balm coming from the Indian Tree Xylo." "There is also a clear whitish Liquor which flows from the bark of the same Tree wounded." Against fevers. Salmon (1707: 22): *Peruanus* "If the Colledge mean the Peruvian Bark, of which the Jesuits Pouder is made, it is an excellent thing against all sorts of Agues." "My own Experience confirms it, for the Cure of the Rickets."

Serpint. virg[a]. *ij*
Serpentaria Virginiana, 'Aristolochia serpentaria, the Virginian snake-root' (Forsyth 1826). Theobald (1761: 24) lists "*Decoctum Serpentariae* A decoction of snake-root for fevers of the more malignant kind".

Althaea ij
2 pounds of *Althaeae* 'marsh-mallow root' (Salmon 1685: 1): ripens swellings, excellent in Pleurisies, Chollick, Bloody Flux, griping of the Guts.

Sant Rubr iij
3 pounds of *Santalum rubrum* 'red saunders root' (Salmon 1707: 25): "They are Exoticks brought from the Indies." Revives the heart in faintings, cools the liver.

Torment ij
2 pounds of *Tormentillae* 'root of tormentil' (Salmon 1685: 19): "resists Poyson, Plague, and all manner of Pestilential Diseases".

Flor: senna vj
6 pounds of *Florae Senae* 'senna flowers' (Woodall 1655: 64): "For purging the belly." Woodall lists the leaves rather than the flowers.

Rhubarb ij
2 pounds of *Rhabarbarum* 'rhubarb root' (Woodall 1655: 64) "good for the stomack and liver, and against the bloody flix."

Bals. Lucatell vj
6 pounds of *Balsamum Lacatelli* 'the Balsam of Lucatellus (Salmon 1707: 735): for "Head-ach, old Aches and Bruises, the Bitings of mad Dogs and other venomous creatures"; gives recipe. *Balsamum lucatelli* "made of oil, turpentine, wax, and red saunders; formerly exhibited in coughs of long standing" (Forsyth 1826).

Terebinth §viij
8 ounces of balsam of *Terebinthinus* 'of Turpentine' (Browne 1685: 222). See *Oleum Terebinthinae* above. Theobald (1761: 56) lists *Enema Terebinthinatum* 'A Turpentine Clyster', made of camomile flowers and turpentine mixed with honey and egg.

Anisat viij (the symbol for 'sulphur' in margin)
Possibly balsam of dill.

Capiua lb ss
Half a pound of *Copaiba* 'balsam capiva'; "from Spanish and Portuguese *copaiba*, from Brazilian *cupauba*. A balsam of aromatic odour and acrid taste, obtained from various S. American trees or shrubs of the genus *Copaifera*; [...] its chief application

is in medicine, as a remedy in diseases of the urinary passages" (*OED*). *Balsam of Copaiva* (Hallet 1819: 6), *Balsami Copaivae* (Pereira 1824).

Herb pr Fotu. M C
1,100 pounds of herbs for poultices. "*Fotus* = *fomentum* that which applied to the Body, cherishes it and warms it." (Blancard 1708).

pr Pectorall C
100 pounds of herbs for the chest and lungs. Salmon (1685: 578) gives a recipe for *Decoctum Pectorale* 'dedicated to the lungs', including liquorice, mayden-hair, hysop, scabious and colts-foot. Theobald (1761: 60) gives a recipe for *Infusum Pectorale* of 2 handfuls of ground-ivy leaves and 2 ounces of liquorice root infused in barley-water.

pr Enemat C
100 pounds of herbs for purging the stomach. Salmon (1685: 577) *Decoctum Commune pro Clystere* 'the Common Decoction for Clysters', gives a recipe including mallows, violets, pellitory, beets, mercury, camomile, sweet fennel seeds and linseed. "It softens the excrements of the Belly, and makes the Guts slippery."

Herb: pr decoct: Amar: C
100 pounds of herbs for a bitter decoction. Blancard (1684: 26): *Decoction* "is a Decoction of Roots, Woods, Barks, Herbs, Flowers, Fruits, Seeds, &c, which is boiled down commonly to Twelve, Fifteen, or Twenty Ounces. It is either Purging, Loosning, Altering, or Drying, *Cephalic*, *Stomachic*, *Diuretic*, *Splenetic*, or *Hepatic*". Salmon (1685: 579) has a recipe for *Decoctum Amarum* 'the Bitter Decoction', good against green sickness in virgins, made from centory, camomile, gentian, senna and carduus.

Centaurius C
100 pounds of *Centaurium* 'centaury' (Salmon 1685: 43): against long agues, biting of mad dogs, scurvy, gout, green sickness, dropsies. Kills worms.

Card. Benedict CC
200 pounds of *Carduus Benedictus* 'blessed thistle' (Woodall 1655: 84): "prevaileth against bitings of Serpents". Salmon (1685: 41): "Cures green wounds to a wonder. Cures old quartans. Helps head-achs and deafness, loss of memory and gripings of the belly."

Flor Rosar Rubr: lb iv
4 pounds of *Flores Rosae Rubrae* 'red rose flowers' (Woodall 1655: 78). Comforts the head, stomack and heart.

Chemama iv
4 pounds of *Flores Chamaemeli* 'chamomile flowers' (Salmon 1685: 120). Against colick and stone; expels wind.

Croc: Ang: iv
4 pounds of *Crocus Anglorum* 'English saffron' (Salmon 1685: 120): "The greatest of all Vegetable Cordials; quickens the senses, exhilerates the heart, provokes sweat, causeth free breathing, prolongs life."

Cochinella §iv
4 ounces of *Cochinella* 'cochineal'. "A dye-stuff consisting of the dried bodies of the insect *Coccus cacti*, which is found on several species of cactus in Mexico and elsewhere. It is used for making carmine, and as a brilliant scarlet dye; also in medicine as an antispasmodic, etc." (*OED*).

Sem 4°. Frigd Maj: lb iv
4 pounds of *Semina quatuor frigida majora* 'the four cold seeds': Cacurbitae, Cucumeris, Citrulli and Melonis (Woodall 1655: 69). They cure heat of blood, choler, fevers, and move urine.

Anisi lb ij
2 pounds of *Anisi* 'aniseeds' (Salmon 1685: 143). See *Ol. Chym Anisi* and *anisi* above.

Carui ij
2 pounds of *Carui* 'caraway seeds' (Salmon 1685: 144). See *Carua* above.

Cymini ij
2 pounds of *Cymini* 'cummin seeds' (Salmon 1685: 145). "Expels wind, helps Headach. Dissolves swellings in the Genitors and Joynts."

Bac: Lauri iv
4 pounds of *Baccae Lauri* 'Bay-berries' (Woodall 1655: 79). Bay berries "resist poyson, help deafnesse, contracted and wearied parts".

Juneperi iv
4 pounds of juniper berries. Sold at 18d an ounce (Salmon 1705). See juniper oil above.

Gum: Gum Aloes j
1 pound of *Gummi Aloes* 'Of Gums Aloe' (Salmon 1685: 154): "Purges the bowels well. Good against Putrefaction, it cleanses wounds, and suddenly heals them."

Myrrha lb j
1 lb of gum of *Myrrha* 'myrrh' (Salmon 1685: 166). See *Myrrh & Aloes* above.

Sang: Dracon ss
Half a pound of gum of *Sanguis Draconis* 'dragon's blood' (Salmon 1685: 172): "It is the Tear of a Tree, red like blood, the Fruit of which is like to a Cherry, whose skin being taken off is like a Dragon. It comes from Portus Sanctus in America. Stops all sorts of Fluxes, and spitting of Blood. Stays Catarrhs." Woodall (1655: 74) *Sanguis Draconis* "closeth up wounds".

Gambog.§vj
6 ounces of gum of *Gambogia* 'juice from an unknown plant 'Gum Cambugia'' (Salmon 1685: 159). "It comes from China to us. Purges and vomits all humors, dropsies, feavers, scabs, Itch, Pox and Gout." Woodall (1655: 62, 66): "Cambogiae is a purging medicine, newly found out in the East-Indies, and thence brought to us." Good against the yellow jaundice.

Vini Benedict lb iv
4 pounds of *Vinum Benedictum* 'blessed wine' (Salmon 1707: 566). Gives recipe: wine, with *Crocus Metallorum*. "A good vomit".

Lixiu Capatal ij
2 pounds of *Lixivium Capitale* "Spirit of Nitre, Vitriol, Salt. A Lixivium prepared of Salt of Tartar and Water in Vegetables, Spirit of Wine in things sulphureous, that is, endued with an oily part" (Blancard 1684: 184). "Water impregnated with alkaline salts extracted by lixiviation from wood ashes; lye. Also, a solution obtained from other substances by lixiviation." (*OED*).

Lap: Contayerve ss
Salmon lists this as a root: *Contrayervae, Radicis Drakenae* 'of the counter-poison', "One of the most excellent of vegetable antidotes against all manner of poysons" (Salmon 1685: 6); "Eminent against Plague, Small Pox, and all Pestilential Fevers" (Salmon 1707: 6). Its etymology is from Spanish *contra* + *hierba* 'plant against poisons': "A name given, in general use, to the root-stock and scaly rhizome of species of *Dorstenia* (*D. Contrayerva* and *D. braziliensis*, family Urticaceæ) native to tropical America, used as a stimulant and tonic, and formerly as an antidote to snake-bites" (*OED*). Grey (1682) also lists *contrayerve* as a stone, so I wonder whether this was Price's source, especially as it is immediately followed by *Gascon powder*, which together with *lapis contra yarvam* forms part of the title page of Grey (1682). Grey lists 22 reasons to use Contra Yerva, no. 22 being "It is a general good upon all occasions, and may be given at all times, when you do not know what the disease is".

Pulo Gasconic §iv
4 ounces of *Gascon's Own Powder* (Grey 1682), with recipe, including "powder of Pearl, of red Corral, of Crabs eyes, of Harts horn, and white Amber" and the black toes of crab's claws. This is the same as the *Powder of Crabs Claws* recipe in the 1650 edition of the *London Dispensatory*. Salmon (1685: 632-3) lists *Pulvis e Chelis*

Cancrorum Compositus ‘Gascoins pouder’, “being a great Benzoartick and Counter-Poyson, resisting the Plague”.

Oc: 69 p p^{l} *lb ss*
Possibly *oculus bovis* ‘ox-eye daisy’, as the *69* symbol signified night and day. Salmon (1685: 82) lists the daisy as good to dissolve cold and hard swellings.

Of the requests for equipment, one item requires comment: *party gold*. This is gold with considerable alloy (*MED*). In London party gold was used in the context of art, being a leaf of gold and silver beaten together, cheaper than gold but dearer than silver, of an intermediate, cool gold colour, which tarnished because of the silver content.[13] Perhaps the doctor required it for medicinal use.

4. Conclusion

In order to discover what sources Price might have consulted, either from his own collection in St Helena, or during his apprenticeship in London, I have surveyed here three kinds of medical works: the authoritative, professional lists of drugs published by accredited apothecaries and doctors (such as Staphorst[14] and Shipton), which were approved by the London Society of Apothecaries, including the works of the East India Company’s own surgeon-general John Woodall; secondly, popular household works bought and used by the populace in general (such as Grey 1682); and thirdly the entrepreneurial, unofficial publications of the unqualified William Salmon. It seems to me that Price used all three kinds. Whether coincidence or not, Price follows the ordering of Shipton (1689: 50, 51, 53, 54) in his listing of *Emp. Epispasticum, Emp. Ad Herniam, Emp. de Mucilaginibus, and Emp. de Sapone*. He follows the ordering of Grey (1682, title page) for *lapis contra yarvam* and *Gascon*

13 British Library, India and Oriental Office, *St Helena Consultation* G/32/5 1711-1717, unpaginated.

14 Staphorst (1686) is a listing of what was then being prepared in the hall laboratories in the Apothecaries’ Hall, London.

powder. And many of the items on his list can be found described in Salmon's various works, referred to more or less exactly as Salmon named them. Although I cannot be entirely certain about this, my perception is that Price found Salmon's works to be useful to him, and that Salmon does deserve to have a place in medical history as a disseminator of medical writing. Given that the London East India Company of the day covered half the globe, I suggest that this influence must have been considerable.

References

Manuscripts

London, Company of Barber-Surgeons, MS 5266/2, *Apprentice Bindings* 1672-1707.

London, Company of Barber-Surgeons, MS 5264, E1, *Lists of Certificates to Navy Surgeons* 1709 to 1744.

London, Company of Barber-Surgeons, MS B/2/1, *Court of Examiners Rough Minute Book.*

London, Company of Barber-Surgeons, MS B/2/2, *Court of Examiners Rough Minute Book.*

London, The Company of Barber-Surgeons, MS, *Quarterage Books* for 1717-1739.

London, Guildhall Library Microfilm, MS 5265/3, *Admissions to Freedom of Barber-Surgeons* 1694-1707.

London, Guildhall Library Microfilm, MS 5257/7, *Company of Barber-Surgeons Court Minute Book* 1707-1731.

London, British Library, India and Oriental Office, *St Helena Consultation* G/32/5 1711-1717.

Books

Blancard (Blanckaert), Steven 1684. *[Lexicon medicum græco-latinum] A Physical Dictionary; in which all the terms relating either to anatomy, chirurgery, pharmacy, or chymistry, are very accurately explain'd.* London: printed by J. D.

Blancard (Blanckaert), Steven [5]1708. *[Lexicon medicum græco-latinum.] A Physical Dictionary; in which all the terms relating either to anatomy, chirurgery, pharmacy, or chymistry, are very accurately explain'd.* London: printed by Sam. Crouch and John Sprint.

Browne, Richard 1685. *Prosodia Pharmacopoeorum: or the Apothecary's prosody, etc.* London: Benj. Billingsley.

Forsyth, J. S. 1826. *The New London Medical and Surgical Dictionary.* London: Sherwood, Gilbert, and Piper.

Fortune, Robert 2001. *The Words of Medicine Sources, Meanings and Delights.* Springfield, Ill.: Charles C. Thomas.

Geshwind, M. 1995. William Salmon, Quack-doctor and Writer of Seventeenth-century London. *Bulletin of the History of Dentistry* 43, 73-6.

Grey, Elizabeth, Countess of Kent 1682. *A Choice Manual, or, Rare and Select Secrets in Physick and Chyrurgery.* London: Henry Mortlock.

Hallet, Job 1819. *De Venereo Morbo, or, a Practical Treatise on Venereal Disease.* Manchester.

MED = Kurath, Hans / Kuhn, Sherman McAllister (eds) 1952-. *Middle English Dictionary.* Ann Arbor: University of Michigan Press.

OED = *Oxford English Dictionary* Online.

Pereira, Jonathan 1824. *A Selection of Prescriptions.* London: John Anderson.

Salmon (Royal College of Physicians (London) and William Salmon) [3]1685. *Pharmacopoeia Londinensis; or, the New London Dispensatory.* London: T. Dawks & Co.

Salmon, William [2]1688. *Doron Medicum: or, A Supplement to the New London Dispensatory.* London: T. Dawks, etc.

Salmon, William 1689. *Phylaxa Medicinae* (bound up with *Collectanea Medica* 1703).

Salmon, William 1698, 1699. *Ars Chirurgica. A Compendium of the Theory and Practice of Chirurgery.* London: J. Dawks.

Salmon, William [7]1703. *Collectanea Medica, the Country Physician, or a Choice Collection of Physick Fitted for Vulgar Use.* London.

Salmon, William 1705. *Gazae Medicae Quinque*. London: Ex Typhis F. C.

Salmon (Royal College of Physicians (London) and William Salmon) [7]1707. *Pharmacopoeia Londinensis; or, the New London Dispensatory.* London: T. Dawks & Co.

Shipton, James 1689. *Pharmacopoeiae Londinensis*. London: T. Basset, R. Chiswell, S. Smith.

Staphorst, Nicholas 1686. *Officina Chymica Londinensis*. Hamburg: Henning Brendek.

Theobald, John [6]1761. *Medulla Medicinae Universae: Or, A New Compendious Dispensatory*. London: J Whiston and B. White.

Wilson, Philip K. 'William Salmon'. *Oxford Dictionary of National Biography Online.*

Woodall, John 1628. *Viaticum: The Pathway to the Surgions Chest.* London.

Woodall, John 1655. *The Surgeons Mate or Military and Domestique Surgery*. London.

Notes on Contributors

MARIA ANGELES ALCARAZ ARIZA holds a BA and an MA in English Studies and a PhD in Linguistics from the University of Alicante (Spain). She is currently teaching English for Tourism and a graduate programme in the analysis of written scientific discourse at the University of Alicante. She has published several articles on the influence of English on medical Spanish and on the discoursal features of medical prose written in different languages. She is a member of the Multidisciplinary and Multilingual Research Group on Scientific Discourse Analysis.

ELLEN BARTON is a Professor in the Linguistics Program at Wayne State University (Detroit, USA). Her research interests in medical communication include end-of-life discussions, recruitment to clinical research, the discourse of specialty medical encounters, and, most recently, the emergence of ethical principles and deliberation in situated interactions like those above. Her work appears in the journals *Communication & Medicine*, *Qualitative Health Research*, *Discourse Studies*, *Discourse and Society*, *The Journal of Applied Linguistics*, *Narrative Inquiry*, *The Journal of Pragmatics*, and *Text*.

HUGO BOWLES is Associate Professor of English at the University of Rome Tor Vergata. His research interests and publications are in many areas of applied linguistics, including genre analysis and LSP, with a particular interest in legal and medical English. He is currently working on the application of conversation analysis to the study of specialist talk.

SALLY CANDLIN is an Adjunct Associate Professor in the School of Nursing and Health at the University of Western Sydney, and Senior Research Fellow in the Department of Linguistics at Macquarie University, Sydney. She is a Registered Nurse, Midwife and Health Visitor. Her academic qualifications include: BA (Hons) in

Linguistics and Psychology, MSc (Public Health), PhD (Linguistics). She has taught in both undergraduate and postgraduate programs in Nursing and Health in Australia and Hong Kong, as well as in postgraduate programs in Communication in Professions and Organisations at Macquarie University, Sydney. Her research and publications are primarily related to issues in health communication.

DIDIER CARNET is a senior Lecturer in the English Department of the Dijon Medical School, University of Burgundy, France. He holds a PhD in English linguistics. His main research is didactics and applied linguistics in English for Medical Purposes. He has published many articles, six books and two CD-Roms on medical English. His latest book is a French-English/English-French dictionary of medical terminology.

LOURDES DIVASSON, PhD, Assistant Professor, belongs to the Department of English and German Philology of the University of La Laguna, Tenerife, Spain. Over the last twenty years she has been teaching Medical English to undergraduates and postgraduates at the Faculty of Medicine of the above mentioned university and has carried out research work in the field of applied linguistics (in the areas of academic and professional discourse analysis and language teaching). Some of her works have been published in *Asp: La Revue du GERAS (Groupe d'Etudes et de Recherches en Anglais de Specialité); Ablex Series,* and *Discourse Analysis and Terminology in Languages for Specific Purposes.*

KJERSTI FLØTTUM is Professor of French Linguistics at the Department of Romance studies and Vice-Rector for international relations at the University of Bergen, Norway. Her general research fields are textlinguistics, discourse analysis, semantics and pragmatics. More specifically her research is related to text summarising, genre theory, linguistic polyphony, academic discourse and political discourse. She is the leader of the KIAP project (Cultural Identity in Academic Prose) and of the multidisciplinary project 'Common European vs. regional/national political discourse'. She is co-author of *La théorie scandinave de la polyphonie linguistique* (Paris 2004).

MAURIZIO GOTTI is Professor of English Linguistics and Director of the Language Centre at the University of Bergamo. He is currently President of the Italian Association of University Language Centres and Director of CERLIS, the research centre on specialized languages based at the University of Bergamo. From 1999 to 2001 he was President of the Italian Association of English Studies. From 2000 to 2004 he was President of the European Confederation of University Language Centres. His main research areas are the features and origins of specialized discourse (*Robert Boyle and the Language of Science* 1996; *Specialized Discourse: Linguistic Features and Changing Conventions* 2003; *Investigating Specialized Discourse* 2005). He is a member of the Editorial Board of national and international journals, and edits the *Linguistic Insights* series for Peter Lang.

MARIA GRAZIA GUIDO is Professor of English Linguistics at the University of Lecce and holds a PhD in English Applied Linguistics from the University of London. Her research interests are in cognitive-functional linguistics applied to intercultural communication and specialized discourse analysis. Her main publications include these volumes: *The Acting Reader* (Legas 1999), *The Imaging Reader* (Legas 2005), *Mediating Cultures* (LED 2004), *Register and Dialect in an Integrated Model of European English* (Bulzoni 1999).

DAVID R. HALL has lived and worked in a number of countries, including Thailand, Malaysia, Iran, Rwanda, France and England, and is currently Associate Professor in the Department of Linguistics at Macquarie University in Sydney, Australia. He teaches curriculum innovation, management, and language for special purposes at postgraduate and doctoral level. With Chris Candlin, he edits the series *Applied Linguistics in Action* (Pearson) and *Research and Practice in Applied Linguistics* (Macmillan). With Sandra Gollin, he is writing a book on Language for Specific Purposes to be published by Macmillan. He coedited, with Ann Hewings, *Innovation in English Language Teaching* (Routledge 2001).

LUCY BROOKES-HOWELL is Research Coordinator for the Health Communication Research Centre, Cardiff University. Her previous research has focused on exploring the process of genetic counselling.

She has worked as Research Associate on a project examining different frames of communication in genetic counselling for predictive testing. Her doctoral research focused on the management of diagnostic uncertainty in talk and in the text of case notes and follow-up letters. She is currently involved in research surrounding medical training and the assessment procedure of both palliative medicine students and refugee doctors seeking to revalidate their medical qualifications, as well as an exploration of prescription practices in primary health care.

RICK IEDEMA is Deputy Director of the Centre for Clinical Governance Research and Associate Professor at the School of Public Health and Community Medicine of the University of New South Wales, Sydney. Prof Rick Iedema's teaching and research centre on clinical communication in hospitals, targeting how doctors, nurses, allied health staff, managers and consumers communicate about the organization of in-hospital work. He publishes across the areas of organization studies, health services research and discourse studies in journals that include *Organization Studies, Social Science and Medicine, The British Medical Journal, Health Services Management Research, Communication and Medicine, Discourse and Society, Text* and *Visual Communication.*

JOHANNA LALOUSCHEK is Assistant Professor of Applied Linguistics at the University of Vienna and Head of the *Gesprächs-Praxis* for systemic coaching, self-management training in communication and scientific counselling. Her fields of research and publication are discourse analysis, communication in institutions (medicine, public health and media), especially doctor-patient-communication, psychosomatic and alternative medicine, health programmes on TV, and the development of linguistically based communication trainings for doctors, medical students and nursing staff.

ISABEL K. LEÓN, PhD, Lecturer of English, belongs to the Department of English and German Philology of the University of La Laguna, Tenerife, Spain. She teaches Medical English to undergraduates and postgraduates at the Faculty of Medicine and has done research in the field of applied linguistics (in the areas of academic and professional discourse analysis and language teaching). She has published in *ASp: La Revue du GERAS (Groupe d'Etudes et de Recherches en Anglais de Specialité), Atlantis. Journal of the Spanish Association for Anglo-American Studies* and *Discourse Analysis and Terminology in Languages for Specific Purposes.*

ANNE MAGNET has founded the English Department of the Life Science Faculty at the University of Burgundy, Dijon, France where she still works as a Senior Lecturer. She holds a PhD in English linguistics (University of Burgundy). Her main interests are scientific discourse analysis and applied linguistics. She has published a number of papers on the discursive and linguistic features of scientific English. Her research focus was first the experimental research article, and is now the minor genres of scientific discourse (Letters to the Editor and Editorials).

SUSAN MCKAY teaches communication, media and cultural studies in the School of English, Media Studies and Art History, at the University of Queensland, Australia. She is the co-author with Lloyd Davis of *Structures and Strategies: An Introduction to Academic Writing*. She holds a degree in Pharmacy (as well as a BA and PhD in English) and has used this health background, together with her academic interest in language in the media, in her research into representations of health issues in the media. Her research into men's health was undertaken as part of the Faculty Fellows Research Program at the Centre for Critical and Cultural Studies at the University of Queensland in 2003.

FLORIAN MENZ, MA (linguistics) and PhD (discourse analysis), is Associate professor at the Department of Linguistics, University of Vienna (Austria). His main research fields are: health communication; language and institutions; language, power and ideology; language and prejudice. He has been working in and leading projects on doctor-patient-interaction, business and organizational communication, legal language, language and politics (prejudice), readability research. His main publications include: *Der geheime Dialog* (Frankfurt 1991), *Die Sprachen der Vergangenheiten* (Frankfurt 1994, with R. Wodak, R.

Mitten and F. Stern), *Selbst- und Fremdorganisation im Diskurs* (Wiesbaden 2000).

PHILIPPA MUNGRA, RSA from UCLES and MSc in cytogenetics from the University of Western Ontario (Canada), is a lecturer in English at the first Medical School of the University of Rome 'La Sapienza'. Her current research priorities revolve around the structure and evolution of specialist medico-scientific publications from a communicative and textual point of view. She has recently investigated the macrostructure of other overviews in Medicine. Other research interests include integration of language and content in tertiary education as well as materials development for writing in an *e-learning* course. She has recently published a textbook for reading and writing skills within the new 5-year syllabus for Italian Medical Schools *(Reading Skills in Medical English*, Rome 2005*)*.

MARYELIS PABÓN BERBESÍ holds a BA in English Language and Literature and an MA in Linguistics from the University of Los Andes, Mérida, Venezuela. She has conducted research in the area of Spanish and English syntax and is currently teaching English at the University of Los Andes.

PÄIVI PAHTA is Fellow of the Helsinki Collegium for Advanced Studies and a member of the Research Unit for Variation, Contacts and Change, both at the University of Helsinki. She has authored and co-edited books and articles on the history of medical and scientific writing, corpus linguistics and language-contact phenomena. Her main publications include *Medieval Embryology in the Vernacular: The Case of De spermate* (1998) and *Medical and Scientific Writing in Late Medieval English* (2004). She is also a co-compiler of the electronic corpora of *Middle English Medical Texts* (CD-ROM, 2005) and *Early Modern English Medical Texts* (in preparation).

DIANA DE SOUZA PINTO is Associate Professor at the Federal University of the Estate of Rio de Janeiro, where she is a researcher at the Graduate Program in Social Memory. Dr. Pinto is also a visiting professor at the Graduate Program in Mental Health at the Institute of Psychiatry of the Federal University of Rio de Janeiro and an

American National Institute of Mental Health researcher. Dr. Pinto has published on the interface between discourse analysis and mental health, on the fields of transcultural psychiatry, ethnography of communication, and narrative studies.

JORDI PIQUÉ-ANGORDANS holds a PhD in language and literature from The Catholic University of America (Washington, DC), where he was also language instructor until 1975. At present he is Senior Lecturer of English for Specific and Academic Purposes at the University of Valencia School of Nursing and Faculty of Philology, and has supervised numerous doctoral dissertations in the area of academic and specific language domains. He is currently editor of *Ibérica*, the journal of the European Association of Languages for Specific Purposes. Among his research interests are corpus-based studies of medical texts, modality and hedging in scientific texts, and translation.

SANTIAGO POSTEGUILLO obtained his PhD/European Doctorate at Universitat de València in 1995. At present, he is a member of the Editorial Board of the journals *English for Specific Purposes* and *Written Communication*, and is Senior Lecturer in English Language and Linguistics at Universitat Jaume I de Castelló, Spain. He is also the President of AELFE (the European Association of Languages for Specific Purposes). His latest publications include *Netlinguistics: Language, Discourse and Ideology in Internet* and the recent Spanish *Computing Dictionary: English-Spanish, Spanish-English.*

BRANCA TELLES RIBEIRO is Associate Professor in Intercultural Relations at Lesley University (Cambridge, USA). She directs a research project in language and communication in mental health at the Institute of Psychiatry of the Federal University of Rio de Janeiro. Dr. Ribeiro has published in the USA and internationally. Among her publications are *Coherence in Psychotic Discourse* (Oxford University Press 1994), 'Erotic Strategies in Powerless Women: Analyzing Psychiatric Interviews' (in J. Sunderland / L. Litosseliti (eds) *Gender Identity and Discourse Analysis*) and 'Frame Analysis' (in J. Verschueren / J. Ostman / J.-Ola Blommaert / C. Bulcaen (eds) *The Handbook of Pragmatics*).

CELIA ROBERTS is a Senior Research Fellow at King's College London. Her publications in intercultural communication and second language socialisation include: *Language and Discrimination* (Longman 1992 with Davies and Jupp), *Achieving Understanding* (Longman 1996 with Bremer *et al.*); in the field of urban discourse, *Talk, Work and Institutional Order* (Mouton 1999 with Sarangi); and in the field of language and cultural learning, *Language Learners as Ethnographers* (Multilingual Matters 2000 with Byram *et al.*). In recent years, she has focused on the medical setting and has researched issues of language, ethnicity and disadvantage among minority ethnic doctors and medical undergraduates and doctor-patient communication in multilingual contexts. She has co-written articles in *The British Medical Journal*, *The Journal of Medical Education* and *The Family Practice Journal*.

FRANÇOISE SALAGER-MEYER holds a BA and an MA in Russian language and literature from the University of Lyons (France) and a PhD in Foreign Language Education from the University of Texas at Austin (USA). She is currently teaching ESP (English for Specific Purposes) and Russian at the University of the Andes (Mérida, Venezuela). She has published several articles on the linguistic, rhetorical and discoursal analysis of medical English prose in international journals such as *System*, *English for Specific Purposes*, *Reading in a Foreign Language*, *Text*, *Interface*, *International Journal of Applied Linguistics*. She created and is currently co-ordinating the Multidisciplinary and Multilingual Research Group on Scientific Discourse Analysis at the University of The Andes, Mérida, Venezuela. She is also the Editor of the Language and Medicine section of the *Encyclopedia of Language and Linguistics* published by Elsevier in 2005.

SRIKANT SARANGI is Professor of Language and Communication and Director of the Health Communication Research Centre at Cardiff University. His research interests are in discourse analysis and applied linguistics; language and identity in public life and institutional/ professional discourse studies. He currently holds several project grants to study various aspects of health communication, e.g., genetic counselling, quality of life in HIV/AIDS, and telemedicine. Other areas of healthcare research include communication in primary care, palliative care, with particular reference to assessment of consulting and communication skills. He is author and editor of six books, guest-editor of five journal special issues and has published over one hundred journal articles and book chapters. He is the editor of *Text & Talk: An Interdisciplinary Journal of Language, Discourse and Communication Studies* as well as the founding editor of *Communication & Medicine* and with (C.N. Candlin) of *Journal of Applied Linguistics*. He is also general editor (with C.N. Candlin) of two book series: *Studies in Applied Linguistics* and *Studies in Language and Communication*.

IRMA TAAVITSAINEN is Professor of English Philology and Director of the Department of English, University of Helsinki, and Deputy Director of the Research Unit for Variation, Contacts and Change in English at the Universities of Helsinki and Jyväskylä. Her research interests cover historical pragmatics, development of specialized discourse, and register and genre studies. She is the co-editor of the *Journal of Historical Pragmatics*. Her recent publications include *Middle English Medical Texts* (an electronic corpus co-compiled with Päivi Pahta and Martti Mäkinen, Benjamins 2005), *Medical and Scientific Writing in Late Medieval English 1375-1500* (co-edited with Päivi Pahta, Cambridge University Press 2004), *Dialogic Language Use: Address in Focus* (co-edited with Juhani Härmä and Jarmo Korhonen, Mémoires de la Société Neophilologique 2006).

LAURA WRIGHT is a Senior Lecturer at the University of Cambridge, and a Fellow of Lucy Cavendish College. She works on the history of the London dialect. She is editor of *The Development of Standard English, 1300-1800: Theories, Descriptions, Conflicts* (Cambridge 2000) and author of several articles on the dissemination of London English, including that taken to Northern America. She also works on code-switching between Medieval Latin, Anglo-Norman and Middle English in London business texts, and has published articles and a book on literary language.

NAHIRANA ZAMBRANO is Professor of English and Anglo-American Culture at the University of Los Andes, Merida, Venezuela. As a member of the Grupo de Investigación Multidisciplinario del Análisis del Discurso Científico, she has contributed to a number of ongoing research projects. She currently is a doctoral student in the Department of American Studies at the University at Buffalo under Fulbright sponsorship. Her main research area is culture and its articulation in written discourse.

Linguistic Insights

Studies in Language and Communication

This series aims to promote specialist language studies in the fields of linguistic theory and applied linguistics, by publishing volumes that focus on specific aspects of language use in one or several languages and provide valuable insights into language and communication research. A cross-disciplinary approach is favoured and most European languages are accepted.

The series includes two types of books:

- **Monographs** – featuring in-depth studies on special aspects of language theory, language analysis or language teaching.
- **Collected papers** – assembling papers from workshops, conferences or symposia.

Vol. 1 Maurizio Gotti & Marina Dossena (eds)
Modality in Specialized Texts. Selected Papers of the 1st CERLIS Conference. 421 pp. 2001.
ISBN 3-906767-10-8. US-ISBN 0-8204-5340-4

Vol. 2 Giuseppina Cortese & Philip Riley (eds)
Domain-specific English. Textual Practices across Communities and Classrooms.
420 pp. 2002.
ISBN 3-906768-98-8. US-ISBN 0-8204-5884-8

Vol. 3 Maurizio Gotti, Dorothee Heller & Marina Dossena (eds)
Conflict and Negotiation in Specialized Texts. Selected Papers of the 2nd CERLIS Conference. 470 pp. 2002.
ISBN 3-906769-12-7. US-ISBN 0-8204-5887-2

Vol. 4 Maurizio Gotti, Marina Dossena, Richard Dury, Roberta Facchinetti & Maria Lima
Variation in Central Modals. A Repertoire of Forms and Types of Usage in Middle English and Early Modern English.
364 pp. 2002.
ISBN 3-906769-84-4. US-ISBN 0-8204-5898-8

Vol. 5 Stefania Nuccorini (ed.)
Phrases and Phraseology. Data and Descriptions.
187 pp. 2002.
ISBN 3-906770-08-7. US-ISBN 0-8204-5933-X

Vol. 6 Vijay Bhatia, Christopher N. Candlin & Maurizio Gotti (eds)
Legal Discourse in Multilingual and Multicultural Contexts. Arbitration Texts in Europe.
385 pp. 2003.
ISBN 3-906770-85-0. US-ISBN 0-8204-6254-3

Vol. 7 Marina Dossena & Charles Jones (eds)
Insights into Late Modern English.
378 pp. 2003.
ISBN 3-906770-97-4. US-ISBN 0-8204-6258-6

Vol. 8 Maurizio Gotti
Specialized Discourse. Linguistic Features and Changing Conventions.
351 pp. 2003, 2005.
ISBN 3-03910-606-6. US-ISBN 0-8204-7000-7

Vol. 9 Alan Partington, John Morley & Louann Haarman (eds)
Corpora and Discourse.
420 pp. 2004.
ISBN 3-03910-026-2. US-ISBN 0-8204-6262-4

Vol. 10 Martina Möllering
The Acquisition of German Modal Particles. A Corpus-Based Approach.
290 pp. 2004.
ISBN 3-03910-043-2. US-ISBN 0-8204-6273-X

Vol. 11 David Hart (ed.)
English Modality in Context. Diachronic Perspectives.
261 pp. 2003.
ISBN 3-03910-046-7. US-ISBN 0-8204-6852-5

Vol. 12 Wendy Swanson
Modes of Co-reference as an Indicator of Genre.
430 pp. 2003.
ISBN 3-03910-052-1. US-ISBN 0-8204-6855-X

Vol. 13 Gina Poncini
Discursive Strategies in Multicultural Business Meetings.
338 pp. 2004.
ISBN 3-03910-222-2. US-ISBN 0-8204-7003-1

Vol. 14 Christopher N. Candlin & Maurizio Gotti (eds)
Intercultural Aspects of Specialized Communication.
369 pp. 2004.
ISBN 3-03910-352-0. US-ISBN 0-8204-7015-5

Vol. 15 Gabriella Del Lungo Camiciotti & Elena Tognini Bonelli (eds)
Academic Discourse. New Insights into Evaluation.
234 pp. 2004.
ISBN 3-03910-353-9. US-ISBN 0-8204-7016-3

Vol. 16 Marina Dossena & Roger Lass (eds)
Methods and Data in English Historical Dialectology.
405 pp. 2004.
ISBN 3-03910-362-8. US-ISBN 0-8204-7018-X

Vol. 17 Judy Noguchi
The Science Review Article. An Opportune Genre in the Construction of Science.
274 pp. 2006.
ISBN 3-03910-426-8. US-ISBN 0-8204-7034-1

Vol. 18 Giuseppina Cortese & Anna Duszak (eds)
Identity, Community, Discourse.
English in Intercultural Settings.
495 pp. 2005.
ISBN 3-03910-632-5. US-ISBN 0-8204-7163-1

Vol. 19 AnnaTrosborg & Poul Erik Flyvholm Jørgensen (eds)
Business Discourse. Texts and Contexts.
250 pp. 2005.
ISBN 3-03910-606-6. US-ISBN 0-8204-7000-7

Vol. 20 Christopher Williams
Tradition and Change in Legal English. Verbal Constructions in Prescriptive Texts.
216 pp. 2005.
ISBN 3-03910-644-9. US-ISBN 0-8204-7166-6

Vol. 21 Katarzyna Dziubalska-Kołaczyk & Joanna Przedlacka (eds)
English Pronunciation Models: A Changing Scene.
476 pp. 2005.
ISBN 3-03910-662-7. US-ISBN 0-8204-7173-9

Vol. 22 Christián Abello-Contesse, Rubén Chacón-Beltrán, M. Dolores López-Jiménez & M. Mar Torreblanca-López (eds)
Age in L2 Acquisition and Teaching.
214 pp. 2006.
ISBN 3-03910-668-6. US-ISBN 0-8204-7174-7

Vol. 23 Vijay K. Bhatia, Maurizio Gotti, Jan Engberg & Dorothee Heller (eds)
Vagueness in Normative Texts.
474 pp. 2005.
ISBN 3-03910-653-8. US-ISBN 0-8204-7169-0

Vol. 24 Paul Gillaerts & Maurizio Gotti (eds)
Genre Variation in Business Letters.
407 pp. 2005.
ISBN 3-03910-674-0. US-ISBN 0-8204-7552-1

Vol. 25 Ana María Hornero, María José Luzón & Silvia Murillo (eds)
Corpus Linguistics. Applications for the Study of English.
526 pp. 2006.
ISBN 3-03910-675-9 / US-ISBN 0-8204-7554-8

Vol. 26 J. Lachlan Mackenzie & María de los Ángeles Gómez-González (eds)
Studies in Functional Discourse Grammar.
259 pp. 2005.
ISBN 3-03910-696-1 / US-ISBN 0-8204-7558-0

Vol. 27 Debbie G.E. Ho
Classroom Talk. Exploring the Sociocultural Structure of Formal ESL Learning.
254 pages. 2006.
ISBN 3-03910-761-5 / US-ISBN 0-8204-7561-0

Vol. 28 Forthcoming.

Vol. 29 Francesca Bargiela-Chiappini & Maurizio Gotti (eds)
Asian Business Discourse(s).
350 pp. 2005.
ISBN 3-03910-804-2 / US-ISBN 0-8204-7574-2

Vol. 30 Nicholas Brownlees (ed.)
News Discourse in Early Modern Britain. Selected Papers of CHINED 2004.
300 pp. 2006.
ISBN 3-03910-805-0 / US-ISBN 0-8204-8025-8

Vol. 31 Roberta Facchinetti & Matti Rissanen (eds)
Corpus-based Studies of Diachronic English.
300 pp. 2006.
ISBN 3-03910-851-4 / US-ISBN 0-8204-8040-1

Vol. 32 Marina Dossena & Susan M. Fitzmaurice (eds)
Business and Official Correspondence: Historical Investigations.
209 pp. 2006.
ISBN 3-03910-880-8 / US-ISBN 0-8204-8352-4

Vol. 33 Forthcoming.

Vol. 34 Forthcoming.

Vol. 35 Vijay K. Bhatia & Maurizio Gotti (eds)
Explorations in Specialized Genres.
316 pp. 2006.
ISBN 3-03910-995-2 / US-ISBN 0-8204-8372-9

Vol. 36 Heribert Picht (ed.)
Modern Approaches to Terminological Theories and Applications.
432 pages. 2006.
ISBN 3-03911-156-6 / US-ISBN 0-8204-8380-X

Vol. 37 Anne Wagner & Sophie Cacciaguidi-Fahy (eds)
Legal Language and the Search for Clarity / Le langage juridique et la quête de clarté. Practice and Tools / Pratiques et instruments.
487 pages. 2006.
ISBN 3-03911-169-8 / US-ISBN 0-8388-5

Vol. 38 Juan Carlos Palmer-Silveira, Miguel F. Ruiz-Garrido & Inmaculada Fortanet-Gómez (eds)
Intercultural and International Business Communication: Theory, Research and Teaching.
343 pages. 2006.
ISBN 3-03910-954-5 / US-ISBN 0-8204-8356-7

Vol. 39 Christiane Dalton-Puffer, Dieter Kastovsky, Nikolaus Ritt & Herbert Schendl (eds)
Syntax, Style and Grammatical Norms: English from 1500–2000.
250 pages. 2006.
ISBN 3-03911-181-7 / US-ISBN 0-8204-8394-X

Vol. 40 Marina Dossena & Irma Taavitsainen (eds)
Diachronic Perspectives on Domain-Specific English.
280 pages. 2006.
ISBN 3-03910-176-0 / US-ISBN 0-8204-8391-5

Vol. 41 John Flowerdew & Maurizio Gotti (eds)
Studies in Specialized Discourse.
293 pages. 2006.
ISBN 3-03911-178-7 / US-ISBN 0-8204-8393-1

Vol. 42 Ken Hyland & Marina Bondi (eds)
Academic Discourse Across Disciplines.
320 pages. 2006.
ISBN 3-03911-183-3 / US-ISBN 0-8204-8396-6

Vol. 43 Paul Gillaerts & Philip Shaw (eds)
The Map and the Landscape: Norms and Practices in Genre.
256 pages. 2006.
ISBN 3-03911-182-5 / US-ISBN 0-8204-8395-4

Vol. 44 Maurizio Gotti & Davide Giannoni (eds)
New Trends in Specialized Discourse Analysis.
301 pages. 2006.
ISBN 3-03911-184-1 / US-ISBN 0-8204-8381-8

Vol. 45 Maurizio Gotti & Françoise Salager-Meyer (eds)
Advances in Medical Discourse Analysis:
Oral and Written Contexts.
492 pages. 2006.
ISBN 3-03911-185-X / US-ISBN 0-8204-8382-6

Editorial address:

Prof. Maurizio Gotti Università di Bergamo, Facoltà di Lingue e Letterature Straniere,
Via Salvecchio 19, 24129 Bergamo, Italy
Fax: 0039 035 2052789, E-Mail: m.gotti@unibg.it

Gabriella Del Lungo Camiciotti / Elena Tognini Bonelli (eds)

Academic Discourse – New Insights into Evaluation

Bern, Berlin, Bruxelles, Frankfurt am Main, New York, Oxford, Wien, 2004.
234 pp., num. tables
Linguistic Insights. Studies in Language and Communication. Vol. 15
Edited by Maurizio Gotti
ISBN 3-03910-353-9 / US-ISBN 0-8204-7016-3 pb.
sFr. 62.– / € 42.80 / €** 40.– / £ 28.– / US-$ 47.95*

* includes VAT – only valid for Germany and Austria ** does not include VAT

This volume assembles a selection of papers presented at an international conference held in Pontignano, Siena, (14-16 June 2003). It discusses the concept of evaluation in academic discourse and the methodological tools most apt to investigate it. All contributions focus on a crucial dimension of academic communication: the epistemic and attitudinal assessment of content and the argumentative and metadiscourse devices used to interact with audiences of scholars or novices. The assembled contributions deal with theoretical and methodological issues including diverse academic genres ranging from written and oral texts. A report of the discussion on evaluation in academic texts concludes the volume.

Contents: Ken Hyland: Engagement and Disciplinarity: The Other Side of Evaluation – John M. Swales: Evaluation in Academic Speech: First Forays – Ellen Valle: «A Nice and Accurate Philosopher»: Interactivity and Evaluation in a Historical Context – Belinda Crawford Camiciottoli: Audience-Oriented Relevance Markers in Business Studies Lectures – Inmaculada Fortanet-Gómez: Verbal Stance in Spoken Academic Discourse – Philip Shaw: How Do We Recognise Implicit Evaluation in Academic Book Reviews? – Marc Silver/Marina Bondi: Weaving Voices: a Study of Article Openings in Historical Discourse – Paul Tucker: Evaluation and Interpretation in Art-Historical Discourse – Pauline Webber: Negation in Linguistics Papers – Anna Mauranen: Where Next? A Summary of the Round Table Discussion – Paul Drew: Integrating Qualitative Analysis of Evaluative Discourse with the Quantitative Approach of Corpus Linguistics.

PETER LANG
Bern · Berlin · Bruxelles · Frankfurt am Main · New York · Oxford · Wien